New Concepts in AIDS Pathogenesis

New Concepts in AIDS Pathogenesis

edited by
Luc Montagnier
Marie-Lise Gougeon

Institut Pasteur
Paris, France

Marcel Dekker, Inc.   New York•Basel•Hong Kong

Library of Congress Cataloging-in-Publication Data

New Concepts in Aids pathogenesis / edited by Luc Montagnier, Marie-
Lise Gougeon.
   p. cm.
   Includes bibliographical references and index.
   ISBN 0-8247-9127-4 (alk. paper)
   1. AIDS (Disease)--Pathogenesis. I. Montagnier, Luc.
II. Gougeon, Marie-Lise.
   [DNLM: 1. Acquired Immunodeficiency Syndrome--etiology. 2. HIV--
pathogenicity. WD 308 N53123 1993]
RC607.A26N484 1993
616.97'92071--dc20
DNLM/DLC
for Library of Congress   93-4765
                                                                 CIP

The publisher offers discounts on this book when ordered in bulk quantities.
For more information, write to Special Sales/Professional Marketing at the address
below.

This book is printed on acid-free paper.

Marcel Dekker, Inc.
270 Madison Avenue, New York, New York 10016

Current printing (last digit):
10 9 8 7 6 5 4 3 2 1

PRINTED IN THE UNITED STATES OF AMERICA

PREFACE

Ten years after the first isolation of HIV, the AIDS epidemic has reached an unprecedented size, following early predictions. Considerable scientific and medical progress has occurred, allowing the early detection of HIV infection in blood transfusions, the implementation of prevention policies, the first clinical effects of viral inhibitors, and the development of candidate vaccines. The viruses have been well characterized, and the function of their genes revealed.

However, it is clear that the status of our scientific knowledge of the disease is not satisfactory, and that many unknowns remain in the multiple facets of the disease.

Did the virus exist prior to the epidemics and where? How is it that a retrovirus that relies on cell activation for establishing a durable infection, and has no genetic information for activating terminally differentiated cells, can find enough target cells to induce a high level of persisting infection of the host? What is the mechanism of CD4 cell depletion, given that the number of HIV-infected cells is small and the bone marrow keeps, at least temporarily, its potential for T-cell renewal?

In a meeting held in June 1992 at Annecy Lake, France, we gathered experts in the field to discuss at length various data and hypotheses. For the first time, partisans of the theory that the virus "does it all by itself" confronted those who believe the virus is helped by the immune system and other factors. The sessions were conducted in a warm and courteous atmosphere.

Those discussions led to this book, which aims at contributing to our understanding of AIDS, a complex disease.

The first part of the book updates the mechanisms of HIV latency and activation of expression, at both the viral and the cellular levels in the human and primate systems. In particular, the role of cytokines in the dysfunction of both the immune system and the central nervous system is underlined. Chapter 7 summarizes the data suggesting that mycoplasma could be a critical cofactor.

The second part is devoted to mechanisms of immune activation that result in anergy and programmed cell death (apoptosis), involving the viral external glycoprotein and possibly other foreign antigens or superantigens.

The third part, more theoretical, includes original hypotheses on pathogenesis in which the virus glycoproteins also play a critical role, by mimicking allogeneic stimulation and disturbing the immune system network.

We hope that the reader will thus find a comprehensive survey of the various data and concepts on AIDS pathogenesis. This is not merely an academic debate, since a global understanding could lead in the future to new approaches of treatment and vaccines.

We would like to thank all the contributors, as well as the Marcel Mérieux Foundation, the European Community AIDS program (contracts MR4-0354-F and MR4-0347-F), and the European Foundation for AIDS Research.

Luc Montagnier
Marie-Lise Gougeon

CONTENTS

AIDS AS AN IMMUNOLOGICAL DISEASE

HYPOTHESES OF AIDS PATHOGENESIS

CONTRIBUTORS

Jean Claude Ameisen, M.D. Associate Professor of Immunology, Unité INSERM U167-CNRS 624, Institut Pasteur, Lille, France

Michael S. Ascher, M.D. Viral and Rickettsial Disease Laboratory, California Department of Health Services, Berkeley, California

Edward W. Bernton Department of Bacterial Diseases, Walter Reed Army Institute of Research, Washington, D.C.

Alessandra Bettinardi, Ph.D. Consorzio per le Biotecnologie, Consiglio Nazionale delle Ricerche (CNR), Institute of Chemistry, School of Medicine, University of Brescia, Brescia, Italy

Salvatore T. Butera, D.V.M., Ph.D. Staff Research Fellow, Retrovirus Diseases Branch, Division of Viral and Rickettsial Diseases, National Center for Infectious Diseases, Centers for Disease Control and Prevention, Atlanta, Georgia

Vittorio Colizzi, M.D., Ph.D. Professor of Immunology, Department of Biology, University of Rome "Tor Vergata," Rome, Italy

Therese A. Cvetkovich, M.D. Instructor and Fellow, Department of Pediatrics, University of Rochester Medical Center, Rochester, New York

Angus G. Dalgleish, B.Sc.(hons), M.B.B.S., M.D.(London), M.R.C.P., M.R.C.Path., F.R.A.C.P. Professor of Oncology, Department of Cell and Molecular Sciences, St. George's Hospital Medical School, University of London, London, England

Charles Dauguet, Ph.D. Scientist, Department of AIDS and Retroviruses, Institut Pasteur, Paris, France

Manuel del Cerro, M.D. Professor of Neurobiology, Anatomy, and Ophthalmology, Department of Neurobiology and Anatomy, University of Rochester Medical Center, Rochester, New York

Silvia Di Cesare, B.Sc. Department of Biology, University of Rome "Tor Vergata," Rome, Italy

Leon G. Epstein Professor of Neurology, Pediatrics, Microbiology, and Immunology, Department of Pediatric Neurology, University of Rochester Medical Center, Rochester, New York

Lucia Ercoli, M.D. Department of Public Health, University of Rome "Tor Vergata," Rome, Italy

Anthony S. Fauci, M.D. Chief, Laboratory of Immunoregulation, and Director, National Institute of Allergy and Infectious Diseases, National Institutes of Health, Bethesda, Maryland

Thomas M. Folks, Ph.D. Chief, Retrovirus Diseases Branch, Division of Viral and Rickettsial Diseases, National Center for Infectious Diseases, Centers for Disease Control and Prevention, Atlanta, Georgia

Patricia N. Fultz, Ph.D. Associate Professor, Department of Microbiology, University of Alabama, Birmingham, Alabama

Sylvie Garcia Viral Oncology Unit, Department of AIDS and Retroviruses, Institut Pasteur, Paris, France

Georg Geissler Department of Hematology, J. W. Goethe University, Frankfurt, Germany

Harris A. Gelbard, M.D., Ph.D. Assistant Professor, Departments of Pediatrics and Neurology, University of Rochester Medical Center, Rochester, New York

Howard E. Gendelman, M.D.* Department of Cellular Immunology, Walter Reed Army Institute of Research, and the Henry M. Jackson Foundation for the Advancement of Military Medicine, Rockville, Maryland

---

Current affiliation: Professor and Chief, Laboratory of Viral Pathogenesis, Department of Pathology and Microbiology, University of Nebraska Medical Center, Omaha, Nebraska

Peter Genis, M.D.* Department of Cellular Immunology, Walter Reed Army Institute of Research, Rockville, Maryland

Jaap Goudsmit, M.D., Ph.D. Professor, Department of Virology, University of Amsterdam, Academic Medical Center, Amsterdam, The Netherlands

Marie-Lise Gougeon, Ph.D. Associate Professor, Viral Oncology Unit, Department of AIDS and Retroviruses, Institut Pasteur, Paris, France

J. A. Habeshaw, Ph.D., M.D., F.R.C.Path. Honorary Lecturer, Department of Academic Virology, London Hospital Whitechapel, London, England

Jonathan Heeney, D.V.M., D.V.Sc.(Path.), Ph.D. Head, Section of Infectious Diseases, Department of Chronic and Infectious Diseases, Laboratory of Viral Pathogenesis, Rijswijk, The Netherlands

Ryszard A. Hermaszewski, M.R.C.P. Clinical Lecturer, Division of Oncology, St. George's Hospital Medical School, University of London, London, England

Dieter Hoelzer Head, Department of Hematology, J. W. Goethe University, Frankfurt, Germany

Geoffrey W. Hoffmann, Ph.D. Associate Professor, Departments of Microbiology and Physics, University of British Columbia, Vancouver, British Columbia, Canada

Elizabeth F. Hounsell, B.Sc., Ph.D., C.Chem., F.R.S.C. Clinical Research Centre, Harrow, England

Ara G. Hovanessian, Ph.D. Director of Research CNRS, Department of AIDS and Retroviruses, Institut Pasteur, Paris, France

Luisa Imberti, M.D. Consorzio per le Biotecnologie, Consiglio Nazionale delle Ricerche (CNR), Institute of Chemistry, School of Medicine, University of Brescia, Brescia, Italy

Marti Jett, Ph.D. Division of Pathology, Walter Reed Army Institute of Research, Washington, D.C.

Marie Paule Kieny, Ph.D. Assistant Scientific Director, Department of Immunology, Transgène S.A., Strasbourg, France

---

Current affiliation: Postdoctorate Research Associate, Department of Pathology and Microbiology, University of Nebraska Medical Center, Omaha, Nebraska

Audrey L. Kinter Laboratory of Immunoregulation, National Institute of Allergy and Infectious Diseases, National Institutes of Health, Bethesda, Maryland

Tracy A. Kion, Ph.D. Postdoctoral Fellow, Department of Microbiology, University of British Columbia, Vancouver, British Columbia, Canada

Bernard Krust, Ph.D. Scientist, Department of AIDS and Retroviruses, Institut Pasteur, Paris, France

Anne G. Laurent-Crawford, Ph.D. Scientist, Department of AIDS and Retroviruses, Institut Pasteur, Paris, France

Eliot S. Lazar, M.D. Scientist in Neurobiology and Anatomy, University of Rochester Medical Center, Rochester, New York

Giorgio Mancino, B.Sc. Department of Biology, University of Rome "Tor Vergata," Rome, Italy

Francesca Mariani, B.Sc. Department of Biology, University of Rome "Tor Vergata," Rome, Italy

Cinzia Mazza, Ph.D. Consorzio per le Biotecnologie, Consiglio Nazionale delle Ricerche (CNR), Institute of Chemistry, School of Medicine, University of Brescia, Brescia, Italy

Linde Meyaard Department of Clinical Viro-Immunology, Central Laboratory of The Netherlands Red Cross Blood Transfusion Service, and Laboratory for Experimental and Clinical Immunology of the University of Amsterdam, Amsterdam, The Netherlands

Frank Miedema, Ph.D. Head, Department of Clinical Viro-Immunology, Central Laboratory of The Netherlands Red Cross Blood Transfusion Service, and Laboratory for Experimental and Clinical Immunology of the University of Amsterdam, Amsterdam, The Netherlands

Luc Montagnier, M.D. Professor, Viral Oncology Unit, and Chief, Department of AIDS and Retroviruses, Institut Pasteur, Paris, France

Sylviane Muller, Ph.D. Research Director, Department of Immunochemistry, Institut de Biologie Moléculaire et Cellulaire du CNRS, Strasbourg, France

Keith E. Nye, Ph.D. Lecturer, Department of Immunology, The Medical College of Saint Bartholomew's Hospital, London, England

Sigrid Otto Department of Clinical Viro-Immunology, Central Laboratory of The Netherlands Red Cross Blood Transfusion Service, and Laboratory for Experimental and Clinical Immunology of the University of Amsterdam, Amsterdam, The Netherlands

Anthony J. Pinching, D.Phil., F.R.C.P. Professor, Department of Immunology, The Medical College of Saint Bartholomew's Hospital, London, England

Roberta Placido, B.Sc. Department of Biology, University of Rome "Tor Vergata," Rome, Italy

Fabrizio Poccia, Ph.D. Department of Biology, University of Rome "Tor Vergata," Rome, Italy

Guido Poli, M.D. Visiting Scientist, Laboratory of Immunoregulation, National Institute of Allergy and Infectious Diseases, National Institutes of Health, Bethesda, Maryland

Daniele Primi, Ph.D. Scientific Director, Consorzio per le Biotecnologie, Consiglio Nazionale delle Ricerche (CNR), Institute of Chemistry, School of Medicine, University of Brescia, Brescia, Italy

Yves Rivière, D.V.M., Ph.D. Chef de Laboratoire, Department of AIDS and Retroviruses, Institut Pasteur, Paris, France

Marijke Roos Department of Clinical Viro-Immunology, Central Laboratory of The Netherlands Red Cross Blood Transfusion Service, and Laboratory for Experimental and Clinical Immunology of the University of Amsterdam, Amsterdam, The Netherlands

Rita Rossol Department of Hematology, J. W. Goethe University, Frankfurt, Germany

Peter Schellekens, Ph.D. Department of Clinical Viro-Immunology, Central Laboratory of The Netherlands Red Cross Blood Transfusion Service, and Laboratory for Experimental and Clinical Immunology of the University of Amsterdam, Amsterdam, The Netherlands

Haynes W. Sheppard, Ph.D. Viral and Rickettsial Disease Laboratory, California Department of Health Services, Berkeley, California

Alessandra Sottini, Ph.D. Consorzio per le Biotecnologie, Consiglio Nazionale delle Ricerche (CNR), Institute of Chemistry, School of Medicine, University of Brescia, Brescia, Italy

Thijs Tersmette, Ph.D. Department of Clinical Viro-Immunology, Central Laboratory of The Netherlands Red Cross Blood Transfusion Service, and Laboratory for Experimental and Clinical Immunology of the University of Amsterdam, Amsterdam, The Netherlands

1

HIV-1 Latency and Activation in the Pathogenesis of AIDS

Salvatore T. Butera and Thomas M. Folks

National Center for Infectious Diseases
Centers for Disease Control and Prevention
Atlanta, Georgia

HIV-1 INFECTION: FROM A CLINICAL TO CELLULAR PERSPECTIVE

Staging of Infection on a Clinical Level

A striking feature of the clinical presentation of AIDS is the discrete stages of disease progression observed in most patients (1). After infection with HIV-1, some patients first undergo an acute influenza-like illness marked by a rapid and transient fall in CD4 T lymphocytes and viral p24 antigenemia. Upon recovery, CD4 T-lymphocyte numbers return to the normal range but do not reach the same circulating level as that prior to HIV-1 infection. The brief acute phase of illness is generally followed by a protracted and variable clinically asymptomatic phase characterized by normal health, normal circulating CD4 T-lymphocyte numbers, and detectable circulating anti-HIV antibody (2). In most cases, the asymptomatic phase eventually gives way to progressive immunosuppression and T-cell dysfunction, resulting in declining CD4 T-lymphocyte numbers, rising viral p24 antigenemia, and the appearance of opportunistic infections; this clinical phase, formally referred to as "AIDS-related complex" (ARC), is known as "symptomatic HIV infection." Without antiretroviral or prophylactic therapies, the symptomatic clinical phase usually progresses to overt AIDS and results in death, generally because of overwhelming opportunistic infections or malignancy in the face of severe immunosuppression.

To date, antiretroviral and supportive therapies have only modestly altered the outcome of AIDS disease progression, and new retroviral targets must be identified to realize full therapeutic potential (3). In general, once an HIV-1+ patient enters the symptomatic phase of disease, steady progression toward lethal immunosuppression rapidly occurs. The damage to the immune system may be so extensive at this point that clinical therapies are unable to reverse and prevent the progressive events resulting in AIDS. It therefore seems logical that the aspect of AIDS that holds the greatest therapeutic potential is the protracted clinically asymptomatic period following HIV-1 infection. During this period, which normally lasts several years, the infected individual remains in good health while the level of circulating CD4 T lymphocytes gradually decline. If novel therapeutic agents and strategies are developed and implemented during the clinically asymptomatic phase to alter the progression toward AIDS, hope may be offered to the estimated millions of individuals worldwide who are HIV-1+ but clinically asymptomatic. The asymptomatic period may be the phase in which our basic understanding of virus-host interactions is best applied.

Staging of Infection on a Cellular Level

Discrete stages of HIV-1 infection can also be observed on a cellular level. After the binding of the HIV-1 envelope protein (gp120) to the host CD4 surface receptor (4), a series of events occurs that results in acute infection at a cellular level and comprises the afferent component of the viral life cycle (Figure 1). Generally, HIV-1 binding results in fusion and penetration, reverse transcription of viral genomic RNA into double-stranded DNA, and integration into the host genome (1,5). Although retroviral integration may rapidly progress to virion production, especially in preactivated target cells (Figure 2), a variable period of viral latency may result in an identifiable population of infected cells (6–8).

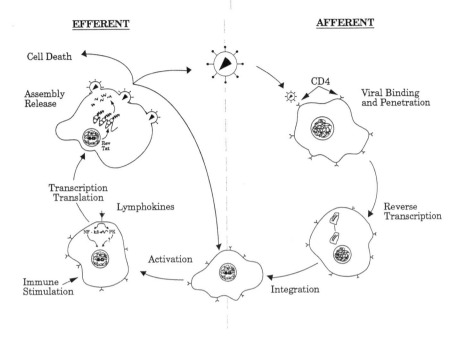

Figure 1 The HIV-1 life cycle can theoretically be divided into afferent and efferent components. The afferent component includes the initial steps of virus binding, penetration, reverse transcription, and integration and occurs fairly rapidly under normal conditions. The efferent component of the HIV-1 life cycle includes those events that produce viral progeny and may require an extracellular signal to activate the integrated provirus after a prolonged period of latency. Although HIV-1 expression could eventually result in cytopathic sequelae, removal of the extracellular stimulus may permit the return of the infected cell to a state of viral latency and therefore repeated episodes of HIV-1 activation. (From Ref. 111.)

Just as the free virion represents the central element in the afferent component of the viral life cycle, the infected cell harboring an integrated but dormant provirus represents the central element of the efferent component of the viral life cycle (Figure 1). On the basis of in vitro observations (9–14), when latently infected cells encounter the right combination of external stimuli, conversion from nonproductive to active HIV-1 expression can occur. This conversion requires those events necessary for the HIV-1 provirus to successfully transcribe, translate, and assemble

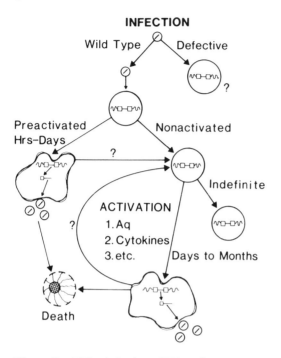

Figure 2   HIV-1 infection of T lymphocytes can proceed in at least two different scenarios. If the cell is preactivated, then acute HIV-1 infection can progress rapidly to complete the life cycle. However, if HIV-1 infects a resting cell, progression through the viral life cycle is prolonged and may involve a latent proviral intermediate. The provirus can remain dormant until immune activation of the infected cell results in concomitant viral activation to complete the viral life cycle.

progeny virions to complete the viral life cycle and permit dissemination to new susceptible target cells. Cytopathic sequelae can result at this point because of the accumulation of unintegrated viral DNA (15,16), immune lysis of infected cells displaying antigenic determinants of the host immune response (17), or fusion of infected cells expressing surface gp120 with noninfected CD4+ target cells (6,7).

The distinction between the clinical and cellular aspects of HIV-1 infection requires that viral latency be defined on two levels. On the clinical level, latency refers to the long and variable asymptomatic period prior to the onset of symptomatic HIV-1 infection. At the cellular level, "microbiological" latency is defined as the postintegrative phase of the viral life cycle when the integrated provirus remains dormant until the proper external stimulus activates viral expression. However, while the distinction between clinical and cellular latency seems to be clearly defined, the interrelationship between latency on these two levels is much less apparent. It could be argued that cellular latency controls the clinically asymptomatic period, and, as dormant cells become activated, HIV-1 disseminates to result in the slow but progressive course of disease. By necessity, this process would identify the latently infected cell as the primary target for therapeutic intervention. Prevention of viral activation on a cellular level might eventually prevent or alter disease progression on a clinical level. However, such an approach to AIDS therapy requires a conclusive link between viral activation at a cellular level and disease progression, as well as an extensive understanding of the events and mechanisms controlling viral dormancy and activation.

Relationship Between Cellular Infection and Clinical Disease Progression

Data to support the possible interrelationship between cellular and clinical latency have been difficult to obtain. Several studies have demonstrated a major discrepancy between the frequency of infected cells in vivo, as measured by the polymerase chain reaction (PCR) for integrated viral genome (18,19), and those actively expressing viral proteins, as measured by in situ hybridization for viral RNA (20). From these studies, it appears that the CD4+ T lymphocyte is the major reservoir in vivo for HIV-1 (18, 21). This observation would imply that the majority of infected cells in vivo harbor a competent but dormant provirus (22) and could potentially be activated upon cellular stimulation (23). Evidence of active viral replication has been obtained at all clinical stages of disease, including the asymptomatic period (24), and the frequency of infected cells increases with progressing disease states (25,26), suggesting a slow but progressive dissemination of virus during the asymptomatic phase as predicted by the model of dormant cell activation and disease progression.

Furthermore, in vitro approaches using both cloned peripheral lymphocytes (27) and transformed cell lines (9–12) have clearly demonstrated that HIV-1 can exist as a stably integrated but transcriptionally dormant provirus (Figure 2). If the cells that survive an acute HIV-1 infection in vitro are expanded and subcloned, populations of cells that harbor an integrated provirus but express little or no viral proteins can be identified. Although some of these clonal populations may represent cells that were infected with replication-defective virions (28), other clones may reflect

Table 1   Cloned Cell Models for Use in Studies of HIV-1 Latency and Activation

Clone derivation	Parental line	CD4	T3-Ti (TCR)	Viral status[a]	Inducible	Ref.
T cells						
ACH-2	A3.01	—	—	Latent	+	9
J1.1	Jurkat	—	+	Latent	+	10
8E5	A3.01	—	—	Constit	NA[b]	29
Promonocytic						
U1	U937	—	—	Latent	+	13
U33	U937	+	—	Constit	NA[b]	5
THP/HIV	THP	?	—	Latent	+/−	30
Promyelocytic						
OM-10.1	HL-60	+	—	Latent	+	11
PLB-IIIB	PLB-985	—	—	Constit	NA[b]	31
B-cell						
LL58	EBV-B	—	—	Latent	?	32

[a]Cells exhibiting either low-level persistent viral expression (Latent) or constitutive viral expression (Constit).
[b]Not applicable.

the state of nonproductive HIV-1 expression exhibited in vivo by the majority of the infected CD4+ cells. When these chronically infected cells encounter the proper external stimulus, they can convert from nonproductive to active HIV-1 expression (Figure 2). This infection and cloning strategy has been used to develop chronically infected cell models of several different lineages, as shown in Table 1, that represent nonproductive infection in several type of natural host target cells. These cell systems have proven to be valuable tools for deciphering intra- and extracellular mechanisms of HIV-1 latency. However, it cannot be overemphasized that all cloned cell models of latency have limitations stemming mainly from their clonal derivation and transformed genotype. Therefore, any particular observation made with a given system must be interpreted cautiously and compared with additional cell models of similar derivation to obtain an appreciation for host cell variation.

CELLULAR MECHANISMS CONTROLLING HIV-1 ACTIVATION AND EXPRESSION

Signaling Pathways Involved in HIV-1 Activation from Latency

Extracellular Stimuli Represent the First Level

The development of in vitro models of cellular latency has permitted a dissection of the pathways leading to HIV-1 activation and expression.

At the first messenger level, several extracellular stimuli appear to be capable of inducing viral activation. As a group, the best-characterized stimuli are cytokines (reviewed in Ref. 33), soluble factors produced by many cell types that function in normal immunological signaling and communication. Viral induction in the latent ACH-2 cell model was originally achieved using supernatant from lipopolysaccharide (LPS)-stimulated macrophages, a rich source of several cytokines (9). Upon further investigation, tumor necrosis factor (TNF)-α and -β were found to be active components of this supernatant. Furthermore, recombinant TNF-α alone was able to induce HIV-1 expression from ACH-2, J1.1, OM-10.1, and U1 cells (9–11, 13). Although TNF-α appears to be nearly universal in its ability to induce HIV-1 expression from a variety of cell types, several other cytokines, including granulocyte-macrophage colony-stimulating factor (GM-CSF) (12) and interleukin-6 (IL-6) (34), have proven to be effective activators of HIV-1 expression in selected cell systems. TNF-α treatment of latently infected cells results in a transcriptional activation of HIV-1, whereas IL-6 treatment results primarily in a translational increase; therefore, the two cytokines may synergize to further HIV-1 expression (34).

In addition to cytokine activation, latently infected T lymphocytes in vivo may increase HIV-1 expression after specific antigen stimulation through the T-cell receptor complex. This possibility is difficult to test in vitro since latently infected T lymphocytes of known antigen specificity are nearly impossible to obtain. However, mitogen or antigen activation of latently infected T cells in vitro does result in HIV-1 expression (35–37). Studies using anti-CD3 cross-linking of the T-cell receptor on latently infected cells have provided mixed results. Anti-CD3 treatment resulted in activation of viral long terminal repeat (LTR)-directed transcription in transient transfection experiments using reported gene constructs (38,39). However, anti-CD3 treatment did not result in viral activation when tested on the CD3 + latently infected T-cell line, J1.1, which contains the entire proviral genome. This latter observation may be due to T-cell receptor uncoupling, a defect observed in J1.1 and other infected T cells as a consequence of HIV-1 infection (40,41).

Protein Kinases Represent the Second Level

The second messenger systems necessary for viral activation still require much further elucidation. Because the phorbol esters are potent activators of HIV-1 expression in several latently infected cell models (11, 13,42,43), activation stimuli mediated via protein kinase C can presumably result in HIV-1 induction. Several agents that directly activate protein kinase C-mediated pathways have proven to act as inducers of HIV-1 expression (44). However, TNF-α stimulation of HIV-1 expression appears to be independent of protein kinase C (45,46), although other protein kinase pathways are certainly involved. We (unpublished observation) and others (reviewed in Ref. 46) have demonstrated that H-7, a broad inhibitor of protein kinase activity (47), can block TNF-α-induced HIV-1 expression whereas staurosporin, a more specific protein kinase C inhibitor, does not. Both H-7 and staurosporin inhibit HIV-1 activation by phorbol esters. Furthermore, in our studies, specific inhibitors of protein kinases A and G had no effect on HIV-1 induction by TNF-α. The second messenger enzyme systems required to mediate the inductive signal of TNF-α may be of key importance in understanding viral activation and designing selective therapies against HIV-1 activation.

Nuclear Factors Represent the Third Level

To generate an effect at the transcriptional level, second messenger enzyme systems must work on a third messenger protein, generally a nuclear factor that alters specific gene regulation. Among the factors recognized to enhance viral LTR-directed transcription (reviewed in Ref. 48), nuclear factor-$\varkappa$B (NF-$\varkappa$B) is the best characterized (45,49–57). Two NF-$\varkappa$B binding motifs are present within the viral LTR (58), and this region has repeatedly been demonstrated to function as a transcriptional enhancer when bound (45,54–57). Removal of the NF-$\varkappa$B motifs from the viral LTR severely restricts, but does not completely eliminate, the capacity for viral replication (59). Preformed cytoplasmic NF-$\varkappa$B remains bound to an inhibitor protein, I-$\varkappa$B (60–62). When an activation signal is generated, NF-$\varkappa$B dissociates from I-$\varkappa$B, migrates to the nucleus, and exerts its effects on transcription by binding to selective regions of upstream gene enhancers. One mechanism—although others have been proposed (reviewed in Refs. 63 and 64)—by which NF-$\varkappa$B can dissociate from I-$\varkappa$B is by the phosphorylation of I-$\varkappa$B (62). Therefore, a potential link between second messenger protein kinase systems and third messenger proteins has been described for NF-$\varkappa$B. The kinases involved and the importance of I-$\varkappa$B phosphorylation in HIV-1 activation are under investigation. An ability to block NF-$\varkappa$B activity via specific kinase inhibitors or other mechanisms may have therapeutic applications that could alter the clinical course to AIDS.

However, evidence has continued to accumulate that suggests that NF-$\varkappa$B is either not sufficient (65) or not involved (66) in HIV-1 activation in certain cell systems. The kinase inhibitor, H-7, was capable of inhibiting TNF-α-stimulated HIV-1 expression from chronically infected cells although TNF-α induction of nuclear NF-$\varkappa$B activity proceeded normally

(67). These observations verify that the presence of active NF-$\varkappa$B is insufficient to result in HIV-1 activation. Therefore, additional third messenger nuclear factors beyond NF-$\varkappa$B may be critically important for HIV-1 activation in certain cell types or following a given stimulus.

Mechanisms Maintaining HIV-1 Latency

Extracellular Influences

Mechanisms must also exist at a cellular level to maintain integrated HIV-1 provirions in a state of nonproductive expression. Several laboratories have demonstrated that the presence of CD8 + cells in culture can repress expression of HIV-1 during an acute infection of CD4 + targets (68,69). This phenomenon is apparently due to soluble factors expressed by the CD8 + population of cells in an HIV-1 antigen-specific manner. Removal of the CD8 + cells from culture releases this suppression and, in some systems, permits the isolation of HIV-1 from CD4 + cell cultures of infected patients. The identity and mechanism of action for this putative natural suppressive factor are unclear. In addition, a natural cytokine, transforming growth factor-β, can inhibit phorbol ester–induced HIV-1 activation in certain chronically infected cell lines (70). Therefore, extracellular signaling events can both positively and negatively influence HIV-1 activation and expression.

Intracellular Influences

Intracellular factors may regulate HIV-1 expression under normal conditions until extracellular stimuli result in both cellular and viral activation due to overlapping activation pathways. At the genomic level, HIV-1 expression can be controlled if viral integration occurs in a region of DNA methylation, a physiological mechanism of gene control (71). In vitro, DNA methylation of the HIV-1 LTR severely restricts LTR-directed gene transcription (72) and chemical demethylation restores transcriptional activity (73). Under physiological conditions, HIV-1 expression may be regulated by methylation of the LTR and demethylation during cellular activation. Viral expression can also be regulated by the binding of negative regulatory proteins to the 5′-region of the viral LTR, a region functionally defined as the negative regulatory element (NRE) (74,75). However, the identity and the functional significance of cellular factors binding to the NRE remain obscure.

Viral Influences

Viral proteins may also participate in the negative regulation of HIV-1 expression. The viral encoded Nef protein was first described as a negative regulatory protein because of the observation that *nef*-mutant viruses grew better than their wild-type counterpart (76). Additional in vitro evidence for negative regulatory action of the Nef protein was obtained from experimental systems in which the addition of Nef reduced LTR-directed chloramphenicol acetyl transferase (CAT) gene expression (77,78). From deletional analysis, the LTR target sequence in this LTR-CAT system was identified within the NRE (77). This putative function of the Nef protein has continued to generate controversy, and the negative regulatory function has not been observed in every system examined (79,80). Furthermore, in vivo studies using *nef*-mutant simian immunodeficiency virus (SIV) infection of rhesus macaques demonstrated an essential role for Nef in enhancing viral replication and disease progression (81). Until the molecular action of the Nef protein is resolved, its contribution to HIV-1 latency will remain controversial.

Control of Viral RNA Splicing

It has long been observed that HIV-1 undergoes selective viral RNA splicing during the course of productive expression and that selective splicing is an important aspect of controlled viral expression (82,83). Recently, using the U1 and ACH-2 cell models of latent infection, studies have demonstrated an altered viral RNA splice pattern during latency (84,85). In uninduced U1 and ACH-2 cultures, the majority of viral RNA was present as doubly spliced 2.0 kb messages encoding the viral regulatory proteins, reminiscent of the viral RNA pattern during the early phases of in vitro infection (83). Latency in these cell lines appears to be relative, more accurately described as "nonproductive expression," whereby low levels of viral message are present but controlled via splicing to prevent productive viral expression. Upon induction, the viral RNA pattern undergoes a temporal splice switch to the full-length and singly spliced messages that encode the genomic and structural proteins. Therefore, in these systems HIV-1 has an inherent ability to regulate its own expression by controlling the amount of structural protein expression via selective RNA splicing.

Although the possibility that Nef is involved in maintaining this state of latency has not been formally excluded, mounting evidence suggests that the viral regulatory protein Rev is the critical element controlling selective RNA splicing during nonproductive and induced expression. First, the known function of the Rev protein is to control viral RNA splicing by protecting the full-length messages from splicing and chaperoning them from the nucleus to the cytoplasmic ribosomes (reviewed in Ref. 86). Second, the viral RNA splicing pattern observed during nonproductive expression in U1 and ACH-2 cells appears identical to that of *rev*-mutant HIV viruses in which only the small spliced messages are produced (82). Third, efficient replication of HIV was recently demonstrated to require a critical threshold of Rev protein (84,87). The requirement for a threshold level of Rev protein may explain the initial accumulation of doubly spliced messages prior to the switch to structural and full-length messages during activated HIV-1 expression. At a molecular level, the threshold requirement may be a direct result of Rev protein multimerization to achieve effective protection against viral RNA splicing (88). Beyond this viral mechanism, cellular proteins have also been demonstrated to be essential for the action of Rev (89). Therefore, in the U1 and ACH-2 systems the level of the Rev protein appears critical in controlling the conversion from nonproductive to productive expression.

However, we have recently described several cellular models that display a distinctly different pattern during latency from that described for U1 and ACH-2 cells. Two additional cellular models, OM-10.1 and J1.1, in the uninduced state show a viral RNA pattern reminiscent of "absolute" latency. In contrast to the nonproductive RNA pattern, the majority of OM-10.1 and J1.1 cells contain undetectable levels of viral RNA as determined by limiting dilutional reverse transcriptase-dependent PCR. However, upon induction the doubly spliced viral messages first accumulate, and a switch to the structural and full-length messages is then temporally observed. This appears to be the first demonstration that absolute latency at a cellular level can still be overcome by exogenous stimuli to result in active viral expression. Therefore, these cells represent a different mechanism of latency, one in which the cell has completely repressed all viral expression until an activation signal is received. A threshold level of Rev protein may still represent a unifying mechanism of viral activation, since an accumulation of regulatory messages was still necessary for the conversion to productive viral expression in the OM-10.1 and J1.1 systems.

Obviously, multiple mechanisms of latency exist with varying degrees of cellular and viral control. These cell systems represent at least two different and distinct mechanisms controlling HIV-1 expression and will serve as important systems of comparison. It will be of continued interest to investigate the molecular mechanisms involved in controlling the state of repressed viral expression and the pathways responsible for viral activation.

APPLICATION OF OM-10.1 CULTURES
TO STUDIES OF HIV-1 ACTIVATION

We have utilized the OM-10.1 cell system as a unique model of viral latency to extend observations along several lines. The OM-10.1 line, which was cloned following an acute HIV-1 (LAI) infection of HL-60 promyelocytes, harbors a single provirion. Unique among models of chronic HIV-1 infection, OM-10.1 cells remain CD4 + under normal culture conditions while expressing a minimal amount of viral proteins. Upon induction by TNF-α, OM-10.1 cultures rapidly become CD4$^-$ and dramatically increase HIV-1 expression (> 30-fold). As previously reported (11), CD4 downmodulation on activated OM-10.1 cells is critically dependent on HIV-1 expression and is the direct result, at least in part, of intracellular complexing between CD4 and viral gp160 translated within the first 6 hours of viral activation.

Oscillation of HIV-1 Activation from Latency

The OM-10.1 cell system was used to demonstrate that latently infected cells could undergo periodic fluctuations in HIV-1 expression, dependent on the external stimuli. OM-10.1 cultures were treated with TNF-α for 36 hours so that maximal HIV-1 activation occurred, as measured by CD4 downmodulation or supernatant reverse transcriptase activity. The exogenous TNF-α stimulus was then removed and the cells were monitored for an additional 10 days while being maintained in normal culture medium. After an initial 3- to 4-day lag period, CD4 surface expression began to return and supernatant reverse transcriptase levels began to decline; both effects were indications of a return to latency in these OM-10.1 cultures. Within 6 to 9 days, these cultures had regained their resting phenotype, with nearly 100% of the cells expressing surface CD4 and the culture supernatant again containing low-level reverse transcriptase activity. However, these OM-10.1 cultures were still inducible by exogenous TNF-α, resulting in the downmodulation of surface CD4 and the rise of reverse transcriptase activity occurring with kinetics similar to those in the first induction cycle (11).

These results support the return to latency, as shown in Figure 1, and indicate an additional feature concerning the activities of CD4 + cells as reservoirs for HIV-1. In vivo, when latently infected cells encounter the proper blend of extracellular stimuli, they may begin to express HIV-1 and actively participate in viral dissemination to new susceptible targets. When that extracellular stimulus is removed, the model would imply that the cell can cycle back into a state of latency and possibly remain hidden from immune surveillance because of low-level or "absent" viral expression. Theoretically, such cycles of activation and latency could contribute to the slow spread of HIV-1 while permitting the infected cells to evade immune surveillance because of the transient nature of their viral expression.

Involvement of Protein Kinases in Continued HIV-1 Expression

This system has been extended to examine the contribution of protein kinases during the period of induced viral expression. As mentioned above, we and others have observed that protein kinases are critical for the initial activation of latent HIV-1, at least via the TNF-α-inducible pathways. However, little is known about the role of these enzyme systems in maintaining active viral expression once induction from latency has occurred. OM-10.1 cells, used in efforts to understand such enzyme systems, were again stimulated for 36 hours with exogenous TNF-α to induce maximal expression. The exogenous TNF-α was then removed and the cells placed back into either normal culture medium or culture medium containing a broad kinase inhibitor, H-7. By following surface CD4 levels as an indirect marker of viral expression, a full return to latency was observed in the normal medium culture after an additional 5- to 6-day culture period. In contrast, OM-10.1 cells cultured in the presence of H-7 returned to latency with greatly enhanced kinetics, with nearly 100% of the cells returning to a state of viral dormancy within 48 hours (11).

Due to the multiple pathways that depend on protein kinase signaling, it is difficult to even speculate at which level these enzyme systems are functioning to maintain active HIV-1 expression. As discussed above, protein kinase-mediated second messenger pathways provide a critical link in viral activation due to extracellular stimuli. The kinase systems involved in maintaining active HIV-1 expression after the removal of the exogenous stimulus may be separate from those responsible for mediating extracellular signaling events. The intracellular targets may involve NF-$\varkappa$B, since phosphorylation is potentially a critical step in its activation (62) and continued exogenous stimulation is required for maintained NF-$\varkappa$B activity (90). Furthermore, the viral regulatory proteins themselves are potential targets for phosphorylation (91), as well as cellular proteins that permit their activity (92).

Relationships Between HIV-1 and Cytokines

HIV-1 has evolved to become intricately entwined with normal immune regulatory networks, and it uses this relationship to enhance its own expression. This effect is especially apparent when considering the relationship between HIV-1 expression and cytokines. Enhanced HIV-1 expression upon cytokine stimulation has been well documented in many systems (reviewed in Ref. 46). Reciprocally, enhanced cytokine expression has been demonstrated upon HIV-1 activation, especially in cells of monocytic or promonocytic origin (31,93,94), although this is not a universal observation (95).

An important implication of these accumulative studies is that HIV-1 can regulate cytokine expression to benefit its own survival. Investigators using the U1 promonocytic model of chronic infection have suggested that TNF-α can function in an autocrine/paracrine manner to activate HIV-1 expression (96); however, these studies have several apparent limitations. First, phorbol ester induction was used to incite TNF-α expression, thereby restricting the physiological implications of the autocrine regulatory network. Second, the possibility of autocrine TNF-α action was based on neutralization by anti-TNF-α antibodies, which might have had untold effects of their own on HIV-1 expression via binding to membrane-bound TNF (97).

Autocrine TNF-α Induction of Latent HIV-1 in OM-10.1 Cells

We have recently applied the OM-10.1 cell system to the investigation of cytokine regulatory networks involved in HIV-1 activation from latency. Because we were able to use CD4 surface expression as a reliable indicator of viral expression, we could examine HIV-1 expression on a cell-by-cell basis in response to various extracellular stimuli. OM-10.1 cells were first stimulated briefly with exogenous TNF-α to induce autocrine TNF-α production. These cells were then placed below a permeable membrane to determine if autocrine TNF-α could function in a paracrine manner to stimulate resting OM-10.1 cells seeded above the membrane. Within 24 hours, >50% of the resting OM-10.1 cells above the membrane had been activated to express HIV-1 and downmodulate surface CD4. Antibody inhibition and absorption experiments further confirmed that autocrine TNF-α was responsible for viral activation of resting cells (116). Therefore, we have conclusively demonstrated that autocrine TNF-α produced after a suboptimal physiological stimulus can function in a panacrine manner to stimulate HIV-1 expression from latently infected cells.

Influence of HIV-1 Expression on TNF Surface Receptors

Cytokine networks can take on several additional levels of complexity, as exemplified by autocrine and paracrine TNF-α pathways (Figure 3). The surface receptors for TNF-α can also participate in self-regulation. Upon cellular activation, TNF-α receptors can be shed into the surrounding medium (98) to either absorb free TNF-α and reduce its bioavailability (99) or stabilize the functional TNF-α trimer molecule and effectively increase its bioactivity (100). TNF-α surface receptors can also directly participate in cellular signaling. Soluble TNF-α receptors can bind to the membrane-bound form of TNF-α expressed on a distant cell, known as a retrocrine interaction, to induce a primary response or modify the respon-

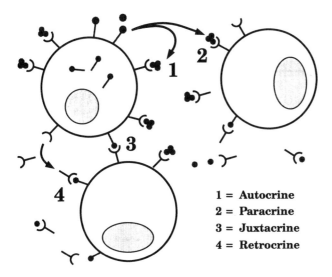

1 = Autocrine
2 = Paracrine
3 = Juxtacrine
4 = Retrocrine

Figure 3 Proposed signaling pathways for regulation of TNF-α responses. Upon transcription, TNF-α is expressed as a membrane-bound molecule that is liberated by proteolytic action. The active trimeric form of TNF-α assembles and can act back upon the secreting cell (autocrine) or upon a distant cell (paracrine) to induce a response. TNF receptors can also participate in modifying TNF-α responses by either contacting membrane-bound TNF-α of an adjacent cell (juxtacrine) or, as a soluble receptor, binding membrane-bound TNF-α of a distant cell (retrocrine). The consequences of these latter two interactions are still not completely understood.

siveness of that cell to subsequent activation (116). Furthermore, if the surface TNF-α receptor contacts the membrane-bound TNF-α molecule of an adjacent cell in a juxtacrine fashion, a series of cellular signals can be generated that potentially alter TNF-α responsive pathways. These signals may be mediated to the cell expressing the receptor, the cell expressing the membrane TNF-α, or both.

Two separate surface TNF receptors (TR) have been identified (101–105, reviewed in Ref. 106). Epithelial cell lines, such as HEp2 and HeLa, express solely a 55-kD TR (TR55) whereas cell lines of myeloid lineage, such as HL-60 and U937, express both the TR55 and a 75-kD TR (TR75) (101). The extracellular domain structure of both TR types is highly homologous (102), attesting to the fact that both bind the same ligand with similar affinities (105). However, the cytoplasmic regions of these receptors are quite divergent (102), presumably mediating the observed differences in intracellular signaling upon ligand binding (103). Although the intracellular signaling pathways may be disparate, ligand binding to either receptor was initially reported to increase nuclear NF-$\varkappa$B activity (104). This association was recently confirmed for the TR55, but NF-$\varkappa$B activation via TR75 binding could not be demonstrated for reasons that remain uncertain (107). The expression of the two TR types appears to be independently regulated (102,104,108–110).

We have begun an investigation of the influence of HIV-1 expression on this complex series of cellular responses by examining TR expression on resting and activated OM-10.1 cells. Expression of TR55 was not influenced by HIV-1 activation in OM-10.1 cultures, and surface levels of this molecule appeared to be nearly identical to those of uninfected parental HL-60 cells. However, surface expression of TR75 was observed to dramatically increase during a 48-hour incubation with TNF-α in HIV-1 expressing OM-10.1 cultures, but not uninfected HL-60 cultures. The upregulation of TR75 expression appeared to be a direct consequence of HIV-1 expression, since it was not observed in any of the uninfected HL-60 subclones examined ($n = 6$) and followed the same TNF-α dose dependency as for HIV-1 activation in OM-10.1 cultures. Therefore, HIV-1 has adapted to influence not only cytokine expression but also cytokine action via specific receptor modulation. How the specific upregulation of TR75 might alter HIV-1 expression is still under active investigation.

APPLICATION OF LATENTLY HIV-INFECTED CELLULAR MODELS TO THERAPEUTIC INTERVENTION

It is becoming more apparent that expressing and nonexpressing infected cells exist in vivo at all stages of disease and that the nonexpressing population represents an inducible reservoir population of cells. It still remains to be resolved how the ratio of these two infected cell populations changes during the clinical course to AIDS and what overall contribution the non-expressing population makes to disease progression. However, it seems reasonable, on the basis of induction experiments with in vitro nonexpressing cellular models, that activation of dormant cells in vivo will aid HIV-1 dissemination to new uninfected targets and a general progression of the disease. Therefore, therapeutic modalities directed against the efferent portion of the viral life cycle and designed to prevent viral activation from the nonexpressing pool of cells may prolong the asymptomatic phase or contribute to the prevention of AIDS development (reviewed in Ref. 111).

Some initial attempts have been made using chronically infected cells to test drug efficacy for altering the efferent viral life cycle (112,113). However, in contrast to classic acute infection systems (114), the development of drugs that perturb the later portion of viral expression has been largely restricted by the development and application of rapid and reliable assay systems that adequately represent in vivo latency. We have recently applied the OM-10.1 cell system to this issue (115). Because OM-10.1 cells remain CD4+ until viral activation and respond to TNF-α induction within 24 hours, these cultures can be conveniently used to examine pharmacologics for an ability to block CD4 downmodulation and HIV-1 expression. We have initially tested >50 antiviral compounds for activity against viral activation in the OM-10.1 system. Several initial compounds, including viral protease and Tat inhibitors, demonstrated modest inhibitory activity. With a better understanding of the cellular pathways involved in controlling viral latency and activation will come an ability to design and develop inhibitors that selectively block critical pathways in the efferent component of the HIV-1 life cycle.

CONCLUSIONS

A hallmark of HIV-1 infection is a slow progressive transition to terminal immunosuppression, a course that includes a clinically asymptomatic period of variable length. This asymptomatic period looms as an enormous opportunity for medical intervention while the infected individual remains in good health and of adequate immune status. However, to therapeutically exploit this period of AIDS progression will require an appreciation of clinical and cellular latency as separate entities. Exactly how these two entities interrelate remains uncertain, but viral activation from cellular latency may well contribute to HIV-1 dissemination and disease progression. Studies using in vitro models of cellular latency indicate that viral activation can occur upon exposure to cytokines or antigens and require still poorly understood second and third messenger pathway systems. These additional signaling components are potential targets for therapeutic intervention if adequate information concerning their role can be obtained. Cloned cellular models of HIV-1 latency developed during the past decade, such as OM-10.1, afford us the opportunity to dissect these mechanisms in great detail. It is equally important to compare responses among different cell models to understand host cell and viral variation in the mechanisms controlling latency. Finally, the application of cellular latency models to drug screening and development will potentially identify therapies to prolong the clinical course to AIDS and give hope to the estimated millions of HIV + asymptomatic individuals worldwide.

REFERENCES

1. Rosenberg ZF, Fauci AS. Immunopathogenesis of HIV infection. FASEB J 1991; 5:2382–2390.
2. Ranki A, Valle SL, Krohn M, Antonen J, Allain JP, Leuther M, Franchini G, Krohn K. Long latency preceded overt seroconversion in sexually transmitted human-immunodeficiency-virus infection. Lancet 1987; ii:589–593.
3. Mitsuya H, Yarchoan R, Kageyama S, Broder S. Targeted therapy of human immunodeficiency virus-related disease. FASEB J 1991; 5:2369–2381.
4. Maddon PJ, Dalgleish AG, McDougal JS, Clapham PR, Weiss RA, Axel R. The T4 gene encodes the AIDS virus receptor and is expressed in the immune system and the brain. Cell 1986; 47:333–348.
5. Bednarik DP, Folks TM. Mechanisms of HIV-1 latency. AIDS 1992; 6:3–16.
6. Folks TM, Kelly J, Benn S, Kinter A, Justement J, Gold J, Redfield R, Sell KW, Fauci AS. Susceptibility of normal human lymphocytes to infection with HTLV-III/LAV. J Immunol 1986; 136:4049–4053.
7. Zagury D, Bernard J, Leonard R, Cheynier R, Feldman M, Sarin PS, Gallo RC. Long-term cultures of HTLV-III-infected T cells: a model of cytopathology of T-cell depletion in AIDS. Science 1986; 231:850–853.
8. Hoxie JA, Haggarty BS, Rackowski JL, Pillsbury N, Levy JA. Persistent noncytopathic infection of normal human T lymphocytes with AIDS-associated retrovirus. Science 1985; 229:1400–1402.
9. Clouse KA, Powell D, Washington I, Poli G, Strebel K, Farrar W, Barstad P, Kovacs J, Fauci AS, Folks TM. Monokine regulation of human immunodeficiency virus-1 expression in a chronically infected human T cell clone. J Immunol 1989; 142:431–438.
10. Perez VL, Rowe T, Justement JS, Butera ST, June CH, Folks TM. An HIV-1-infected T cell clone defective in IL-2 production and Ca^{2+} mobilization after CD3 stimulation. J Immunol 1991; 147:3145–3148.

11. Butera ST, Perez VL, Wu B-Y, Nabel GJ, Folks TM. Oscillation of the human immunodeficiency virus surface receptor is regulated by the state of viral activation in a CD4$^+$ cell model of chronic infection. J Virol 1991; 65:4645–4653.
12. Folks TM, Justement J, Kinter A, Dinarello CA, Fauci AS. Cytokine-induced expression of HIV-1 in a chronically infected promonocytic cell lune. Science 1987; 238:800–802.
13. Folks TM, Justement J, Kinter A, Schnittman S, Orienting J, Poli G, Fauci AS. Characterization of a promonocyte clone chronically infected with HIV and inducible by 13-phorbol-12-myristate acetate. J Immunol 1988; 140:1117–1122.
14. Folks TM, Clouse K, Justement J, Rabson A, Duh E, Kehrl JH, Fauci AS. Tumor necrosis factor-alpha induces expression of human immunodeficiency virus in a chronically infected T-cell clone. Proc Natl Acad Sci USA 1989; 86:2365–2368.
15. Pauza CD, Galindo JE, Richman DD. Reinfection results in accumulation of unintegrated viral DNA in cytopathic and persistent human immunodeficiency virus type 1 infection of CEM cells. J Exp Med 1990; 172:1035–1042.
16. Robins HL, Zinkus DM. Accumulation of human immunodeficiency virus type 1 DNA in T cells: result of multiple infection events. J Virol 1990; 64:4836–4841.
17. Fauci AS, Schnittman SM, Poli G, Koenig S, Pantaleo G. Immunopathogenic mechanisms in human immunodeficiency virus (HIV) infection. Ann Intern Med 1991; 114:678–693.
18. Schnittman SM, Psallidopoulos MC, Lane HC, Thompson L, Baseler M, Massari F, Fox CH, Salzman NP, Fauci AS. The reservoir for HIV-1 in human peripheral blood is a T cell that maintains expression of CD4. Science 1989; 245:305–308.
19. Bagasra O, Hauptman SP, Lischner HW, Sachs M, Pomerantz RJ. Detection of human immunodeficiency virus type 1 provirus in mononuclear cells by *in situ* polymerase chain reaction. N Engl J Med 1992; 326:1385–1391.
20. Harper ME, Marselle LM, Gallo RC, Wong-Stall F. Detection of lymphocytes expressing human T-lymphotropic virus type III in lymph nodes and peripheral blood from infected individuals by *in situ* hybridization. Proc Natl Acad Sci USA 1986; 83:772–776.
21. Psallidopoulos MC, Schnittman SM, Thompson L III, Baseler M, Fauci AS, Lane HC, Salzman NP. Integrated proviral human immunodeficiency virus type 1 is present in CD4$^+$ peripheral blood lymphocytes in healthy seropositive individuals. J Virol 1989; 63:4626–4631.
22. Brinchman JE, Albert J, Vartdal F. Few infected CD4$^+$ T cells but a high proportion of replication-competent provirus copies in asymptomatic human immunodeficiency virus type 1 infection. J Virol 1991; 65:2019–2023.

23. Bukrinsky MI, Stanwick TL, Dempsey MP, Stevenson M. Quiesent T lymphocytes as an inducible virus reservoir in HIV-1 infection. Science 1991; 254: 423–427.

24. Schnittman SM, Greenhouse JJ, Lane HC, Pierce PF, Fauci AS. Frequent detection of HIV-1-specific mRNA in infected individuals suggests ongoing active viral expression in all stages of disease. AIDS Res Hum Retrovir 1991; 7:361–367.

25. Schnittman SM, Greenhouse JJ, Psallidopoulos MC, Baseler M, Salzman NP, Fauci AS, Lane HC. Increasing viral burden in CD4$^+$ T cells from patients with human immunodeficiency virus (HIV) infection reflects rapidly progressive immunosuppression and clinical disease. Ann Intern Med 1990; 113:438–443.

26. Hsia K, Spector SA. Human immunodeficiency virus DNA is present in a high percentage of CD4$^+$ lymphocytes of seropositive individuals. J Infect Dis 1991; 164:470–475.

27. Chapel A, Bensussan A, Vilmer E, Dormont D. Differential human immunodeficiency virus expression in CD4$^+$ cloned lymphocytes: from viral latency to replication. J Virol 1992; 66:3966–3970.

28. Boulerice F, Bour S, Geleziunas R, Lvovich A, Wainberg MA. High frequency of isolation of defective human immunodeficiency virus type 1 and heterogeneity of viral gene expression in clones of infected U-937 cells. J Virol 1990; 64:1745–1755.

29. Folks TM, Powell D, Lightfoote M, Koenig S, Fauci AS, Benn S, Rabson A, Daugherty D, Gendelman HE, Hoggan MD, Venkatesan S, Martin MA. Biological and biochemical characterization of a cloned Leu-3$^-$ cell surviving infection with the acquired immune deficiency syndrome retrovirus. J Exp Med 1986; 64:280–290.

30. Mikovits JA, Raziuddin, Gonda M, Ruta M, Lohrey NC, King HF, Ruscetti FW. Negative regulation of human immune deficiency virus replication in monocytes. Distinction between restricted and latent expression in THP-1 cells. J Exp Med 1990; 171:1705–1720.

31. D'Addario M, Wainberg MA, Hiscott J. Activation of cytokine genes in HIV-1 infected myelomonoblastic cells by phorbol esters and tumor necrosis factor. J Immunol 1992; 148:1222–1229.

32. Dahl KE, Burrage T, Jones F, Miller G. Persistent nonproductive infection of Epstein-Barr virus–transformed human B lymphocytes by human immunodeficiency virus type 1. J Virol 1990; 64:1771–1783.

33. Poli G, Fauci AS. The effect of cytokines and pharmacologic agents on chronic HIV infection. AIDS Res Hum Retrovir 1992; 8:191-197.

34. Poli G, Bressler P, Kinter A, Duh E, Timmer WC, Rabson A, Justement JS, Stanley S, Fauci AS. Interleukin 6 induces human immunodeficiency virus expression in infected monocytic cells alone and in synergy with tumor necrosis factor α by transcriptional and post-transcriptional mechanisms. J Exp Med 1990; 172:151–158.

35. Gruters RA, Otto SA, Al BJM, Verhoeven AJ, Verweij CL, van Lier RAW, Miedema F. Non-mitogenic T cell activation signals are sufficient for induction of human immunodeficiency virus transcription. Eur J Immunol 1991; 21:167–172.

36. Margolick JB, Volkman DH, Folks TM, Fauci AS. Amplification HTLV-III/LAV infection by antigen-induced activation of T cells and direct suppression by virus of lymphocyte blastogenic responses. J Immunol 1987; 138: 1719–1723.

37. Siekevitz M, Josephs SF, Dukovich M, Peffer N, Wong-Staal F, Greene WC. Activation of the HIV-1 LTR by T cell mitogens and the trans-activator protein of HTLV-1. Science 1987; 238:1575–1578.

38. Tong-Starken SE, Luciw PA, Peterlin BM. Signaling through T lymphocyte surface proteins, TCR/CD3 and CD28, activates the HIV-1 long terminal repeat. J Immunol 1989; 142:702–707.

39. Tong-Starksen SE, Luciw PA, Peterlin BM. Human immunodeficiency virus long terminal repeat responds to a T-cell activation signals. Proc Natl Acad Sci USA 1987; 84:6845–6849.

40. Linnette GP, Hartzman RJ, Ledbetter JA, June C. HIV-infected T cells show a selective signaling defect after perturbation of CD3-antigen receptor. Science 1988; 241:573.

41. Gupta S, Vayuvegula B. Human immunodeficiency virus-associated changes in signal transduction. J Clin Immunol 1987; 7:486–489.

42. Kaufman JD, Valandra G, Roderiquez G, Bushar G, Giri C, Norcross MA. Phorbol ester enhances human immunodeficiency virus–promoted gene expression and acts on a repeated 10-base-pair functional enhancer element. Mol Cell Biol 1987; 7:3759–3766.

43. Harada S, Koyanagi Y, Nakashima H, Kobayashi N, Yamamoto N. Tumor promoter, TPA, enhances replication of HTLV-III/LAV. Virology 1986; 154:249–258.

44. Kinter AL, Poli G, Maury W, Folks TM, Fauci AS. Direct and cytokine-mediated activation of protein kinase C induces human immunodeficiency virus expression in chronically infected promonocytic cells. J Virol 1990; 64: 4306–4312.

45. Osborn L, Kunkel S, Nabel GJ. Tumor necrosis factor α and interleukin 1 stimulate the human immunodeficiency virus enhancer by activation of the nuclear factor κB. Proc Natl Acad Sci USA 1989; 86:2336–2340.

46. Matsuyama T, Kobayashi N, Yamamoto N. Cytokines and HIV infection: is AIDS a tumor necrosis factor disease? AIDS 1991; 5:1405–1417.

47. Hidaka H, Inagaki M, Kawamote S, Sasaki Y. Isoquinolinesulfonamides, novel and potent inhibitors of cyclic nucleotide dependent protein kinase protein kinase and protein kinase C. Biochemistry 1984; 23:5036–5041.

48. Gaynor R. Cellular transcription factors involved in the regulation of HIV-1 gene expression. AIDS 1992; 6:347–363.

49. Nabel G, Baltimore D. An inducible transcription factor activates expression of human immunodeficiency virus in T cells. Nature 1987; 326:711–713.

50. Sen R, Baltimore D. Inductibility of k immunoglobulin enhancer-binding protein NF-xB by a posttranslational mechanism. Cell 1986; 47:921–928.

51. Nolan GP, Ghosh S, Liou HC, Tempset P, Baltimore D. DNA binding and IkB inhibition of the cloned p65 subunit of NF-xB, a rel-related polypeptide. Cell 1991; 64:961–969.

52. Kieran M, Blank V, Logeat F, Vandekrckhove J, Lottspeich F, LeBail O, Urban MB, Kourilsky P, Baeuerle PA, Isreal A. The DNA binding subunit of NF-xB is identical to factor KBF1 and homologous to the rel oncogene product. Cell 1990; 62:1007–1018.

53. Ghosh S, Gifford AM, Riviere LR, Tempst P, Nolan GP, Baltimore D. Cloning of the p50 DNA binding subunit of NF-xB: homology to rel and dorsal. Cell 1990; 62:1019–1029.

54. Bohnlein E, Lowenthal JW, Siekevitz M, Ballard DW, Franza BR, Greene WC. The same inducible nuclear proteins regulates mitogen activation of both the interleukin-2 receptor-alpha gene and type 1 HIV. Cell 1988; 53: 827–836.

55. Duh EJ, Maury W, Folks TM, Fauci As, Rabson AB. Tumor necrosis factor-alpha activates human immunodeficiency virus-1 through induction of nuclear factor binding to the NF-xB sites in the long terminal repeat. Proc Natl Acad Sci USA 1989; 86:5974–5978.

56. Griffin GE, Leung K, Folks TM, Kunkel S, Nabel GJ. Activation of HIV gene expression during monocytic differentiation by induction of NF-xB. Nature 1989; 339:70–73.

57. Vlach J, Pitha PM. Activation of human immunodeficiency virus type 1 provirus in T cells and macrophages is associated with induction of inducer-specific NF-xB binding proteins. Virology 1991; 187:63–72.

58. Jones KA, Luciw PA, Duchange N. Structural arrangements of transcriptional control domains within the 5'-untranslated leader regions of the HIV-1 and HIV-2 promoters. Genes Dev 1988; 2:1101–1114.

59. Leonard J, Parrott C, Buckler-White A, Turner W, Ross E, Martin M, Rabson A. The NF-xB binding sites in the human immunodeficiency virus type 1 long terminal repeat are not required for virus infectivity. J Virol 1989; 63: 4919–4924.

60. Mitchell PJ, Tjian R. Ikb: A specific inhibitor of the NF-xB transcription factor. Science 1989; 245:371–378.

61. Baeuerle PA, Baltimore D. Ikb: A specific inhibitor of the NF-xB transcription factor. Science 1988; 242:540–546.

62. Ghosh S, Baltimore D. Activation *in vitro* of NF-xB by phosphorylation of its inhibitor IxB. Nature 1990; 344:678–682.

63. Karin M. Signal transduction from cell surface to nucleus in development and disease. FASEB J 1992; 6:2581–2590.

64. Baeuerle PA. The inducible transcription activator NF-xB: regulation by distinct protein subunits. Biochim Biophys Acta 1991; 1072:63–80.

65. Doppler C, Schalasta G, Amtmann E, Sauer G. Binding of NF-xB to the HIV-1 LTR is not sufficient to induce HIV-1 LTR activity. AIDS Res Hum Retrovir 1992; 8:245–252.

66. Sakaguchi M, Zenzie-Gregory B, Groopman JE, Smale ST, Kim S. Alternative pathway for induction of human immunodeficiency virus gene expression: involvement of the general transcription machinery. J Virol 1991; 65: 5448–5456.

67. Meichle A, Schutze S, Hensel G, Brunsing D, Kronke M. Protein kinase C-independent activation of nuclear factor xB by tumor necrosis factor. J Biol Chem 1990; 265:8339–8343.

68. Walker CM, Moody DJ, Sittes DP, Levy JA. CD8$^+$ lymphocytes can control HIV infection *in vitro* by suppressing virus replication. Science 1986; 234: 1563–1566.

69. Brinchman JE, Gaudernack G, Vartdal F. CD8$^+$ T cells inhibit HIV replication in naturally infected CD4$^+$ T cells. J Immunol 1990; 144:2961–2966.

70. Poli G, Kinter AL, Justement JS, Bressler P, Kehrl JH, Fauci AS. Transforming growth factor β suppresses human immunodeficiency virus expression and replication in infected cells of monocyte/macrophage lineage. J Exp Med 1991; 173:589–597.

71. Doerfler W. DNA methylation and gene activity. Annu Rev Biochem 1983; 52:93–124.

72. Bednarik DP, Cook JA, Pitha PM. Inactivation of the HIV LTR by DNA CpG methylation: evidence for a role in latency. EMBO J 1990; 9:1157–1164.

73. Bednarik DP, Mosca JD, Raj NBK. Methylation as a modulator of the HIV LTR. J Virol 1987; 61:1253–1257.

74. Rosen CA, Sodroski JG, Haseltine W. The location of the cis-acting regulatory sequences in the human T cell lymphotropic virus type III (HTLV-III/LAV) long terminal repeat. Cell 1985; 41:813–823.

75. Kato H, Horikoshi M, Roeder R. Repression of HIV-1 transcription by a cellular protein. Science 1991; 251:1476–1479.

76. Luciw PA, Chen-Mayer C, Levy JA. Mutational analysis of the human immunodeficiency virus: The orf-B down-regulates virus replication. Proc Natl Acad Sci USA 1987; 84:1434–1438.

77. Ahmad N, Venkatesan S. Nef protein of HIV-1 is a transcriptional repressor of HIV-1 LTR. Science 1988; 241:1481–1485.

78. Niederman TMJ, Thielan BJ, Ratner L. Human immunodeficiency virus type 1 negative factor is a transcriptional silencer. Proc Natl Acad Sci USA 1989; 86:1128–1132.

79. Cheng-Mayer C, Iannello P, Shaw K, Luciw PA, Levy JA. Differential effects of nef on HIV replication: implications for viral pathogenesis in the host. Science 1989; 246:1629–1632.

80. Hammes SR, Dixon EP, Malim MH, Cullen BR, Greene WC. Nef protein of human immunodeficiency virus type 1: evidence against its role as a transcriptional inhibitor. Proc Natl Acad Sci USA 1989; 86:9549–9553.
81. Kestler HW III, Ringler DJ, Mori K, Panicali DL, Sehgal PK, Daniel MD, Desrosiers RC. Importance of the *nef* gene for maintenance of high virus loads and for development of AIDS. Cell 1991; 65:651–662.
82. Feinberg MB, Jarrett RF, Aldovini A, Gallo RC, Wong-Staal F. HTLV-III expression and production involve complex regulation at the levels of splicing and translation of viral RNA. Cell 1986; 46:807–817.
83. Kim S, Byrn R, Groopman J, Baltimore D. Temporal aspects of DNA and RNA synthesis during human immunodeficiency virus infection: evidence for differential gene expression. J Virol 1989; 63:3708–3713.
84. Pomerantz RJ, Trono D, Feinberg MB, Baltimore D. Cells nonproductively infected with HIV-1 exhibit an aberrant pattern of viral RNA expression: a molecular model for latency. Cell 1990; 61:1271–1276.
85. Michael NL, Morrow P, Mosca J, Vahey M, Burke DS, Redfield RR. Induction of human immunodeficiency virus type 1 expression in chronically infected cells is associated primarily with a shift in RNA splicing patterns. J Virol 1990; 65:1291–1303.
86. Rosen CA, Pavlakis GN. Tat and Rev: positive regulators of HIV gene expression. AIDS 1990; 4:499–509.
87. Pomerantz RJ, Seshamma T, Trono D. Efficient replication of human immunodeficiency virus type 1 requires a threshold level of Rev: potential implications for latency. J Virol 1992; 66:1809–1813.
88. Malim MH, Cullen BR. HIV-1 structural gene expression requires the binding of multiple Rev monomers to the viral RRE: implications for HIV-1 latency. Cell 1991; 65:241–248.
89. Trono D, Baltimore D. A human cell factor is essential for HIV-1 Rev action. EMBO J 1990; 9:4155–4160.
90. Hohmann H-P, Remy R, Scheidereit C, van Loon APGM. Maintenance of NF-$\varkappa$B activation is dependent on protein synthesis and the continuous presence of external stimuli. Mol Cell Biol 1991; 11:259–266.
91. Cochrane AW, Golub E, Volsky D, Ruben S, Rosen CA. Functional significance of phosphorylation to the human immunodeficiency virus Rev protein. J Virol 1989; 63:4438–4440.
92. Jakobovits A, Rosenthal A, Capon DJ. Trans-activation of HIV-1 LTR-directed gene expression by Tat requires protein kinase C. EMBO J 1990; 9:1165–1170.
93. D'Addario M, Roulston A, Wainberg MA, Hiscott J. Coordinate enhancement of cytokine gene expression in human immunodeficiency virus type-1 infected promonocytic cells. J Virol 1990; 64:6080–6089.
94. Molina JM, Scadden DT, Byrn R, Dinarello CA, Groopman JF. Production of tumor necrosis factor α and interleukin 1β by monocytic cells infected with human immunodeficiency virus. J Clin Invest 1990; 84:733–737.

95. Molina JM, Scadden DT, Amirault C, Woon A, Vannier E, Dinarello CA, Groopman JF. Human immunodeficiency virus does not induce interleukin 1, interleukin 6, or tumor necrosis factor in mononuclear cells. J Virol 1990; 64:2901–2906.

96. Poli G, Kinter A, Justement JS, Kehrl JH, Bressler P, Stanley S, Fauci AS. Tumor necrosis factor α functions in an autocrine manner in the induction of human immunodeficiency virus expression. Proc Natl Acad Sci USA 1990; 87:782–785.

97. Tadmori W, Mondal D, Tadmori I, Prakash O. Transactivation of human immunodeficiency virus long terminal repeats by cell surface tumor necrosis factor α. J Virol 1991; 65:6425–6429.

98. Porteu F, Nathan C. Shedding of tumor necrosis factor receptors by activated human neutrophils. J Exp Med 1990; 172:599–607.

99. Seckinger P, Zhang J-H, Hauptmann B, Dayer J-M. Characterization of a tumor necrosis factor α (TNFα) inhibitor: evidence of immunological cross-reactivity with the TNF receptor. Proc Natl Acad Sci USA 1990; 87:5188–5192.

100. Aderka D, Engelmann H, Maor Y, Brakebusch C, Wallach D. Stabilization of the bioactivity of tumor necrosis factor by its soluble receptor. J Exp Med 1992; 175:323–329.

101. Brockhaus M, Schoenfeld H-J, Schlaeger E-J, Hunziker W, Lesslauer W, Loetscher H. Identification of two types of tumor necrosis factor receptors on human cells lines by monoclonal antibodies. Proc Natl Acad Sci USA 1990; 87:3127–3131.

102. Dembic Z, Loetscher H, Gubler U, Pan Y-CE, Lahm H-W, Gentz R, Brockhaus M, Lesslauer W. Two human TNF receptors have similar extracellular, but distinct intracellular, domain sequences. Cytokine 1990; 2:231–237.

103. Tartaglia LA, Weber RF, Figari IS, Reynolds C, Palladino MA Jr, Goeddel DV. The two different receptors for tumor necrosis factor mediate distinct cellular responses. Proc Natl Acad Sci USA 1991; 9292–9296.

104. Hohmann H-P, Brockhaus M, Baeuerle PA, Remy R, Kolbeck R, van Loon APGM. Expression of the types A and B tumor necrosis factor (TNF) receptors is independently regulated, and both receptors mediate activation of the transcription factor NF-xB. TNF-α is not needed for induction of a biologic effect via TNF receptors. J Biol Chem 1990; 265:22409–22417.

105. Hohmann H-P, Remy R, Poschl B, van Loon APGM. Tumor necrosis factors -α and -β bind to the same two types of tumor necrosis factor receptors and maximally activate the transcription factor NF-xB at low receptor occupancy and within minutes after receptor binding. J Biol Chem 1990; 265:15183–15188.

106. Loetscher H, Steinmetz M, Lesslauer W. Tumor necrosis factor: receptors and inhibitors. Cancer Cells 1991; 3:221–226.

107. Kruppa G, Thoma B, Machleidt T, Wiegmann K, Kronke M. Inhibition of tumor necrosis factor (TNF)-mediated NF-xB activation by selective blockade of the human 55-kDa TNF receptor. J Immunol 1992; 148:3152–3157.

108. Erikstein BK, Smeland EB, Blomhoff HK, Funderud S, Prydz K, Lesslauer W, Espevik T. Independent regulation of 55-kDa and 75 kDa tumor necrosis factor receptors during activation of human peripheral blood B lymphocytes. Eur J Immunol 1991; 21:1033–1037.

109. Thoma B, Grell M, Pfizenmaier K, Scheurich P. Identification of a 60-kD tumor necrosis factor (TNF) receptor as the major signal transducing component in TNF responses. J Exp Med 1990; 172:1019–1023.

110. Espevik T, Brockhaus M, Loetscher H, Nonstad U, Shalaby R. Characterization of binding and biological effects of monoclonal antibodies against human tumor necrosis factor receptors. J Exp Med 1990; 171:415–426.

111. Butera ST, Folks TM. Application of latent HIV-1 infected cellular models to therapeutic intervention. AIDS Res Hum Retrovir 1992; 8:991–995.

112. Craig JC, Grief C, Mills JS, Hockley D, Duncan IB, Roberts NA. Effects of a specific inhibitor of HIV proteinase (Ro 31-8959) on virus maturation in a chronically infected promonocytic cell line (U1). Antiviral Chem Chemother 1991; 2:181–186.

113. Lambert DM, Petteway SR Jr, McDanal CE, Hart TK, Leary JJ, Dreyer GB, Meek TD, Bugelski PJ, Bolognesi DP, Metcalf BW, Matthews TJ. Human immunodeficiency virus type 1 protease inhibitors irreversibly block infectivity of purified virions from chronically infected cells. Antimicrob Agents Chemother 1992; 36:982–988.

114. Mitsuya H, Broder S. Inhibition of the *in vitro* infectivity and cytopathic effect of human T-lymphotropic virus type III/lymphadenopathy virus-associated virus (HTLV-III/LAV) by 2',3'-dideoxynucleosides. Proc Natl Acad Sci USA 1986; 83:1911–1915.

115. Feorino PM, Butera ST, Folks TM, Schinazi RF. Prevention of activation of HIV-1 by antiviral agents in OM-10.1 cells. Antiviral Chem Chemother 1992; 4:55–63.

116. Butera ST, Roberts BD, Folks TM. Regulation of HIV-1 expression by cytokine networks in a CD4 + model of chronic infection. J Immunol 1993; 150:625–634.

2

Determinants of HIV-1 Virulence In Vitro and In Vivo Localized in the Envelope V3 Domain

Jaap Goudsmit

University of Amsterdam
Academic Medical Center
Amsterdam, The Netherlands

INTRODUCTION

Human immunodeficiency virus type 1 (HIV-1) appears to cause the acquired immunodeficiency syndrome (AIDS) through a combination of direct HIV-1 cytopathic effects and systemic effects of HIV-1 particles, infected cells, or HIV-1 proteins. The targets of both of these host-cell virus interactions are cells of the immune system, carrying the CD4 molecule on their surface. Recent evidence indicates that the emergence of syncytium-inducing (SI), fast-replicating viruses in a given host heralds rapid CD4 + cell decline and disease progression (Tersmette, Koot, and Miedema, personal communication). This shift from non-SI to SI virus phenotype follows an equally remarkable shift in antigenic virus phenotype, approximately 1–2 years prior to the biological phenotype shift (1). I propose, in accordance with colleagues (2), that antigenic variation allows for increased replication resulting in the acquisition of mutations associated with the SI phenotype. I will try to demonstrate that those mutations are localized primarily in the third variable (V3) domain of the virus envelope.

THE CONCEPT OF THE ASYMPTOMATIC
HIV-1 CARRIER STATE

The natural history of HIV-1 in humans is characterized by the extreme variability in time passed between seroconversion and AIDS diagnosis. Almost all HIV-1-infected individuals experience a period, mostly a few years, that I call an "asymptomatic HIV carrier state" (Table 1). Some individuals may be in this phase of infection for decades and others only for years or months, depending on the virulence of the virus population, the susceptibility of the host, and the immune competence of the host.

Prior to the detection of HIV-1-specific antibodies, a peak of p24 antigen is the first sign of virus expression in the newly infected host (3–5). This antigen peak lasts only a week or two and has vanished by the time p24 antibodies rise. Only in one instance did we observe among the many seroconverters we studied that p24 antigen was below detection level without p24 antibodies having yet been detected. In that one case, no antigen and no antibody were detected for about a week, although the PBMCs were positive for HIV-1 DNA throughout that period (Goudsmit and Jurriaans, unpublished observations). The original assays for detection of p24 antigen in serum detected free p24 antigen exclusively. Neither p24 antigen/antibody complexes nor antigen hidden in a virion were detected. Acid treatment of the samples prior to assaying for antigen revealed that, especially in p24 antibody-negative individuals, a varying proportion of

Table 1   Virological Characterization of the Asymptomatic HIV-1 Carrier State

---

1. Cytoplasmic, linear unintegrated DNA in all (or most) DNA + cells (0.07–0.4% of PBMCs)
   No or little nuclear, integrated or circular unintegrated DNA in any DNA + cell (0.4–1% of PBMCs)
2. Low levels of or no genomic RNA in serum
3. Low or no p24 antigen in serum (± acid/triton); high p24 antibody titers
4. Low yield of or no virus from plasma
5. Coculture of PBMCs yields virus of the non-syncytium-inducing phenotype that is *not* transmissible to cell lines (MT-2)

---

p24 antigen is trapped in antigen/antibody complexes (6–9), resulting in low or absent p24 antibody titers. p24 antibody positivity, in particular with high titers, is a characteristic of asymptomatic individuals not progressing to AIDS rapidly. Detergent treatment of the samples prior to assaying for antigen revealed that a large proportion of antigen during the early antigen peak is virion-associated (10).

This notion is confirmed by the ability to isolate HIV-1 readily from the plasma at or prior to seroconversion (5,11–14). This plasma viremia (15) is cleared during the first year of seropositivity. In a separate experiment, Wolfs and coworkers (1) titrated genomic HIV-1 RNA levels in serum during the course of infection of two seroconverters and showed that HIV-1 RNA levels are highest at or prior to seroconversion, again declining to baseline levels in the first year of seropositivity.

From these results it may be concluded that, following a burst of uncontrolled virus replication in the host resulting in the production of large amounts of cell-free virus, the host is able to limit the virus production to relatively low levels within the first year of seropositivity. During this asymptomatic stage of HIV-1 infection, apparently little cell-free virus is produced. This notion is confirmed by the demonstration of very low levels of infected PBMCs (0.01–0.001%) that express viral RNA (16,17). In contrast, the number of PBMCs harboring viral DNA is about 10–40 times higher (0.07–0.4%) in the asymptomatic stage and 40–100 times higher (0.4–1%) in the symptomatic stage (18). Recently an elegant study by Bukrinsky and co-workers elucidated in part the state of the viral genome during the asymptomatic and symptomatic stages of HIV-1 infection.

Only activated T cells appear to be able to produce virus particles, and this virion multiplication appears to be related to integration of HIV-1 genome in the cellular genome (18). This implies that the number of activated T cells in the asymptomatic stage of infection has to be low since very little virus is produced. Stevenson et al. (19) and Zack et al. (20) postulated that quiescent cells predominating during the asymptomatic stage of infection form a latent and inducible reservoir for HIV-1 in vivo.

In a first set of experiments, Bukrinsky et al. (18) analyzed the arrangement of viral DNA in single infected cells. This method allowed them to distinguish between restricted integration versus superinfection as an explanation for the accumulation of unintegrated viral DNA. Analysis of PBMCs of AIDS patients with 0.4–1% of cells infected showed that between 59 and 80% of the infected cells contained exclusively integrated DNA, and, in the remaining cells, either exclusively unintegrated DNA or both integrated *and* unintegrated DNA was present. Analysis of

PBMCs of asymptomatic individuals with 0.07–0.4% of cells infected showed that between 50 and 88% of the infected cells contained uninte-grated DNA exclusively. In the remaining minority of cells, either inte-grated DNA exclusively or both integrated *and* unintegrated DNA was present. From these data one may conclude, as the authors suggest, that superinfection is not widespread in PBMCs of HIV-1-infected individ-uals and that in asymptomatic individuals low level of virus production is due to the restricted integration in quiescent cells. Depletion of activated T cells by using a monoclonal antibody to HLA class II increased the per-centage of cells harboring unintegrated viral DNA from 20–35% to 80–100%. In addition, PHA stimulation of PBMCs of an asymptomatic in-dividual increased the number of cells with integrated DNA from 20 to 100%.

The question that comes to mind is which virus mutations drive these HIV-1 replication kinetics. I propose the mutations are associated with, first, antigenic variation and, second, the SI phenotype.

BIOLOGICAL PHENOTYPE OF VIRUS ISOLATED DURING EARLY PHASES OF HIV-1 INFECTION

Åsjö and coworkers (21–23) were the first to show that HIV-1 isolates recovered from PBMCs of asymptomatic individuals multiplied in PHA-stimulated donor PBMCs, but were not transmissible to permanent cell lines. Isolates recovered from AIDS patients replicate faster than isolates obtained from PBMCs in asymptomatic individuals and are generally transmissible to cell lines. Subsequently, Tersmette and coworkers (24–26) showed that HIV-1 isolates may be distinguished according to their ability to form syncytia in primary PBMC cultures. As a rule, HIV-1 is-olates that induce syncytia in PBMC cultures can be transmitted to per-manent cell lines, while HIV-1 isolates that do not induce syncytia in PBMC cultures cannot. This latter category of viruses can be divided into those that replicate fast and those that replicate slowly in PBMC cultures. These rules have exceptions: some non-syncytium-inducing viruses will replicate in SupT1 cells but not in H9 cells.

PBMCs contain both T cells and monocytes. Monocytotropic strains appear to be a subset of the viruses that show the non-SI phenotype in PBMCs and are not transmissible to cell lines (27,28). The phenotypes described are found in primary isolates that are not biologically cloned.

Clonal analysis of primary isolates suggested that viruses cultured in bulk and showing the non-SI phenotype (no syncytia in PBMCs and non-transmissible to cell lines) exclusively contain clones with the non-SI phenotype (29,30). On the other hand, viruses cultured in bulk and showing the SI phenotype (syncytia in PBMCs and transmissible to cell lines) may contain a whole range (from 10 to 100%) of clones of SI viruses in the midst of clones of the non-SI phenotype.

The next questions are:

1. What is the phenotype of viruses recovered from either PBMCs or plasma during the initial years of seropositivity?
2. Are viruses with distinct biological phenotypes antigenically different?

Most pertinent to these questions are, again, studies of seroconverters either progressing to AIDS or remaining asymptomatic for a given time period (31). The findings of these studies can be summarized by stating that viruses of the SI phenotype are not detectable throughout the course of infection but emerge prior to the progression to disease. Apparently, as a consequence, infection with a swarm of viruses of either the SI or non-SI phenotype results in the predominance of viruses of the non-SI phenotype during the asymptomatic stage of infection. Unfortunately, no conclusive data are available at present on whether culture of the plasma or the PBMCs prior to or at seroconversion yields viruses of the SI phenotype that may be subsequently suppressed by immune mechanisms.

Virologically, therefore, the asymptomatic stage is characterized by the isolation of viruses of the non-SI phenotype (a subset being monocytotropic) that exhibit low infectivity and appear to be relatively resistant to neutralization by antibodies and sCD4 (32–37).

Preliminary genetic evidence indicates that the virus initiating the infection in a new host is genetically homogeneous (see below), with the same applying to PBMCs, plasma, and serum (Wolfs and Goudsmit, unpublished observations). The biological phenotype of these PBMC- and plasma-initiating virus populations is predicted to be non-SI. It is not known, however, whether infection is possible from cells harboring virus genome but not expressing the virus envelope, or if infection is initiated exclusively by cell-free virus and/or virus-expressing cells. In both instances, determinants within the external envelope coding region appear to play a major role, in particular localized in the V3 region.

EVOLUTION OF V3 MUTATIONS ASSOCIATED WITH ANTIGENIC AND BIOLOGICAL VARIATION DURING THE COURSE OF INFECTION

The V3 domain of the external envelope glycoprotein (gp120) of HIV-1 contains determinants of virus cytopathicity, cell tropism, and virus infectivity (38–46) (Figure 1).

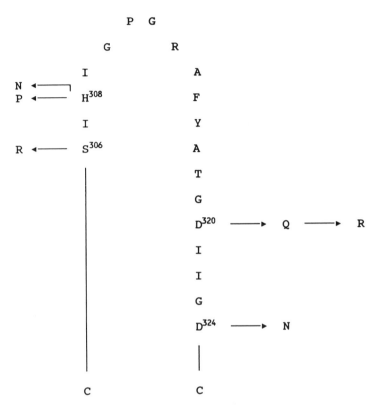

Figure 1 Map of virulence and antigenic determinants within the third variable (V3) envelope domain of HIV-1. *Note*: H^{308} → P/N: antigenic variant; S^{306} → R: incomplete SI; R^{306} + D^{320} → Q: complete SI; R^{306} + D^{324} → N: complete SI; Q^{320} → R: complete SI phenotype.

A general increase in genomic heterogeneity is observed during persistently high neutralizing and V3-specific antibody titers in genomic RNA (1). The continuous increase in genomic diversity over a period of years resulting in an increasing genomic distance from the initial genome population appears to be independent of both the rapidity of disease progression and the virus copy number (1). Shortly after virus transmission, around the time of antibody seroconversion, the HIV-1 V3 RNA population is extremely homogeneous. This appears to be generally true for both extracellular HIV-1 RNA and intracellular HIV-1 DNA populations. Also seen in both HIV-1 RNA and HIV-1 DNA populations is a decrease in the Hamming distances later in the course of infection and related to disease development. However, it is still unresolved if the homogeneity rate in infection is due to virus phenotype, use of a drug such as AZT, or another pathogenic factor. Nowak and coworkers (2) explain this observation by the existence of an antigenicity threshold that is passed at a certain time due to overwhelming of the immune system by a myriad of HIV variants.

The second major form of genomic variation occurs in a more discontinuous fashion. This concerns mutations that are fixed in all molecular clones within a very limited time span of a few months. Two to four years after the acquisition of HIV-1 infection, an amino acid–changing mutation occurs at position 308 within the V3 loop. This change has direct impact on the binding of patients' antibodies in both specificity and affinity to V3 peptides exclusively distinct at position 308. From these data one may conclude that naturally occurring mutations within HIV-1 V3 genomic RNA lead to antigenetic variation dependent on this one particular amino acid substitution.

A second set of fixed mutations in the V3 region occurs approximately 2 years prior to disease development and is associated with the emergence of SI viruses. These changes at positions 306, 320, and 324 (45–47) may also have impact on the antigenicity of the V3 domain although such data have not yet been gathered.

In conclusion, one may say that during the course of HIV-1 infection, despite the continuous genomic diversification, two distinct events occur: a fixation of mutations at position 308 related to antigenicity of HIV-1 and a subsequent fixation of mutations at positions 306 and 320, in particular, related to the biological phenotype of the virus.

IN VIVO RELEVANCE OF THE PHENOTYPE-ASSOCIATED V3 MUTATIONS

How relevant is this selection process for the in vivo situation? This question was addressed by Kuiken and coworkers (47), studying the evolution of the V3 envelope domain in proviral sequences and isolates of HIV-1 during transition of the viral biological phenotype.

Isolation of SI viruses—which form syncytia in donor PBMCs, grow rapidly, and are transmissible to transformed T-cell lines—heralds progression to AIDS (24,26,33). Primary isolates showing the non-SI phenotype exclusively contain clones with the non-SI phenotype. In contrast, SI isolates nearly always constitute a mixed population of clones with and without SI capacity (27,30). Apparently, the phenotype of the primary isolate is determined by the phenotype of the most virulent clone present. It is argued that non-SI monocytotropic clones are responsible for the persistence of HIV-1 infection. Progression of disease is associated with a selective increase of T-cell-tropic, nonmonocytotropic clones (27).

Convincing evidence has emerged that the SI (T-cell-tropic) phenotype of HIV-1 strains is associated, if not determined in total, by the V3 domain of that particular isolate (45,46). Kuiken and coworkers (47) generated V3 sequences from DNA of samples taken 3 months apart, over a period of 24 and 30 months, from PBMCs of two individuals, both before and after cocultivation with uninfected donor PBMCs. The isolated virus shifted from the non-SI phenotype to the SI phenotype during the study period. This shift was associated with distinct changes in the V3 domain of both patients. The association of the phenotype shift with the V3 sequence changes was confirmed by construction of viruses with chimeric V3 loops. The shift from non-SI to SI-associated V3 variants was also seen in the uncultured PBMCs of both patients, but not until 3 and 9 months after the detection of SI virus in culture.

To further investigate the evolution of the SI phenotype, multidimensional scaling can be done on the matrix of Hamming distances between consensus sequences of all samples. This statistical method can be used to assess the number of mathematical dimensions that are minimally required to give an accurate description of the data. If one dimension is sufficient, the datum points can be represented as lying on a straight line. If the sequences are very heteroplasious, meaning that many acquired mutations are lost again and there is no unidirectional evolutionary line, more than one dimension is needed to accurately represent the Hamming distance matrix. Kuiken's experiments show that the V3 sequence population in the uncultured material moves in sequence space in the same direction as the V3 sequence population in the cultured material—however, with a time lag of about 9 months.

One uncultured sample was the main cause of deviation from a one-dimensional representation. This pattern looks like a "fitness landscape." Several fitness peaks (concentrations of similar variants) are formed by viruses that are almost as fit as the "master" virus. Variants in the fitness lowlands between the peaks generate fewer offspring and exist only at low frequency. In crossing the lowlands, it may be advantageous for a variant to take a longer route, if that enables it to avoid a particularly crippling mutation. If this concept, put forward by Kuiken, is right, neither the calculation of a minimum-length phylogenetic tree nor the computation of evolutionary rates for the V3 domain is justified. Still, fixation of particular biologically significant mutations within the V3 domain may help in interpreting the evolution of the V3 domain during the course of infection.

CONCLUDING REMARKS

From our results and those of others, I conclude that fixed V3 mutations— mainly at position 308—lowering the ability of neutralizing antibodies to bind the virus, followed by another set of fixed V3 mutations—particularly at positions 306, 320, and 324—enhancing virus infectivity, in particular for T cells, are major contributing factors to the AIDS progression rate in natural HIV-1 infection.

REFERENCES

1. Wolfs TFW, Zwart G, Bakker M, Valk M, Kuiken CL, Goudsmit J. Naturally occurring mutations within HIV-1 V3 genomic RNA lead to antigenic variation dependent on a single amino acid substitution. Virology 1991; 185:195–205.
2. Nowak MA, Anderson RM, McLean AR, Wolfs TFW, Goudsmit J, May RM. Antigenic diversity thresholds and the development of AIDS. Science 1991; 254:963–969.
3. Goudsmit J, de Wolf F, Paul DA, Epstein LG, Lange JMA, Krone WJA, Speelman H, Wolters EC, van der Noordaa, Oleske JM, van der Helm, Coutinho RA. Expression of human immunodeficiency virus antigen (HIV-Ag) in serum and cerebrospinal fluid during acute and chronic infection. Lancet 1986; ii: 177–180.
4. Lange JMA, Paul DA, Huisman JG, de Wolf F, van den Berg H, Coutinho RA, Danner SA, van der Noordaa J, Goudsmit J. Persistent HIV antigenaemia and decline of HIV core antibodies associated with transition to AIDS. Br Med J 1986; 293:1459–1462.
5. Gaines H, Albert J, von Sydow M, Sönnerborg A, Chiodi F, Ehrnst F, Strannegård, O, Åsjö B. HIV antigenaemia and virus isolation from plasma during primary HIV infection. Lancet 1987; i:1317.
6. Carini C, Mezzaroma I, Scano G, D'Amelio R, Matricardi P, Aiuti F. Characterization of specific immune complexes in HIV-related disorders. Scand J Immunol 1987; 26:21–28.
7. Lange JMA, Paul DA, de Wolf F, Coutinho RA, Goudsmit J. Viral gene expression, antibody production and immune complex formation in human immunodeficiency virus infection. AIDS 1987; 1:15–20.
8. McHugh TM, Sittes DP, Busch MP, Krowka JF, Stricker RB, Hollander H. Relation of circulating levels of human immunodeficiency virus (HIV) anti-

gen, antibody to p24, and HIV-containing immune complexes in HIV-infected patients. J Infect Dis 1988; 158:1088–1091.

9. Morrow WJW, Wharton M, Stricker RB, Levy JA. Circulating immune complexes in patients with acquired immune deficiency syndrome contain the AIDS-associated retrovirus. Clin Immunol Immunopathol 1986; 40:515–524.

10. Mulder JW, Lange JMA, de Wolf F, Houweling JTM, Bakker M, Coutinho RA, Goudsmit J. Serum p24 antigen levels in untreated and zidovudine-treated HIV-1 infected subjects. Neth J Med 1990; 37:4–10.

11. Albert J, Gaines H, Sönnerborg A, Nyström G, Pehrson PO, Chiodi F, von Sydow M, Moberg L, Lidman K, Christensson B, Åsjö B, Fenyö EM. Isolation of HIV from plasma during primary HIV infection. J Med Virol 1987; 23:67–73.

12. Cooper DA, Gold J, Maclean P, Donovan B, Finlayson R, Barnes TG, Michelmore HM, Brooke P, Penny R. Acute AIDS retrovirus infection. Definition of a clinical illness associated with seroconversion. Lancet 1985; i: 537–540.

13. Clark SJ, Saag MS, Decker WD, Campbell-Hill S, Roberson JL, Veldkamp PJ, Kappes JC, Hahn BH, Shaw GM. High titers of cytopathic virus in plasma of patients with symptomatic primary HIV-1 infection. N Engl J Med 1991; 324:954–960.

14. Daar ES, Moudgil T, Meyer RD, Ho DD. Transient high levels of viremia in patients with primary human immunodeficiency virus type 1 infection. N Engl J Med 1991; 324:961–964.

15. Baur A, Schwarz N, Ellinger S, Korn K, Harper T, Mang K, Jahn G. Continuous clearance of HIV in a vertically infected child. Lancet 1989; ii:1045.

16. Harper ME, Marselle LM, Gallo RC, Wong-Staal F. Detection of lymphocytes expressing HTLV-III in lymph nodes and peripheral blood from infected persons by in situ hybridization. Proc Natl Acad Sci USA 1986; 83: 772–776.

17. Ho DD, Moudgil T, Alam M. Quantitation of human immunodeficiency virus type 1 in the blood of infected persons. N Engl J Med 1989; 321:1621–1625.

18. Bukrinsky MI, Stanwick TL, Dempsey MP, Stevenson M. Quiescent T lymphocytes as an inducible virus reservoir in HIV-1 infection. Science 1991; 254:423–427.

19. Stevenson M, Stanwick TL, Dempsey MP, Lamonica CA. HIV-1 replication is controlled at the level of T cell activation and proviral integration. EMBO J 1990; 9(5):1551–1560.

20. Zack JA, Arrigo SJ, Weitsman SR, Go AS, Haislip A, Chen ISY. HIV-1 entry into quiescent primary lymphocytes: molecular analysis reveals a labile, latent viral structure. Cell 1990; 61:213–222.

21. Åsjö B, Morefeldt-Månson L, Albert J, Biberfeld G, Karlsson A, Lidman K, Fenyö EM. Replicative capacity of human immunodeficiency virus from patients with varying severity of HIV infection. Lancet 1986; ii:660–662.

22. Fenyö EM, Albert J, Åsjö B. Replicative capacity, cytopathic effect and cell tropism of HIV. AIDS 1989; 3(suppl 1):S5–S12.

23. Fenyö EM, Morfeld-Manson L, Chiodi F, Lind B, von Gegerfelt A, Albert J, Olausson E, Åsjö B. Distinct replicative and cytopathic characteristics of human immunodeficiency virus isolates. J Virol 1988; 62:4414–4419.

24. Tersmette M, Goede de REY, Al BJM, Winkel IN, Coutinho RA, Cuypers HThM, Huisman JG, Miedema F. Differential syncytium-inducing capacity of HIV isolates. Frequent detection of syncytium-inducing isolates in patients with AIDS and ARC. J Virol 1988; 62:2026–2032.

25. Tersmette M, Gruters RA, de Wolf F, de Goede REY, Lange JMA, Schellekens PTH, Goudsmit J, Huisman JG, Miedema F. Evidence for a role of virulent human immunodeficiency virus (HIV) variants in the pathogenesis of acquired immunodeficiency syndrome: studies on sequential HIV isolates. J Virol 1989; 63(5):2118–2125.

26. Tersmette M, Lange JMA, de Goede REY, de Wolf F, Eeftinck Schattenkerk JKM, Schellekens PTH, Coutinho RA, Huisman JG, Goudsmit J, Miedema F. Association between biological properties of human immunodeficiency virus variants and risk for AIDS and AIDS mortality. Lancet 1989; i:983–985.

27. Schuitemaker H, Kootstra NA, de Goede REY, de Wolf F, Miedema F, Tersmette M. Monocytotropic human immunodeficiency virus type 1 (HIV-1) variants detectable in all stages of HIV-1 infection lack T-cell line tropism and syncytium-inducing ability in primary T-cell culture. J Virol 1991; 65(1):356–363.

28. Boucher CAB, Krone WJA, Goudsmit J, Meloen RH, Naylor PH, Goldstein AL, Sun DK, Sarin PS. Immune response and epitope mapping of a candidate HIV-1 p17 vaccine HGP30. J Clin Lab Anal 1990; 4(1):43–47.

29. Tersmette M, de Goede REY, de Wolf F, et al. Clonal analysis of changes in biological phenotype of sequential HIV isolates from seroconverting and seropositive individuals. J Cell Biochem 1990; suppl 14D:170.

30. Tersmette M, Miedema F. Interactions between HIV and the host immune system in the pathogenesis of AIDS. AIDS 1990; 4(suppl 1):S57–S66.

31. Gruters RA, Terpstra FG, de Goede REY, Mulder JW, de Wolf F, Schellekens PT, van Lier RAW, Tersmette M, Miedema F. Immunological and virological markers in individuals progressing from seroconversion to AIDS. AIDS 1991; 5:837–844.

32. Cheng-Mayer C, Quiroga M, Tung JW, Dina D, Levy JA. Viral determinants of human immunodeficiency virus type 1 T-cell or macrophage tropism, cytopathogenicity, and CD4 antigen modulation. J Virol 1990; 64(9):4390–4398.

33. Cheng-Mayer C, Seto D, Tateno M, Levy JA. Biologic features of HIV-1 that correlate with virulence in the host. Science 1988; 240:80–82.

34. Cheng-Mayer C, Weiss C, Seto D, Levy JA. Isolates of human immunodeficiency virus type 1 from the brain may constitute a special group of the AIDS virus. Proc Natl Acad Sci USA 1989; 86:8575–8579.

35. von Briesen H, Becker WB, Henco K, Helm EB, Gelderblom HR, Brede HD, Rübsamen-Waigmann H. Isolation frequency and growth properties of HIV variants: multiple simultaneous variants in a patient demonstrated by molecular cloning. J Med Virol 1987; 23:51–66.

36. Cheng-Mayer C, Homsy J, Evans LA, Levy JA. Identification of human immunodeficiency virus subtypes with distinct patterns of sensitivity to serum neutralization. Proc Natl Acad Sci USA 1988; 85:2815–2819.

37. Daar ES, Li XL, Moudgil T, Ho DD. High concentrations of recombinant soluble CD4 are required to neutralize primary HIV-1 isolates. Proc Natl Acad Sci USA 1990; 87:6574–6578.

38. Hwang SS, Boyle TJ, Lyerly HK, Cullen BR. Identification of the envelope V3 loop as the primary determinant of cell tropism in HIV-1. Science 1991; 253:71–74.

39. Takeuchi Y, Akutsu M, Murayama K, Shimizu N, Hoshino H. Host range mutant of human immunodeficiency virus type 1: modification of cell tropism by a single point mutation at the neutralization epitope in the env gene. J Virol 1991; 65:1710–1718.

40. Ivanoff LA, Looney DJ, McDanal C, Morris JF, Wong-Staal F, Langlois AJ, Petteway SR Jr, Matthews TJ. Alteration of HIV-1 infectivity and neutralization by a single amino acid replacement in the V3 loop domain. AIDS Res Hum Retrovir 1991; 7:595–603.

41. Cheng-Mayer C, Shioda T, Levy J. Host range, replicative, and cytopathic properties of human immunodeficiency virus type 1 are determined by very few amino acid changes in tat and gp120. J Virol 1991; 65:6931–6941.

42. Chesebro B, Nishio J, Perryman S, Cann A, O'Brien W, Chen ISY, Wehrly K. Identification of human immunodeficiency virus envelope gene sequences influencing viral entry into CD4-positive HeLa cells, T-leukemia cells, and macrophages. J Virol 1991; 65:5782–5789.

43. Freed EO, Myers DJ, Risser R. Identification of the principal neutralizing determinant of human immunodeficiency virus type 1 as a fusion domain. J Virol 1991; 65:190–194.

44. Freed EO, Risser R. Identification of conserved residues in the human immunodeficiency virus type 1 principal neutralizing determinant that are involved in fusion. AIDS Res Hum Retrovir 1991; 7:807–811.

45. Fouchier RAM, Groenink M, Kootstra NA, Tersmette M, Huisman HG, Miedema F, Schuitemaker H. Phenotype associated sequence variation in the third variable domain of the human immunodeficiency virus type 1 gp120 molecule. J Virol 1992; 66:3183–3187.

46. de Jong JJ, Goudsmit J, Keulen W, Klaver B, Krone W, Tersmette M, de Ronde A. Human immunodeficiency virus type 1 clones chimeric for the envelope V3 domain differ in syncytium formation and replication capacity. J Virol 1992; 66:757–765.

47. Kuiken CL, de Jong JJ, Baan E, Keulen W, Tersmette M, Goudsmit J. Evolution of the V3 envelope domain in proviral sequences and isolates of human immunodeficiency virus type 1 during transition of the viral biological phenotype. J Virol 1992; 66:4622–4627.

3

Membrane Expression of HIV Envelope Glycoproteins Triggers Apoptosis in CD4 Cells

A Direct Mechanism for T4 Cell Depletion Mediated by Virus Replication

Ara G. Hovanessian, Bernard Krust, and Yves Rivière

Institut Pasteur
Paris, France

Sylviane Muller

Institut de Biologie Moléculaire et Cellulaire du CNRS
Strasbourg, France

Marie Paule Kieny

Transgène S.A.
Strasbourg, France

Charles Dauguet and Anne G. Laurent-Crawford

Institut Pasteur
Paris, France

Apoptosis, or programmed cell death, is a physiological cell suicide mechanism occurring in normal tissue turnover (1,2). The mechanisms leading to apoptosis have not been completely elucidated and may be different

---

This work was carried out at Institut Pasteur, Unité de Virologie et Immunologie Cellulaire, UA CNRS 1157, Paris, France.

from one system to another. In most cases, cells undergoing apoptosis manifest profound modifications of their cytoskeleton, showing blebbing of the plasma membrane (3). However, one of the ubiquitous effects of apoptosis is the Ca^{2+}-mediated activation of a nuclear endonuclease, which cleaves the chromatin at internucleosomal junctions and thus generates oligonucleosomal-length DNA fragments. Consequently, the detection of low-molecular-weight (LMW) DNA made up of multimers of a nucleosomal length unit of 200 bp DNA is considered a marker of apoptosis. This LMW DNA, when analyzed by electrophoresis, is revealed as a DNA ladder made of 200 bp DNA multimers. Using an alternative method, we have recently demonstrated that the analysis of histones (H2A, H2B, H3, and H4) recovered from the LMW DNA fragments can be used as a sensitive marker to monitor apoptosis (4). It should be emphasized that degradation of the chromatin during apoptosis occurs in metabolically active cells (1,2). Under electron microscopy, apoptosis can be demonstrated by the condensation of the chromatin at the periphery of the nuclear membrane in characteristic peripheral crescent forms.

Recently we and others reported that the cytopathic effect of HIV-1 and HIV-2 in CD4 cell cultures is associated with apoptosis (4,5). In a more recent work we demonstrated that the expression of the HIV envelope glycoprotein gene is sufficient for apoptosis (6). These observations indicate that the CD4 T-cell depletion occurring in HIV-contaminated patients during the development of AIDS (7) might be due—at least in part—to the expression of the HIV envelope gene, probably during massive viral production. However, this alone cannot account for the CD4 T-cell depletion. Accordingly, several authors have reported that apoptosis independent of virus replication might be occurring in AIDS patients (8–12). HIV infection therefore results in apoptotic mechanisms mediated either directly by virus replication or indirectly by priming uninfected cells. Such mechanisms should account in great part for the T4-cell depletion observed in patients during the development of AIDS. In addition to these, a complementary cytopathic effect is probably provided by the immune system (13), since infected cells may be killed by HIV-specific cytotoxic cells (CTLs) or antibody-dependent cell-mediated cytotoxicity (ADCC) (14–17).

APOPTOSIS AND THE CYTOPATHIC EFFECT OF HIV

HIV infects lymphocytes, monocytes, and macrophages by binding to its principal receptor, the CD4 molecule (18). This binding, mediated by the external envelope glycoprotein of HIV, is essential for the viral envelope and cell membrane fusion and thus for viral entry (19).

In general, HIV infection of cell cultures results in the generation of an acute and/or chronic infection. In both cases virus is produced and becomes released by budding at the cellular membrane. Acute infection is characterized by a typical cytopathic effect manifested by ballooning of cells and formation of syncytia and subsequently by cell death. On the other hand, chronically infected cells do not show this typical cytopathic effect despite their constant capacity to produce infectious HIV particles. This difference between cultures of acute and chronic infection has been reported to be due in part to a lower number of virus particles produced and downregulation of CD4 receptors in chronically infected cells (20).

In Figure 1, we analyze in parallel chronically and acutely infected CEM cells. Both cell types produced comparable levels of HIV-1 proteins. However, analysis of LMW DNA in the nucleoplasm indicated that the oligonucleosomal DNA ladder was found only in acutely infected cells. Similarly, histones were detectable only in acutely, not chronically infected cells. These results indicate that apoptosis does not occur in chronically infected cells. This is probably due to downregulation of CD4 receptor expression (less than 7%) in our chronically infected cells compared to acutely infected cells, since both cell types produced equivalent amounts of viral proteins.

APOPTOSIS IN THE LATER STAGES OF HIV INFECTION

In a single-cycle acute infection, all cells become infected by the input HIV. At 48 hours postinfection (p.i.), more than 90% of cells become producers of HIV proteins detectable by immunofluorescence using anti-p25 or anti-gp120 antibodies. Examination of infected cultures under light microscope reveals that most cells become aggregated at 24 hours p.i.; syncytia formation becomes detectable 30 hours p.i. At 48 hours p.i., almost no single cells are observed, as giant syncytia are formed. All cells become lysed by the third day of infection. At 48 hours p.i., when cells are viable and actively synthesizing viral proteins, apoptosis is clearly indicated by the presence of histones and the typical oligonucleosomal DNA ladder (Figure 2).

At 1 hour p.i., considerable amounts of viral core protein p25 is found inside cells. Addition of AZT at 1 hour results in 90% inhibition of virus production and apoptosis occurring at 48 hours p.i. (Figure 3). These ob-

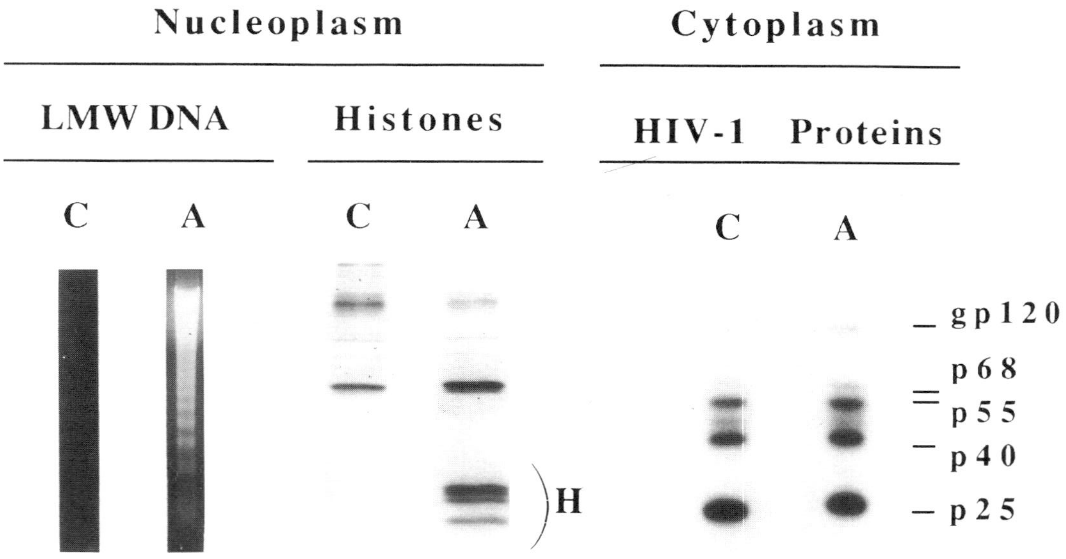

Figure 1   Chronically infected CEM cells produced continuously infectious HIV-1 particles without showing any apparent cytopathic effect. Extracts from these chronically infected cells (lanes C) in parallel with CEM cells acutely infected (4 days p.i.) with HIV-1 were analyzed here. Histones and LMW DNA (phenol/chloroform/isoamyl) extracts from the nucleoplasm of chronically (lanes C) or acutely (lanes A) infected CEM cells were analyzed by electrophoresis on SDS-polyacrylamide gel followed by Coomassie blue staining and on 1.4% agarose gel, respectively. The presence of HIV-1 proteins in cytoplasmic extracts was assayed by immunoblotting using HIV-1-positive serum. In this autoradiograph, the positions of HIV-1 gp120, p68, p55, p40, and p25 are indicated on the right. All experimental procedures were described in Ref. 4.

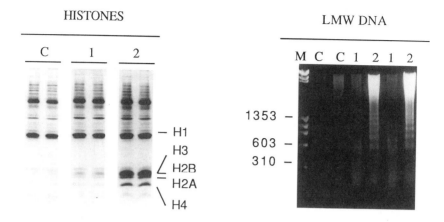

Figure 2 Apoptosis during a single-cycle HIV infection. CEM cells were infected with 500 TCID$_{50}$ of HIV-1 per cell and analyzed at 24 and 48 hours p.i. Experimental procedures were described in Ref. 6. Apoptosis was assayed by the accumulation of histones (left panel) and by the profile of LMW DNA (right panel). Lanes C, 1, and 2 represent uninfected control cells and infected cells at 1 and 2 days p.i., respectively. The positions of histones (constituents of nucleosomes), H1, H2A, H2B, H3, and H4 are as indicated. Lane M gives the HaeIII digest of ϕx174 used as a DNA marker.

servations indicate that virus adsorption and entry do not induce apoptosis and that virus replication is required in order to produce viral proteins.

NECESSITY OF HIV REPLICATION BUT NOT ACCUMULATION OF UNINTEGRATED HIV DNA FOR APOPTOSIS IN ACUTE INFECTION

In the single-cycle infection, we blocked replication of HIV by the addition of AZT at different times after virus adsorption. The production of virus, accumulation of unintegrated HIV DNA, development of syncytia, and apoptosis were then analyzed at 48 hours p.i. Addition of AZT together with the virus, or 1 hour after virus adsorption, resulted in a dramatic inhibition of virus production, development of syncytia, and apoptosis. On the other hand, AZT added from 6 hours onward, did not cause any apparent modification in the kinetics and the production of virus or in the development of syncytia and apoptosis. Treatment with AZT was effective, since accumulation of the unintegrated HIV DNA was almost

Histones   LMW DNA

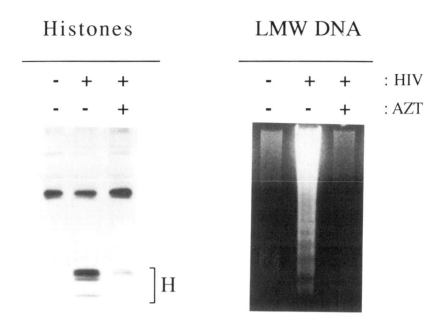

| - | + | + | | - | + | + | : HIV |
| - | - | + | | - | - | + | : AZT |

]H

Figure 3 HIV replication is required for the onset of apoptosis during an acute infection. CEM cells were infected with HIV-1 as in Figure 2, but AZT (5 μM) was added at 1 hour p.i. At 48 hours p.i., all cultures were examined under a light microscope for the development of CPE (ballooning of cells and formation of syncytia) and nuclear extracts were prepared. Apoptosis was monitored by the accumulation of histones (left panel) and by the profile of LMW DNA (right panel). No apoptosis was observed in HIV-1-infected cells in the presence of AZT as is the case in uninfected cells.

completely inhibited. These results indicate that an interval of about 6 hours was required during which time the input viral RNA was transcribed into the proviral DNA to initiate the single cycle infection. Accordingly, AZT added until 6 hours p.i. inhibited transcription of the input viral RNA and blocked virus infection and apoptosis. Without replication, therefore, the input virus has no capacity by itself to mediate apoptosis. The fact that, when added at 6 hours p.i., AZT did not modify the kinetics of virus infection but drastically inhibited the accumulation of unintegrated HIV DNA suggested that this latter phenomenon might be due to superinfection of cells, as has been reported previously (21,22). Whatever the case, our data rule out any correlation between the accumulation of unintegrated HIV DNA and HIV infection–induced cytopathic effect as suggested previously (21).

INTERACTION BETWEEN gp120 AND THE CD4 RECEPTOR AS FIRST STEP IN APOPTOSIS INDUCTION DURING ACUTE HIV INFECTION

For further characterization of apoptosis occurring during a single-cycle HIV infection, we studied the effect of monoclonal antibodies (Mabs) specific for gp120 and the CD4 receptor:

> Mab 110/4 recognizes the principal neutralization epitope (V3) on gp 120. This Mab inhibits virus infection and syncytia formation without much affecting the binding of gp120 to the CD4 receptor (23,24).
>
> Mabs specific for the CD4 receptor: Mab OKT4a, which blocks gp120 binding to the CD4 receptor and thus syncytia formation, and Mab OKT4, which blocks neither. The epitope recognized by Mab OKT4 seems to be close to the cell membrane since it is resistant to trypsin treatment (24–26).

For a control, we used a Mab specific for the major core protein p25 of HIV (27). The different Mabs were added 6 hours after virus adsorption, and apoptosis was analyzed at 48 hours (Figure 4). In the presence of these different Mabs, no apparent alteration was observed in the kinetics of one-cycle HIV infection or any significant modification in the synthesis and production of gp120 and other viral proteins (data not shown). MAB 110/4 and Mab OKT4a blocked syncytia formation and also prevented apoptosis. On the other hand, Mab OKT4, which only slightly affected syncytia formation, inhibited apoptosis by more than 80%. These observations indicate that the binding of gp120 to CD4 might represent the first step required but is not by itself sufficient for inducing apoptosis, since Mab 110/4, which does not prevent binding, inhibits apoptosis. The observation that Mab OKT4 inhibits apoptosis without much effect on syncytia formation suggests that the OKT4 epitope is probably an essential component of CD4 that is implicated in the mechanism of apoptosis.

CHRONICALLY INFECTED CELLS EXPRESSING CELL-SURFACE ENVELOPE GLYCOPROTEINS AS A TRIGGER OF APOPTOSIS IN UNINFECTED CELLS

The results presented above indicated that apoptosis is not simply triggered during HIV RNA and protein synthesis, but is the consequence of

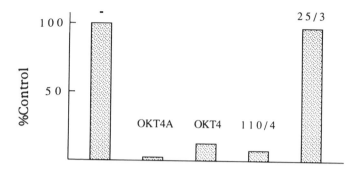

Acute HIV Infection, 48 hr p.i.

Figure 4   Inhibition of apoptosis by anti-CD4 and anti-gp120 antibodies. CEM cells were infected with HIV-1 (as in Figure 2), and at 20 hours p.i. different monoclonal antibodies were added: Mab OKT4A, OKT4, 110/4, and 25/3 (see text for details). At 48 hours p.i. cultures were analyzed for the accumulation of LMW DNA–associated histones. The histone bands H2A, H2B, H3, and H4 were quantitated by scanning the Coomassie blue stained gels. The ordinate represents the percentage of histones (as a marker of apoptosis) found in each culture (the abscissa). The 100% value corresponds to the amount of histones found in infected cells (10^6) without any antibody. These histograms were estimated from the results described in Ref. 1.

cell membrane expression of the envelope glycoproteins that bind CD4 receptors on neighboring cells. Accordingly, chronically infected cells that express cell-surface envelope glycoproteins were shown to be efficient effector cells to induce apoptosis in CD4+ uninfected target cells. For these experiments, we cocultured chronically infected H9 cells (10^6 cells) with uninfected MOLT4-T4 cells (10^7 cells). As expected, coculturing of such cells resulted in syncytia formation within a few hours and also led to cell-to-cell spreading of HIV (28,29). At 16 to 20 hours, when almost no single cells were present, apoptosis was clearly observed in MOLT4-T4 cells cocultured with chronically infected cells (Figure 5, lane 3). No apoptosis was observed in uninfected cells or in cocultures at time 0 hr (Figure 5, lanes 1 and 2). The levels of HIV proteins were significantly increased during the 24-hour coculture as a consequence of infection of MOLT4-T4 cells (6). Accordingly, reduced levels of viral proteins were observed in the presence of AZT, which blocks proviral DNA synthesis, a step essential for the initiation of HIV infection in newly infected cells. Interestingly, the presence of AZT interfered with neither the formation of giant syncy-

 urpose, vaccinia virus (VV) recombinants expressing the different HIV genes were employed to infect CEM cells, which were then assayed for apoptosis. The VV recombinants used in this experiments encoded the following HIV proteins: Gag, the precursor of the core proteins; Pol, the precursor encoded by the polymerase gene which is then processed by its N-terminal protease to produce the reverse transcriptase and the endo-nuclease/integrase; Env, the envelope glycoprotein precursor which is processed intracellularly to produce mature envelope glycoproteins; Tat, the transactivating protein; Nef, the negative regulatory factor which is still not well defined; and Vif, the virion infectivity factor (for a review see Ref. 30). At 16 hours p.i. of CEM cells with these different VV recombinants, nuclei were prepared and histones associated to LMW DNA were analyzed by polyacrylamide gel electrophoresis. Apoptosis was observed only in CEM cells in which the envelope glycoproteins were expressed (Table 1). It should be noted that at 16 hours p.i. the different VV-infected cells were viable and metabolically active in synthesizing vaccinia and HIV proteins. Examination of these infected cultures under a light microscope revealed the presence of giant syncytia only in cells expressing HIV envelope glycoproteins. This is in agreement with previously published reports, indicating that the mature HIV envelope glycoproteins are responsible for cell aggregation and syncytium formation (31).

Table 1 Apoptosis in CEM Cells Infected with VV Recombinants (100 p.f.u./cell) Expressing HIV-1 Envelope Glycoproteins

HIV-1 gene	Fusion	Apoptosis
gag	−	−
pol	−	−
env	+	+
tat	−	−
nef	−	--
vif	−	−

At 16 hours p.i. nuclear extracts were prepared for the analysis of histones associated with LMW DNA. Cell fusion (monitored by light microscopy) and apoptosis (monitored by histones) were observed only in cells expressing the env gene. Source: Refs. 6 and 30.

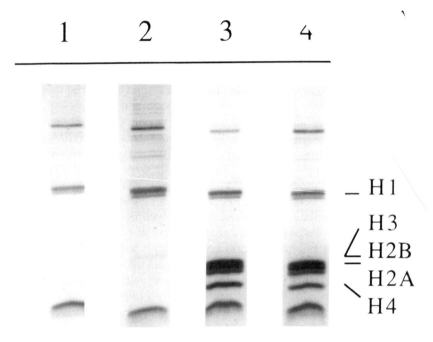

Figure 5 Chronically infected cells induce apoptosis in uninfected cells. Chronically HIV-1 infected H9/IIIB cells (10^6) were cocultured for 24 hours with uninfected MOLT4-T4 cells (10^7). Apoptosis was monitored by the presence of histones associated with LMW DNA (6). Lane 1: uninfected MOLT4/T4 cells (10^6). Lane 2: coculture of chronically infected H9/IIIB (10^5) and uninfected MOLT4/T4 (10^6) cells at time 0. Lane 3: as in lane 2 but at 24 hours of coculture. Lane 4: as in lane 2 but at 24 hours of coculture in the presence of AZT (5 μM).

tia nor the induction of apoptosis (Figure 5, lane 4). Chronically infected cells, therefore can induce apoptosis in uninfected CD4+ cells simply due to their capacity to cause membrane fusion through interactions between the gp120-gp41 complex and the CD4 receptor.

EXPRESSION OF THE HIV ENVELOPE AND INDUCTION OF APOPTOSIS

To characterize the contribution of the different HIV genes in the mechanism of induction of apoptosis during viral infection, we investigated the effect of each individual gene when expressed alone in CEM cells. For this

Apoptosis in CEM cells expressing HIV envelope glycoproteins was confirmed by monitoring for chromatin condensation by electron microscopy. CEM cells expressing HIV proteins other than the envelope were found to have normal nuclei. In the culture of CEM cells expressing HIV envelope glycoproteins, some small syncytia with somewhat normal nuclei were found in this culture (Figure 6, upper panel), but there were mainly giant syncytia that manifested compacted chromatin either in characteristic peripheral crescent forms or distributed throughout the cross-sectional area (Figure 6, lower panel).

APOPTOSIS INDUCTION REQUIRES EXPRESSION OF BOTH gp120 AND gp41

The HIV-1 envelope gene codes for a 160-kDa glycoprotein precursor that is cleaved by a cellular protease to yield the extracellular and transmembrane glycoproteins, gp120 and gp41, respectively (19). The gp120 is responsible for binding to the CD4 receptor (32) whereas gp41 is involved in the fusion process (33) essential for syncytium formation. For further characterization of the respective role of the two components of gp160, we used VV recombinants (31,34) containing HIV *env* genes with specific modifications (Figure 7). The results of these experiments (shown in Ref. 6) indicated that the HIV envelope-mediated apoptosis requires the production of both gp120 and gp41. Both components are also required for syncytia formation. However, apoptosis and syncytia did not occur with the uncleaved gp160, indicating that the specific cleavage eliciting some conformational changes in the resulting gp120-gp41 complex is necessary. With gp120 alone, no apoptosis was observed in spite of the capacity of this virus to cause aggregation of CEM cells, i.e., binding to the CD4 receptors. Similarly, expression of gp41 was not sufficient by itself to cause apoptosis. This may be due to the lack of close contact between cell membranes, which is normally realized by the interaction of gp120 molecules and CD4 receptors.

CONCLUSION

Using different experimental models, we were able to demonstrate that the induction of apoptosis requires cell membrane expression of mature HIV envelope glycoproteins, the gp120-gp41 complex, and accessible CD4

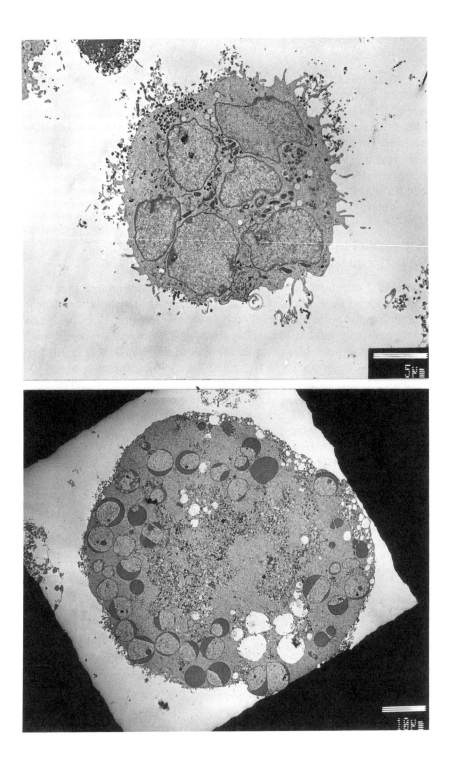

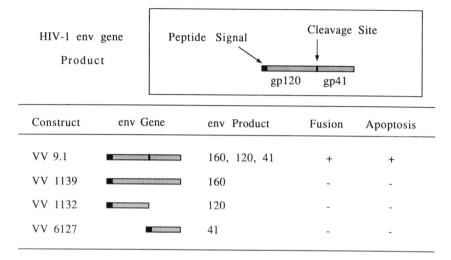

Construct	env Gene	env Product	Fusion	Apoptosis
VV 9.1		160, 120, 41	+	+
VV 1139		160	-	-
VV 1132		120	-	-
VV 6127		41	-	-

Figure 7   CEM cells were infected with different VV recombinations (100 pfu/cell) as described in Ref. 6. At 16 hours p.i., cell cultures were examined under a light microscope for aggregation and syncytia formation (fusion). The VV 9.1 construct produces a gp160, which is then cleaved into gp120 and gp41. VV 1139 construct expresses gp160, which cannot be cleaved because of mutations in the cleavage site. VV 1132 construct expresses only the gp120 portion of the HIV envelope, whereas the VV 6127 construct expresses the gp41 portion. The different VV recombinants besides VV6127 were described before (16,31,34). Apoptosis was assayed by the presence of histones and LMW DNA (as in Figure 2).

Figure 6   CEM cells were infected with VV recombinant VVTG 9.1 (34) expressing the HIV-1 *env* gene products gp120-gp41. At 16 hours p.i., cell cultures were processed for electron microscopy; ultrathin sections were stained with uranyl acetate and lead citrate. The top panel on facing page shows a syncytium, the small black spots being VV particles. The bottom panel on facing page shows a giant syncytium with apoptotic nuclei. Compacted chromatin appears as peripheral crescents in the nuclei or distributed throughout the nuclei. Experimental procedures were described in Ref. 6.

receptor molecules (6). In general, syncytia formation and apoptosis induction were closely associated; both events require proper processing of
HIV envelope precursor and proper folding of the gp120-gp41 complex.
Indeed, the formation of syncytia is a direct consequence of interactions
of gp120 with the CD4 receptor on one hand and gp41 with a cell membrane component on the other hand. The onset of apoptosis might occur
during or after syncytia formation. Accordingly, apoptosis but not syncytia formation is suppressed by a monoclonal antibody (MAb OKT4)
directed toward an epitope in the CD4 receptor that is distal to the gp120
binding domain. This suggests that during the fusion process a specific
region in the gp120-gp41 complex might become unmasked and thus mediate the onset of apoptosis.

Evidence that no HIV-coded proteins other than the gp120-gp41 complex were involved in triggering apoptosis was demonstrated by the use
VV recombinants expressing individual structural or regulatory genes of
HIV. In agreement with this, chronically infected cells expressing the gp120-
gp41 complex were shown to be potent effector cells for the induction of
syncytia and apoptosis in uninfected T4 target cells. Our results indicate
that cell death during HIV infection is not simply the consequence of toxic
damage occurring during massive virus production, but it is due to a specific chain of events initiated by the gp120-gp41 complex programming
death in metabolically active cells. Such a mechanism could represent one
of the pathways responsible for the depletion of T4 lymphocytes during
the course of AIDS disease.

Dramatically reduced T4 cell counts are observed in AIDS patients
with high virus titers (7). In general there is a very good correlation between the gradual decrease of T4 lymphocytes and the increase of viremia
during the development of AIDS (35), indicating that virus replication
might play an important role. Accordingly, the apoptotic mechanism triggered by the HIV envelope should provide at least one of the pathways
through which T4 cells become eliminated. In asymptomatic individuals,
it has been reported that less than 1% of T4 circulating lymphocytes harbor HIV DNA (36,37). As AIDS develops, this frequency is increased to
at least 1% and in some cases 10% (35,38,39). These values should be considered estimations for the steady-state levels of HIV DNA since they simply
reflect the relative differences between asymptomatic and AIDS patients.
Also, it should be emphasized that the half-life of HIV-producing cell is
probably several-fold less than that of uninfected cells. Consequently, an
infected T4 cell will die very rapidly after fusioning with a great number
of cells and inducing apoptosis. In support of this, rapidly replicating and

highly syncytium-inducing virus isolates have been reported to be present in greater numbers in AIDS patients with low T4 lymphocyte counts compared to asymptomatic individuals (40,41). The HIV-producing cell or the syncytium may also be quickly eliminated by the CTL or/and ADCC responses (14). It should also be noted that HIV-induced apoptotic cells may be eliminated very rapidly by macrophages. For example, it has recently been reported that apoptosis-induced alterations in plasma membranes lead to recognition of apoptotic bodies by macrophages and their rapid phagocytosis (42). Therefore, it is almost impossible to obtain a true image of the number of infected T4 lymphocytes in the circulation at a given time. Furthermore, it has been reported that the number of infected cells in lymphoid tissue is at least 10-fold higher than that found in the circulation (43).

Finally, it should be emphasized that envelope-mediated apoptosis represents one of the pathways implicated in T4-cell depletion in AIDS patients. Particularly interesting is the priming of HIV patients' lymphocytes to undergo apoptosis by a mechanism that appears to be independent of HIV replication. In this case, T lymphocytes become programmed in vivo in HIV-infected patients and undergo apoptosis either spontaneously or after activation by mitogens, superantigens, and calcium ionophores (10–12,44; Chapter 10). Indirect evidence for the occurrence of apoptosis in AIDS patients might be the presence of high-affinity antibodies directed against histones and DNA (45). Thus, nucleosomes released during apoptosis might stimulate a pathological state manifested by abnormal B-cell proliferation and autoantibody formation.

ACKNOWLEDGMENTS

This work was supported in part by a grant from Agence Nationale de la Recherche sur le SIDA in France. We thank Luc Montagnier for discussion and advice during this work.

REFERENCES

1. Duvall E, Wyllie AH. Death and the cell. Immunol Today 1986; 7:115–119.
2. McConkey DJ, Orrenius S, Jondal M. Cellular signaling in programmed cell death (apoptosis). Immunol Today 1990; 11:120–121.
3. Sanderson CJ. Morphological aspects of lymphocyte mediated cytotoxicity. In: Clark WR, Goldstein P, eds. Mechanisms of Cell Mediated Cytotoxicity. New York: Plenum, 1982:3–31.

4. Laurent-Crawford AG, Krust B, Muller S, Rivière Y, Rey-Cuillé MA, Béchet
    JM, Montagnier L, Hovanessian AG. The cytopathic effect of HIV is asso-
    ciated with apoptosis. Virology 1991; 185:829–839.
5. Terai C, Kornbluth RS, Pauza CD, Richman DD, Carson DA. Apoptosis as
    as mechanism of cell death in cultured T lymphoblasts acutely infected with
    HIV-1. J Clin Invest 1991; 87:1710–1715.
6. Laurent-Crawford AG, Krust B, Rivière Y, Muller S, Dauguet C, Hovanes-
    sian AG. Membrane expression of HIV envelope glycoproteins triggers apop-
    tosis in CD4 cells. Submitted.
7. Stein DS, Korvick JA, Vermund SH. CD4+ lymphocyte cell enumeration
    for prediction of clinical course of human immunodeficiency virus disease: A
    review. J Infect Dis 1992; 165:352–363.
8. Ameisen J, Capron A. Cell dysfunction and depletion in AIDS: The pro-
    grammed cell death hypothesis. Immunol Today 1991; 12:102–105.
9. Montagnier L, Gougeon ML, Olivier R, Garcia S, Dauguet C, Adams M,
    Béchet JM, Guétard D, Laurent A, Hovanessian AG, Kirstetter M, Roué
    R, Pialoux G, Dupont B. Factors and mechanisms of AIDS pathogenesis in
    science challenging AIDS. In: Rossi GB, Beth-Giraldo E, Chieco-Bianchi L,
    Dianzani F, Giraldo G, Verani P, eds. Basel: Karger, 1991:51–70.
10. Gougeon ML, Olivier R, Garcia S, Guetard D, Dragic T, Dauguet C, Mon-
    tagnier L. Mise en évidence d'un processus d'engagement vers la mort cellu-
    laire par apoptose dans les lymphocytes de patients infectés par le VIH. CR
    Acad Sci 1991; 312:529–537.
11. Groux H, Monte D, Bourrez JM, Capron A, Ameisen JC. L'activation des
    lymphocytes T CD4+ de sujets asymptomatiques infectés par le VIH en-
    traîne le déclenchement d'un programme de mort lymphocytaire par apop-
    tose. CR Acad Sci 1991; 312:599–606.
12. Groux H, Torpier G, Monté D, Mouton Y, Capron A, Ameisen JC. Acti-
    vation-induced death by apoptosis in CD4+ T cells from human immuno-
    deficiency virus-infected asymptomatic individuals. J Exp Med 1992; 175:
    331–340.
13. Janossy G. Immune parameters in HIV infection—practical guide. Immunol
    Today 1991; 12:255–256.
14. Walker BD, Plata F. Cytotoxic T lymphocytes against HIV. AIDS 1990; 4:
    177–184.
15. Rivière Y, Tanneau-Salvadori F, Regnault A, Lopez O, Sansonetti P, Guy B,
    Kieny MP, Fournel JJ, Montagnier L. Human immunodeficiency virus-specific
    cytotoxic responses of seropositive individuals: distinct types of effector cells
    mediate killing of targets expressing gag and env proteins. J Virol 1989; 63:
    2270–2277.
16. McChesney M, Tanneau F, Regnault A, Sansonetti P, Montagnier L, Kieny
    MP, Rivière Y. Detection of primary cytotoxic T lymphocytes specific for the
    envelope glycoprotein of HIV-1 by deletion of the env amino-terminal signal
    sequence. Eur J Immunol 1990; 20:215–220.

17. Tanneau F, McChesney M, Lopez O, Sansonetti P, Montagnier L, Rivière Y. Primary cytotoxicity against the envelope glycoprotein of human immunodeficiency virus-1: Evidence for antibody-dependent cellular cytotoxicity in vivo. J Infect Dis 1990; 162:837–843.
18. Marsh M, Dalgleish A. How do human immunodeficiency viruses enter cells? Immunol Today 1987; 8:369–371.
19. McKeating JA, Willey RL. Structure and function of the HIV envelope. AIDS 1989; 3:S35–S41.
20. Besansky NJ, Butera ST, Sinha S, Folks TM. Unintegrated human immunodeficiency virus type 1 DNA in chronically infected cell lines is not correlated with surface CD4 expression. J Virol 1991; 65:2695–2698.
21. Pauza CD, Galindo JE, Richman DD. Reinfection results in accumulation of unintegrated viral DNA in cytopathic and persistent human immunodeficiency virus type 1 infection of CEM cells. J Exp Med 1990; 172:1035–1042.
22. Robinson HL, Zinkus DM. Accumulation of human immunodeficiency virus type 1 DNA in T cells: result of multiple infection events. J Virol 1990; 64: 4836–4841.
23. Kinney-Thomas E, Weber JN, McClure J, Clapham PR, Singhal MC, Shriver MK, Weiss R. Neutralising monoclonal antibodies to the AIDS virus. AIDS 1988; 2:25–29.
24. Linsley PS, Ledbetter JA, Kinney-Thomas E, Hu SL. Effects of anti-gp120 monoclonal antibodies on CD4 receptor binding by the env protein of human immunodeficiency virus type 1. J Virol 1988; 62:3695–3702.
25. Rao PR, Talle MA, Kung PC, Goldstein G. Five epitopes of a differentiation antigen on human inducer T cells distinguished by monoclonal antibodies. Cell Immunol 1983; 80:310–319.
26. Sattentau QJ, Dalgleish AG, Weiss RA, Beverley PCL. Epitopes of the CD4 antigen and HIV infection. Science 1986; 234:1120–1123.
27. Laurent AG, Krust B, Rey MA, Montagnier L, Hovanessian AG. Cell surface expression of several species of human immunodeficiency virus type 1 major core protein. J Virol 1989; 63:4074–4078.
28. Sato H, Orenstein J, Dimitrov D, Martin M. Cell-to-cell spread of HIV-1 occurs within minutes and may not involve the participation of virus particles. Virology 1992; 186:712–724.
29. Li P, Burrell CJ. Synthesis of human immunodeficiency virus DNA in a cell-to-cell transmission model. Aids Res Hum Retrovir 1992; 8:253–259.
30. Cann AJ, Karn J. Molecular biology of HIV: New insights into the virus life-cycle. AIDS 1989; 3:S19–S34.
31. Kieny MP, Lathe R, Rivière Y, Dott K, Schmitt D, Girard M, Montagnier L, Lecocq JP. Emproved antigenecity of the HIV env protein by cleavage site removal. Protein Engineering 1988; 2:219–225.
32. McDougal JS, Kennedy S, Sligh JM, Cort SP, Mawle A, Nicholson JKA. Binding of HTLV-III/LAV to T4+ cells by a complex of the 110K viral protein and the T4 molecule. Science 1986; 231:382–385.

33. Kowalski M, Bergeron L, Dorfman T, Haseltine W, Sodroski J. Attenuation of human immunodeficiency virus type 1 cytopathic effect by a mutation affecting the transmembrane envelope glycoprotein. J Virol 1991; 65:281–291.

34. Kieny MP, Rautmann G, Schmitt D, Dott K, Wain-Hobson S, Alizon M, Girard M, Chamaret S, Laurent A, Montagnier L, Lecocz JP. AIDS virus *env* protein expressed from a recombinant vaccinia virus. Bio/Technology 1986; 4:790–795.

35. Ho DD, Moudgil T, Alam M. Quantitation of human immunodeficiency virus type 1 in the blood of infected persons. N Engl J Med 1989; 321:1621–1625.

36. Simmonds P, Balfe P, Peutherer JF, Ludlam CA, Bishop JO, Leigh Brown AJ. Human immunodeficiency virus infected individuals contain provirus in small numbers of peripheral mononuclear cells and at low copy numbers. J Virol 1990; 64:864–872.

37. Brinchmann JE, Albert J, Vartdal F. Few infected CD4 + T cells but a high proportion of replication-competent provirus copies in asymptomatic human immunodeficiency virus type 1 infection. J Virol 1991; 65:2019–2023.

38. Schnittman SM, Psallidopoulos MC, Lane HC, Thompson L, Baseler M, Massari F, Fox CH, Salzman NP, Fauci AS. The reservoir for HIV-1 in human peripheral blood is a T cell that maintains expression of CD4. Science 1989; 245:305–308.

39. Bagasra O, Hauptman SP, Lischner HW, Sachs M, Pomerantz RJ. Detection of human immunodeficiency virus type 1 provirus in mononuclear cells by in situ polymerase chain reaction. N Engl J Med 1992; 326:1385–1391.

40. Tersmette M, de Goede REY, Al BJM, Winkel IN, Gruters RA, Cuypers HT, Huisman HG, Miedema F. Differential syncytium-inducing capacity of human immunodeficiency virus isolates: frequent detection of syncytium inducing isolates in patients with acquired immunodeficiency syndrome (AIDS) and AIDS-related complex. J Virol 1988; 62:2026–2032.

41. Cheng-Mayer C, Shioda T, Levy JA. Host range, replicative, and cytopathic properties of human immunodeficiency virus type 1 are determined by very few amino acid changes in tat and gp 120. J Virol 1991; 65:6931–6941.

42. Savill J, Dransfield I, Hogg N, Haslett C. Vitronectin receptor-mediated phagocytosis of cells undergoing apoptosis. Nature 1990; 343:170–173.

43. Fauci AS. Immunopathogenic mechanisms of HIV infection. In: Girard M, Valette L, eds. Retroviruses of Human AIDS and Related Animal Diseases. 1991:5–8, France: Pasteur Mérieux.

44. Meyaard L, Otto SA, Jonker RR, Mijnster MJ, Keet RPM, Miedema F. Programmed death of T cells in HIV-1 infection. Science 1992; 257:217–219.

45. Muller S, Richalet P, Laurent-Crawford A, Barakat S, Rivière Y, Porrot F, Chamaret S, Briand JP, Montagnier L, Hovanessian AG. Presence in HIV-seropositive patients of autoantibodies typically found in non-organ specific autoimmune diseases. AIDS 1992; 933–942.

4

The Pathobiology of SIV Infection of Macaques

Patricia N. Fultz

University of Alabama
Birmingham, Alabama

INTRODUCTION

The most valuable animal model for providing insight into the natural history and pathogenesis of the human immunodeficiency virus (HIV) is infection of macaques with various isolates of the simian immunodeficiency virus (SIV). Because individual SIV isolates can exhibit distinct molecular and biological properties in different macaque species, e.g., rhesus (*Macaca mulatta*), pig-tailed (*M. nemestrina*), and cynomolgus (*M. fascicularis*), it is possible to manipulate the model system to obtain the maximum amount of information. Although many aspects of HIV infection and virus-host cell interactions can be characterized in vitro with HIV isolates or peripheral blood mononuclear cells (PBMCs) from HIV-infected persons, these studies are compromised because, in general, the actual time of infection and the nature of the infecting inoculum [i.e., the extent of variation among the quasispecies (1)] is not known. Based on the purpose of a study (e.g., natural history of infection, determinants of pathogenicity, therapeutic effects of antiviral drugs, or immunogenicity and efficacy of vaccines), one can select a particular SIV isolate or defined molecularly cloned virus and a macaque species that together optimize conditions for the specific parameters to be monitored.

DIVERSITY OF PRIMATE LENTIVIRUSES

Although multiple Old World simian species have been shown to be seropositive for antibodies to SIV/HIV-related viruses, thus far isolates have been obtained from only eight simian species (Table 1) (2–13). In addition to monkeys, distinct HIV-like viruses have been isolated from two chimpanzees (*Pan troglodytes*) (14,15). [Since chimpanzees are great apes, not simians, these viruses should be designated CIV (chimpanzee immunodeficiency virus).] Among the simian species tested to date, only those animals indigenous to Africa appear to be naturally infected with SIV (6,8, 16), and these natural hosts appear not to develop an AIDS-like disease as a result of infection (16–18). In contrast, all SIVs obtained from Asian macaque species have the potential to induce disease in macaques (19,20).

Table 1 Nonhuman Primate Species from Which HIV/SIV-related Viruses Have Been Isolated

Genus/species	Common name	Designation	Disease[a]
Asian simian species			
Macaca mulatta	Rhesus macaque	SIV_{mac}	Yes
M. nemestrina	Pig-tailed macaque	SIV_{mne}	Yes
M. fascicularis	Cynomolgus monkey	SIV_{mac}	Yes
M. arctoides	Stump-tailed macaque	SIV_{stm}	Yes
African simian species			
Cercocebus atys	Sooty mangabey monkey	SIV_{smm}	No
Cercopithecus			
aethiops	African green monkey	SIV_{agm}	No
C. mitis	Sykes' monkey	SIV_{syk}	No
Papio sphinx	Mandrill (baboon)	SIV_{mnd}	?[b]
African great ape			
Pan troglodytes	Chimpanzee	CIV[c]	?[b]

[a]Experimental infection results in AIDS-like disease in species from which viruses were isolated.
[b]Potential to induce disease is not known.
[c]Proposed.

Because the original SIV_{mac} isolates were from animals in a domestic colony (2), and no macaques in their native countries appear to be infected, it is assumed that Asian species are not natural hosts for SIV.

At the molecular level, the SIV, HIV, and CIV isolates form five distinct groups that exhibit similar degrees of nucleotide sequence divergence (approximately 45–55% overall) (21–28). There are also differences in the number and identity of auxiliary genes encoded by these virus groups (21–28), but whether the auxiliary genes, individually or in concert, have a major influence on pathogenesis is not clear. There is convincing evidence that the *nef* gene is required for high levels of SIV_{mac239} gene expression and disease development in rhesus macaques (29). However, whether this virus requires a functional *nef* gene to elicit disease in other macaque species is not known. Furthermore, it is possible that other SIVs, with distinct genetic features, may not require the *nef* gene product for pathogenicity in any species.

The previous conclusion regarding the influence of *nef* must be qualified because, as mentioned above, different SIV isolates in the same species exhibit varying pathogenicities (Table 2) (30–36). Thus, one must be cautious about making generalizations regarding characteristics of SIV infection of monkeys.

Table 2 Differences in Pathogenicity of SIV Isolates in Various Macaque Species

Isolate	Species	Time to death	Ref.
SIV_{mac}	*M. mulatta*	1.4–12 mo (68%)	35
		1–3.3 yr (32%)	
$SIV_{mac1A11}$	*M. mulatta*	>3 yr[a]	36
SIV_{smm9}	*C. atys*[b]	Natural causes	4,16
	M. nemestrina	7–14 mo	34
	M. mulatta	14–>60 mo	34
$SIV_{smmPBj14}$	*C. atys*	10–13 days (75%)	33
	M. nemestrina	6–14 days (>90%)	33,51
	M. mulatta	14–>40 mo (67%)	51,52
		7–14 days (33%)	33
$SIV_{smmB670}$	*M. mulatta*	1–7 mo (75%)	32

[a]After more than 3 years of follow-up, no animals infected with this isolate have developed disease or died.
[b]Natural host.

SIV-INDUCED DISEASE MANIFESTATIONS

Part of the value of SIV infection of macaques as a model for HIV pathogenesis is that many of the sequelae following inoculation of monkeys
with various SIV isolates resemble or exactly parallel those observed in
HIV-infected people. The similarities include pathological consequences,
opportunistic infections, neoplastic disease, viral burdens, and development of immunity.

Although the pathophysiology of SIV infection is varied, some of the
more common aspects of disease involve the lymphoid, nervous, and respiratory systems (13,19,20,30,34,35,37–39). Early after infection, lymphadenopathy with follicular hyperplasia is often detected in lymph nodes.
Later stages of infection are characterized by follicular depletion with a
normal or expanded cortex, followed by diffuse atrophy and lymphoid
depletion in terminal stages. One feature of lymphadenopathy is the presence of SIV antigen-positive multinucleated giant cells in the parenchyma,
but these cells are not found in all animals. In addition, regardless of the
age of the animal, the thymus becomes atrophied. In the nervous system,
SIV-induced AIDS is often accompanied by a perivascular accumulation
of macrophages (often multinucleated) in meninges and gray matter of
the cerebrum, cerebellum, brain stem, and spinal cord. There is frequently
encephalitis with multinucleated cells and/or foci of gliosis in the neuro-
pil. One of the most common pathologies associated with the respiratory
system is granulomatous interstitial and alveolar pneumonia with infiltrates of foamy macrophages, multinucleated giant cells, and lymphocytes. In all tissues, the multinucleated giant cells are the primary cells
expressing SIV antigens and appear to be derived from macrophages.

Some of the major opportunistic infectious agents seen in SIV-infected
macaques include *Pneumocystis carinii* (pulmonary), *Trichomonas* (cecum
and colon), disseminated *Mycobacterium avium/intracellulare*, disseminated cytomegalovirus, adenovirus (pancreas), *Candida* and *Cryptospor-
idium* (13,19,20,34,37–39). Observed differences in the types of opportunistic infections identified in immunodeficient macaques appear to be
a function of the specific research facility where a study was performed
and not of the SIV isolate.

In general, the incidence of lymphomas in SIV-infected macaques
has been low, with one exception. Biberfeld and colleagues (40,41) reported that approximately 40% of cynomolgus macaques infected with
the SIV_{smm3} isolate developed aggressive high-grade malignant lymphomas
that have many of the same characteristics as lymphomas seen in HIV-
infected persons (Table 3). Although the macaques used at this one facility

Table 3 Common Characteristics of HIV- and SIV-Associated Lymphomas

Appearance preceded by marked immunosuppression
Extranodal manifestations, including CNS involvement
Almost exclusively B-cell non-Hodgkin's lymphomas
Most associated with EBV-like herpes viruses
Aggressive high-grade malignant lymphomas
Heterogeneous morphology

Source: Refs. 40, 41.

are naturally infected with a herpes virus, it is not yet known whether the herpes virus is necessary for neoplastic disease or whether the high incidence of lymphomas is specific for the SIV_{smm3} strain. Irrespective of this, infection of cynomolgus macaques with SIV_{smm} provides a valuable model system for identifying factors that influence the development of lymphomas in HIV-infected persons.

SIV_{smm}-MACAQUE MODEL SYSTEMS

Multiple SIV_{smm} isolates have been obtained from naturally infected sooty mangabey monkeys, which rarely develop diseases that can be attributed to these viruses (16). However, because these SIV isolates do induce progressive AIDS-like disease in various macaque species, infection of both mangabeys and macaques provides a mechanism for comparing virus-host interactions and natural histories of infection in hosts for which the virus is either apathogenic or pathogenic. It is hoped that such studies will lead to the identification of specific viral and host factors that induce or exacerbate disease.

In general, the natural history of SIV infection of macaques during the first few weeks and months parallels that of HIV infection of humans. Rapid increases in plasma viremia are followed by a rise in SIV-specific antibody titers with an accompanying decrease in viremia, often to undetectable levels (17,20,31). To illustrate the diversity of SIV infection of monkeys, this report will present results from three model systems that we have studied: 1) natural and experimental asymptomatic infection of sooty mangabeys, 2) chronic AIDS-like disease induced in pig-tailed and rhesus macaques by SIV_{smm9}, and 3) an acute fatal disease induced in pig-tailed macaques and sooty mangabeys by a variant of SIV_{smm9}, designated $SIV_{smmPBj14}$.

SIV$_{smm}$Infection of Mangabeys Versus Macaques

One hypothesis to explain the differential pathogenicity of SIV$_{smm}$ for mangabeys and macaques is that the anti-SIV immune response of mangabeys is more effective. Both in the spectrum of antibodies to specific viral proteins and in the functional activities of those antibodies, humoral immune responses to SIV$_{smm}$ infection in naturally infected mangabeys and experimentally infected macaques are similar. Since antiviral immunity to SIV$_{smm}$ appeared to be comparable, it was possible that the virus replicated more efficiently and to higher titers in macaques than in mangabeys. However, comparison of viral burdens yielded unexpected results (17). Virus was easily recovered from 100% of PBMCs and 88% of plasma samples of all SIV$_{smm}$-infected mangabeys tested; this analysis included PBMCs from 70 and plasma samples from eight seropositive animals. In contrast, isolation of virus from PBMCs or plasma samples from asymptomatic macaques was either infrequent (15 of 48 successful attempts with PBMCs) or impossible (none of eight plasma samples). However, macaques that had obvious AIDS-like symptoms had viral burdens comparable to those of the asymptomatic mangabeys. Thus, lack of disease in mangabeys is not due to limited virus replication or to immune control of the infection.

It is clear, however, that increased expression of SIV$_{smm}$ in macaques correlates with disease (17,31), which is also true of HIV infection of humans (42,43). As mentioned above, a characteristic of asymptomatic infection of macaques is an inability to isolate cell-free infectious virus from plasma. Those macaques that rapidly progress to disease following initial infection usually have detectable plasma viremia at all times. Sporadic success at isolating cell-free virus often corresponds to transient episodes of disease, such as rash or lymphadenopathy. In general, increased viral burdens and exposure of the immune system to increased levels of viral antigen results in high serum titers of SIV-specific antibodies (17). This contrasts with some reports of relatively rapid progression (2 to 3 months) to AIDS-like disease in macaques following inoculation with other SIV isolates, such as SIV$_{mac}$ (44), SIV$_{smmB670}$ (31), or SIV$_{smmF236}$ (45). In these cases, SIV-specific antibodies were never detected. The correlation between failure to generate SIV-specific antibodies and rapid progression to disease and death strongly supports the idea that the immune system does have a major impact on retarding disease development.

Since the major feature of HIV or SIV infection that predicts disease progression is loss of CD4+ lymphocytes, the effect of replication of SIV$_{smm}$ in mangabey and macaque PBMCs on this cell population was assessed in vitro. Multiple prototype SIV_{smm} isolates (that were not associated with disease in mangabeys) replicated equally well in PBMCs from both mangabeys and macaques. However, replication of virus in mangabey PBMCs was not associated with loss of CD4 + lymphocytes, whereas in macaque PBMC cultures infected with SIV_{smm}, preferential loss of CD4 + cells occurred (46,47). These results indicated that, despite efficient replication and high virus production, SIV_{smm} was not cytopathic for mangabey CD4 + lymphocytes. Since these same viruses are cytopathic for macaque CD4 + lymphocytes, it implies that there is a cellular component that either inhibits (mangabeys) or facilitates (macaques) cell death. Thus, it will be important to identify the specific cellular protein or regulatory region that mediates (or inhibits) this function as well as specific regions or gene products of the virus that may influence cytopathicity.

SIV_{smm9} Versus $SIV_{smmPBj14}$ Infection of Macaques

A variant of SIV_{smm9} designated $SIV_{smmPBj14}$ was isolated from a pig-tailed macaque that died of AIDS 14 months after infection (33). This latter isolate was subsequently shown to induce a rapidly fatal disease, characterized by profuse, bloody diarrhea and death within 6 to 12 days, in not only pig-tailed macaques but also sooty mangabeys. In vitro experiments also identified at least eight biological properties that differed between the smm9 and smmPBj14 viruses (Table 4). Although smmPBj14 acquired unique mutations compared to smm9, there was an average of 1.6% nucleotide sequence divergence between the two viruses (46,48-50). In addition to 57 specific point mutations, which resulted in 36 amino acid changes

Table 4 Biological Properties of SIV_{smm9} and $SIV_{smmPBj14}$

Property	smm9	smmPBj14
Enhanced replication in cell lines	−	+
Replication in chimpanzee PBMC	−	+
Neutralized by serum from macaque PBj	+	−
Syncytia formation with SupT1 cells	−	+
Infection blocked by OKT4a	+	−
Replication in resting macaque PBMCs	−	+
Activation/induction of PBMC proliferation	−	+
Cytopathicity for mangabey CD4 + cells	−	+
Induction of acute diarrhea and death	−	+

Source: Refs. 33, 46; Fultz, unpublished data.

(48), there were two insertions/duplications: one duplication of 22 nucleotides was in the U3 region of the LTR and resulted in a second NF-$\varkappa$B binding site; the second duplication consisted of 15 nucleotides (five amino acids) in the *env* gene. It is likely that both of these insertions, in conjunction with one or more of the point mutations, are required for the virulent phenotype of smmPBj14, but this has not been demonstrated. A chimeric virus in which the LTR duplication was inserted into the SIV$_{smmH4}$ molecular clone did not induce acute disease or death in pig-tailed macaques (50). This result indicates that two functional NF-$\varkappa$B sites are not sufficient to confer increased pathogenicity to viruses in the SIV$_{smm}$/SIV$_{mac}$/HIV-2 subgroup.

Pathological features indicative of acute death induced by smmPBj14 include extensive lymphadenopathy and splenomegaly, with extensive enlargement of gut-associated lymphoid tissues due to the presence of large numbers of proliferating lymphocytes or lymphoblasts (33,51). Numerous retrovirus particles were detected by electron microscopy in the lymphoid tissue, especially within Peyer's patches. Despite the massive increase of both CD4 + and CD8 + lymphocytes in lymph nodes and spleen, significant decreases in absolute numbers of both B and T cells in the peripheral blood occur within 4 or 5 days after infection (46,51). Interestingly, in vitro infection of simian PBMC by smmPBj14 results in preferential loss of both macaque and mangabey CD4 + lymphocytes, which strengthens the correlation between this property and pathogenicity of SIV isolates.

A majority of the animals infected with SIV$_{smmPBj14}$ developed profuse bloody diarrhea 2 to 3 days before death, leading to the speculation that death was due to dehydration and electrolyte imbalance (33,46). However, fluid therapy rarely prevents death, and the rapid decline and abrupt death of some animals in the absence of diarrhea (Fultz, unpublished) are reminiscent of toxic shock syndrome. The presence of large numbers of activated lymphocytes that may be elaborating numerous inflammatory cytokines may be a major factor in the acute deaths. To support this, elevated levels of interleukin (IL)-1 and tumor necrosis factor (TNF)-α were detected in serum from animals that died acutely (Fultz, unpublished). Furthermore, in an unrelated study, high levels of IL-6, the expression of which is induced by IL-1 or TNF, correlated directly with susceptibility to acute death (52). All three of these cytokines are part of acute-phase inflammatory responses elicited by many pathogens.

Despite the extreme virulence of smmPBj14, the immune system, if given an advantage, appears able to control virus replication and prevent acute disease and death. This was shown by smmPBj14 superinfection of pig-tailed macaques that had been infected for different lengths of time with the parent virus, smm9 (Fultz, DC Anderson, and HM McClure, unpublished). Even when macaques had been inoculated with smm9 only 3 weeks before exposure to smmPBj14, all animals survived, and none developed the acute disease syndrome, characterized by severe diarrhea. In addition, these superinfected animals had no detectable increase in viral burden after smmPBj14 inoculation. This apparent lack of replication was of special interest since this virus generally replicates to high titers following infection of naive animals. Because the SIV-specific antibody response at 3 weeks is presumed to be immature, with no neutralizing antibodies detectable, it is unlikely that humoral immunity was responsible for the obvious inhibition of viral replication and dissemination. However, whether the protective effect was due to specific (cytotoxic T lymphocytes) or nonspecific (e.g., natural killer cells) cell-mediated immunity is not known. It is also not known whether previous infection with an unrelated SIV would influence smmPBj14 replication and disease induction.

The extensive lymphoid proliferation seen in tissues of infected animals at necropsy correlates with unusual in vitro properties of smmPBj14. Unlike other SIV and HIV isolates, smmPBj14 does not require prior mitogenic stimulation of PBMCs in order to replicate (53). The ability to replicate in resting lymphocytes is probably related to another unusual property of the virus: the ability to activate and induce proliferation of both CD4 + and CD8 + lymphocytes. Using dual-label immunofluorescence analysis of cells from macaque PBMC cultures, the activation markers CD25 (IL-2 receptor) and TfR (transferrin receptor) were detected on CD4 + and (primarily) CD8 + lymphocytes *after* virus production (reverse transcriptase activity) peaked (Fultz and R Schwiebert, unpublished). This result suggests that activation and proliferation of lymphocytes are a consequence of, rather than a prerequisite for, viral replication. Furthermore, unlike most antigen-specific or mitogen-induced stimulation, activation of lymphocytes by smmPBj14 was not affected by depletion of antigen-presenting cells before infection. Thus, the smmPBj14-mediated activation of lymphocytes may not occur via normal cellular activation pathways. This hypothesis is supported by the finding that exogenous IL-2 is not required in cultures of resting lymphocytes in which smmPBj14 is actively replicating (53). Furthermore, smmPBj14 can replicate in macaque PBMC cultures to which antibodies to both IL-2 and IL-2R have been added (Fultz and Schwiebert, unpublished).

Although both the acute disease and replicative properties of smmPBj14 are unique among SIV and HIV isolates characterized to date, viruses from all the primate lentivirus subgroups probably have the potential to acquire these properties. It is also possible that the smmPBj14-induced disease reflects, albeit in a more severe form, events that occur during acute HIV-1 infections. Even if no virulent HIV-1 analogous to smmPBj14 is ever identified, in-depth analysis of this isolate's specific interactions with lymphocytes and other cell types may provide valuable insight into mechanisms whereby lentiretroviruses disrupt normal cellular processes and cause disease.

CONCLUSIONS

The diversity of the SIVs and the disease syndromes they induce in different simian species range from asymptomatic infections to slowly progressive, long-term disease to rapid progression and AIDS to acute death. Some characteristics of each of these states resemble or closely mimic those found in HIV-infected persons. Thus, information derived from specific SIV-macaque models probably can be extrapolated to human HIV infections.

The value of these model systems is further enhanced by the ability to identify and define specific biological and molecular characteristics of variant viruses in vitro and to test the effects of such variation on pathogenesis and virulence in vivo. This approach is the most direct way to identify viral determinants of pathogenicity and host protective responses. This knowledge is required to target specific viral functions and genomic regions when designing new intervention and prevention strategies to control HIV infections.

REFERENCES

1. Goodenow M, Huet T, Saurin W, Kwok S, Sninsky J, Wain-Hobson S. HIV-1 isolates are rapidly evolving quasispecies: evidence for viral mixtures and preferred nucleotide substitutions. J AIDS 1989; 2:344–352.
2. Daniel MD, Letvin NL, King NW, Kannagi M, Sehgal PK, Hunt RD, Kanki PJ, Essex M, Desrosiers RC. Isolation of T-cell tropic HTLV-III-like retrovirus from macaques. Science 1985; 228:1201–1204.
3. Benveniste RE, Arthur LO, Tsai C-C, Sowder R, Copeland TD, Henderson LE, Oroszlan S. Isolation of a lentivirus from a macaque with lymphoma: comparison with HTLV-III/LAV and other lentiviruses. J Virol 1986; 60:483–490.

4. Fultz PN, McClure HM, Anderson DC, Swenson RB, Anand R, Srinivasan A. Isolation of a T-lymphotropic retrovirus from naturally infected sooty mangabey monkeys (*Cercocebus atys*). Proc Natl Acad Sci USA 1986; 83: 5286–5290.

5. Murphey-Corb M, Martin LN, Rangan SRS, Baskin GB, Gormus BJ, Wolf RH, Andes WA, West M, Montelaro RC. Isolation of an HTLV-III-related retrovirus from macaques with simian AIDS and its possible origin in asymptomatic mangabeys. Nature 1986; 321:435–437.

6. Lowenstine LJ, Pedersen NC, Higgins J, Pallis KC, Uyeda A, Marx P, Lerche NW, Munn RJ, Gardner MB. Seroepidemiologic survey of captive old-world primates for antibodies to human and simian retroviruses, and isolation of a lentivirus from sooty mangabeys (*Cercocebus atys*). Int J Cancer 1986; 38: 563–574.

7. Kestler HW, Li Y, Naidu YM, Butler CV, Ochs MF, Jaenel G, King NW, Daniel MD, Desrosiers RC. Comparison of simian immunodeficiency virus isolates. Nature 1988; 331:619–622.

8. Ohta Y, Masuda T, Tsujimoto H, Ishikawa K, Kodama T, Morikawa S, Nakai M, Honjo S, Hayami M. Isolation of simian immunodeficiency virus from African green monkeys and seroepidemiologic survey of the virus in various non-human primates. Int J Cancer 1988; 41:115–122.

9. Tsujimoto H, Cooper RW, Kodama T, Fukasawa M, Miura T, Ohta Y, Ishikawa K-I, Nakai M, Frost E, Roelants GE, Roffi J, Hayami M. Isolation and characterization of simian immunodeficiency virus from mandrills in Africa and its relationship to other human and simian immunodeficiency viruses. J Virol 1988; 62:4044–4050.

10. Emau P, McClure HM, Isahakia M, Else JG, Fultz PN. Isolation from African Sykes' monkeys (*Cercopithecus mitis*) of a lentivirus related to human and simian immunodeficiency viruses. J Virol 1991; 65:2135–2140.

11. Allan JS, Kanda P, Kennedy RC, Cobb EK, Anthony M, Eichberg JW. Isolation and characterization of simian immunodeficiency viruses from two subspecies of African green monkeys. AIDS Res Hum Retrovir 1990; 6:275–285.

12. Khan AS, Galvin TA, Lowenstine LJ, Jennings MB, Gardner MB, Buckler CE. A highly divergent simian immunodeficiency virus (SIV_{stm}) recovered from stored stump-tailed macaque tissues. J Virol 1991; 65:7061–7065.

13. Lowenstine LJ, Lerche NW, Yee JL, Uyeda A, Jennings MB, Munn RJ, McClure HM, Anderson DC, Fultz PN, Gardner MB. Evidence for a lentiviral etiology in an epizootic of immune deficiency and lymphoma in stump-tailed macaques (*Macaca arctoides*). J Med Primatol 1992; 21:1–14.

14. Peeters M, Honore C, Huet T, Bedjabaga L, Ossari S, Bussi P, Cooper RW, Delaporte E. Isolation and partial characterization of an HIV-related virus occurring naturally in chimpanzees in Gabon. AIDS 1989; 3:625–630.

15. Vanden Haesevelde M, Peeters M, Willems B, Saman E, van der Groen G, van Heuverswyn H. Molecular cloning and sequence analysis of a variant immunodeficiency virus isolated from a wild captured chimpanzee. VIII International Conference on AIDS, Amsterdam, 1992. Abstr. WeA1081.

16. Fultz PN, Gordon TP, Anderson DC, McClure HM. Prevalence of natural infection with SIVsmm and STLV-I in a breeding colony of sooty mangabey monkeys. AIDS 1990; 4:619–625.

17. Fultz PN, Stricker RB, McClure HM, Anderson DC, Switzer WM, Horaist C. Humoral response to SIV/SMM infection in macaque and mangabey monkeys. J AIDS 1990; 3:319–329.

18. Norley SG, Kraus G, Ennen J, Bonilla J, Konig H, Kurth R. Immunological studies of the basis for the apathogenicity of simian immunodeficiency virus from African green monkeys. Proc Natl Acad Sci USA 1990; 87:9067–9071.

19. Letvin NL, Daniel MD, Sehgal PK, Desrosiers RC, Hunt RD, Waldron LM, Mackey JJ, Schmidt DK, Chalifoux LV, King NW. Induction of AIDS-like disease in macaque monkeys with T-cell tropic retrovirus STLV-III. Science 1985; 230:71–73.

20. Benveniste RE, Morton WR, Clark EA, Tsai C-C, Ochs HD, Ward JM, Kuller L, Knott WB, Hill RW, Gale MJ, Thouless ME. Inoculation of baboons and macaques with simian immunodeficiency virus/Mne, a primate lentivirus closely related to human immunodeficiency virus type 2. J Virol 1988; 62: 2091–2101.

21. Chakrabarti L, Guyader M, Alizon M, Daniel MD, Desrosiers RC, Tiollais P, Sonigo P. Sequence of simian immunodeficiency virus from macaque and its relationship to other human and simian retroviruses. Nature 1987; 328: 543–547.

22. Fukasawa M, Miura T, Hasegawa A, Morikawa S, Tsujimoto H, Miki K, Kitamura T, Hayami M. Sequence of simian immunodeficiency virus from African green monkey, a new member of the HIV/SIV group. Nature 1988; 333:457–461.

23. Hirsch VM, Olmsted RA, Murphey-Corb M, Purcell RH, Johnson PR. An African primate lentivirus (SIVsm) closely related to HIV-2. Nature 1989; 339:389–392.

24. Tsujimoto H, Hasegawa A, Maki N, Fukasawa M, Miura T, Speidel S, Cooper RW, Moriyama EN, Gojobori T, Hayami M. Sequence of a novel simian immunodeficiency virus from a wild-caught African mandrill. Nature 1989; 341:539–541.

25. Huet T, Cheynier R, Meyerhans A, Roelants G, Wain-Hobson S. Genetic organization of a chimpanzee lentivirus related to HIV-1. Nature 1990; 345: 356–359.

26. Johnson PR, Hirsch VM, Myers G. Genetic diversity and phylogeny of non-human primate lentiviruses. In: Koff WC, Wong-Staal F, Kennedy RC, eds. AIDS Research Reviews, Vol. 1. New York: Marcel Dekker, 1991:47–62.

27. Novembre FJ, Hirsch VM, McClure HM, Fultz PN, Johnson PR. SIV from stump-tailed macaques: molecular characterization of a highly transmissible primate lentivirus. Virology 1992; 186:783–787.

28. Hirsch VM, Dapolito GA, Goldstein S, McClure H, Emau P, Fultz PN, Isahakia M, Lenroot R, Myers G, Johnson PR. A distinct African lentivirus from Sykes' monkeys. J Virol 1993; 67. In press.

29. Kestler HW, Ringler DJ, Mori K, Panicali DL, Sehgal PK, Daniel MD, Desrosiers RC. Importance of the *nef* gene for maintenance of high virus loads and for development of AIDS. Cell 1991; 65:651–662.

30. Baskin GB, Murphey-Corb M, Watson EA, Martin LN. Necropsy findings in rhesus monkeys experimentally infected with cultured simian immunodeficiency virus (SIV)/Delta. Vet Pathol 1988; 25:456–467.

31. Zhang J, Martin LN, Watson EA, Montelaro RC, West M, Epstein L, Murphey-Corb M. Relationship of antibody response and viral antigenemia to SIV/Delta-induced immunodeficiency disease in the rhesus monkey. J Infect Dis 1988; 158:1277–1286.

32. Murphey-Corb M, Martin LN, Davison-Fairborn B, Montelaro RC, Miller M, Ohkawa S, Baskin GB, Zhang J-Y, Putney SD, Allison AC, Eppstein DA. A formalin-inactivated whole SIV vaccine confers protection in macaques. Science 1989; 246:1293–1297.

33. Fultz PN, McClure HM, Anderson DC, Switzer WM. Identification and biologic characterization of an acutely lethal variant of simian immunodeficiency virus from sooty mangabeys (SIV/SMM). AIDS Res Hum Retrovir 1989; 5: 397–409.

34. McClure HM, Anderson DC, Fultz PN, Ansari AA, Lockwood E, Brodie A. Spectrum of disease in macaque monkeys chronically infected with SIV/SMM. Vet Immunol Immunopathol 1989; 21:13–24.

35. King NW, Chalifoux LV, Ringler DJ, Wyand M, Sehgal PK, Daniel MD, Letvin NL, Desrosiers RC, Blake BJ, Hunt RD. Comparative biology of natural and experimental SIVmac infection in macaque monkeys: a review. J Med Primatol 1990; 19:109–118.

36. Marthas ML, Sutjipto S, Higgins J, Lohman B, Torten J, Luciw PA, Marx PA, Pedersen NC. Immunization with a live, attenuated simian immunodeficiency virus (SIV) prevents early disease but not infection in rhesus macaques challenged with pathogenic SIV. J Virol 1990; 64:3694–3700.

37. Letvin NL, King NW. Immunologic and pathologic manifestations of the infection of rhesus monkeys with simian immunodeficiency virus of macaques. J AIDS 1990; 3:1023–1040.

38. Baskerville A, Ramsay A, Cranage MP, Cook N, Cook RW, Dennis MJ, Greenaway PJ, Kitchin PA, Stott EJ. Histopathological changes in simian immunodeficiency virus infection. J Pathol 1990; 162:67–75.

39. Simon MA, Chalifoux LV, Ringler DJ. Pathologic features of SIV-induced disease and the association of macrophage infection with disease evolution. AIDS Res Hum Retrovir 1992; 8:327–337.

40. Feichtinger H, Putkonen P, Parravicini C, Li S-L, Kaaya EE, Bottiger D, Biberfeld G, Biberfeld P. Malignant lymphomas in cynomolgus monkeys infected with simian immunodeficiency virus. Am J Pathol 1990; 137:1311–1315.

41. Feichtinger H, Kaaya E, Putkonen P, Li S-L, Ekman M, Gendelman R, Biberfeld P. Malignant lymphoma associated with human AIDS and with SIV-induced immunodeficiency in macaques. AIDS Res Hum Retrovir 1992; 8: 339–348.

42. Coombs RW, Collier AC, Allain J-P, Nikora B, Leuther M, Gjerset GF, Corey I. Plasma viremia in human immunodeficiency virus infection. N Engl J Med 1989; 321:1626–1631.

43. Ho DD, Moudgil T, Alam M. Quantitation of human immunodeficiency virus type 1 in the blood of infected persons. N Engl J Med 1989; 321:1621–1625.

44. Kannagi M, Kiyotaki M, Desrosiers RC, Reimann KA, King NW, Waldron LM, Letvin NL. Humoral immune responses to T cell tropic retrovirus simian T lymphotropic virus type III in monkeys with experimentally induced acquired immune deficiency-like syndrome. J Clin Invest 1986; 78:129–1236.

45. Hirsch VM, Zack PM, Vogel AP, Johnson PR. Simian immunodeficiency virus infection of macaques: end-stage disease is characterized by widespread distribution of proviral DNA in tissues. J Infect Dis 1991; 163:976–988.

46. Dewhurst S, Embretson JE, Anderson DC, Mullins JI, Fultz PN. Sequence analysis and acute pathogenicity of molecularly cloned $SIV_{SMM-PBj14}$. Nature 1990; 345:636–640.

47. Fultz PN, Anderson DC, McClure HM, Dewhurst S, Mullins JI. SIVsmm infection of macaque and mangabey monkeys: correlation between *in vivo* and *in vitro* properties of different isolates. Develop Biol Standard 1990; 72: 253–258.

48. Courgnaud V, Laure F, Fultz PN, Montagnier L, Brechot C, Sonigo P. Genetic differences accounting for evolution and pathogenicity of simian immunodeficiency virus from a sooty mangabey after cross-species transmission to a pig-tailed macaque. J Virol 1992; 66:414–419.

49. Dewhurst S, Embretson JE, Fultz PN, Mullins JI. Molecular clones from a non-acutely pathogenic derivative of SIVsmmPBj14: characterization and comparison to acutely pathogenic clones. AIDS Res Hum Retrovir 1992; 8: 1179–1187.

50. Novembre FJ, Hirsch VM, McClure HM, Johnson PR. Molecular diversity of SIVsmm/PBj and a cognate variant, SIVsmm/PGg. J Med Primatol 1991; 20:188–192.

51. Zack PM, Hall WC, Vogel AP, Brown CR, Lewis MG, Jahrling PB. Pathology and immunopathology of $SIV_{SMM-PBj}$ associated gastroenteritis in macaques. Symposium on Nonhuman Primate Models for AIDS, Portland, OR, 1989. Abstr. 85:99.

52. Lewis MG, Birx DL, Zack PM, Vahey MA, Redfield RR, Burke DS, Jahrling PB. Elevated levels of circulating interleukin-6 are associated with an acutely fatal simian immunodeficiency virus isolate (SIVsm/pbj). III Annual Meeting of the NIH Cooperative Drug Discovery Groups for the Treatment of AIDS, Washington, DC, 1990. Abstr. 43:105.

53. Fultz PN. Replication of an acutely lethal simian immunodeficiency virus activates and induces proliferation of lymphocytes. J Virol 1991; 65:4902–4909.

5

Cytokines and HIV Expression

Guido Poli, Audrey L. Kinter, and Anthony S. Fauci

National Institute of Allergy and Infectious Diseases
National Institutes of Health
Bethesda, Maryland

INTRODUCTION

Several questions remain unanswered concerning the immunopathogenesis of human immunodeficiency virus (HIV) infection leading to the clinical disease termed the acquired immunodeficiency syndrome (AIDS) (1). The causative agents of this disease, HIV type 1 or type 2, utilize as their cell surface receptor the CD4 molecule, which normally plays an important role in immune recognition and cell signaling (reviewed in Ref. 2). The identification of CD4 as the viral receptor has explained the selective tropism of this virus for a discrete functional subset of T lymphocytes with helper/inducer function and for mononuclear phagocytes (MPs) (1). One peculiar aspect of HIV infection is the long period of clinical latency (approximately 10 years) following primary infection, which is characterized by high levels of virus replication in the peripheral blood (PB) compartment occurring within weeks of inital infection and lasting 1 to 3 weeks with or without the presence of acute symptoms (1,3). In contrast, during the clinically asymptomatic phase, the levels of HIV replication in PB are low to undetectable, and the viral burden as determined by polymerase chain reaction (PCR) analysis of proviral DNA is quite low in PB CD4 + T cells (1,3,4). Nonetheless, levels of CD4 + T cells progressively decline during this period. In this regard, recent studies have highlighted that active viral replication occurs at any stage of HIV disease, including the clinically asymptomatic phase, in lymph nodes and other lymphoid organs that are anatomical sites of important immunological events (3–5).

Earlier observations have demonstrated that viral replication occurs in tissue macrophages infiltrating the brain of HIV-infected individuals, usually in association with an inflammatory reaction despite the fact that PB monocytes are an infrequent target of HIV infection (1,6). These findings support the concept that both the state of relative or absolute viral latency (as seen in the PB compartment during the asymptomatic period) and the ability of HIV to replicate and spread to new target cells (as observed in lymphoid tissues and in the brain) are profoundly influenced by factors that also govern the state of activation of T lymphocytes and MP during immunological and/or inflammatory reactions. In this regard, the network of functional cytokines has become a major focus of investigation. In particular, a number of studies have demonstrated that HIV infection in vivo and in vitro can cause production of important cytokines such as tumor necrosis factor (TNF), interleukin-1 (IL-1), and IL-6 (7–10). Other studies have demonstrated that the same cytokines can profoundly affect the replicative state of HIV in vitro, and this particular aspect will be further considered in the following discussion. Finally, several cytokines seem to play an important role in the pathophysiology of HIV disease by acting as autocrine/paracrine growth factors for AIDS-associated malignancies, such as B-cell lymphomas and Kaposi's sarcoma (KS) (reviewed in Refs. 11 and 12).

CYTOKINES UPREGULATE HIV EXPRESSION

Since the earlier attempts to identify the causative agent of AIDS, cytokines or cytokine-enriched supernatants have been important experimental tools (13,14). The addition of IL-2 to mitogen-stimulated PB mononuclear cells (PBMCs) represented a key element for the isolation of HIV, and provided a first example of the importance of cell activation and proliferation (in the case of T lymphocytes) for the propagation of virus in culture. It has been subsequently shown that although resting T cells are susceptible to infection with HIV, proper cell activation is required to complete the process of reverse transcription of the viral genome followed by integration of linear proviral DNA into the host chromosomes (15). On the other hand, cell proliferation does not seem to be required to obtain a productive infection of MPs (16). Furthermore, during earlier attempts to isolate the virus from infected people, it was also noted that addition to the cell cultures of either anti-IFN-α neutralizing antibodies (Ab) or glucocorticoid (GC) hormones, which are known to exert profound immunosuppressive effects, increased both the frequency of positive viral isolation from infected individuals and the levels of HIV replication (13,14,17), suggesting that certain cytokines, such as IFN-α, could exert a negative regulatory role on virus expression.

Among the numerous cytokines described to date as being capable of upregulating the expression of HIV (summarized in Table 1), TNF-α and -β are the best-defined in terms of their mechanism of action. Both TNF-α (also known as cachectin) and TNF-β (or lymphotoxin) are produced by a variety of cell types, including MP and T lymphocytes and exert multiple effects on the immune system as well as on the metabolism of proteins and lipids via interaction with two types of cell surface receptors (p55 and p75) (reviewed in Ref. 44). At the cellular level, both TNF-α and -β exert similar effects in most of the systems studied. Although earlier observations described a negative regulatory effect of TNF on HIV-infected cells (42), further studies have demonstrated that these cytokines are strong activators of HIV replication in both T lymphocytes and MPs.

Table 1 Cytokines Known to Regulate
HIV Expression In Vitro

Cytokine	Effect	Cell type	Ref.
IL-1	↑	MP	18,19
IL-2	↑	T	13–15
IL-3	↑	MP	19,20
IL-4	↑↓	MP,T[a]	19,21–23
IL-6	↑	MP	24,25
TNF-α/-β	↑	MP,T	18,19,24–30
TGF-β	↑↓	MP,T	25,31–34
GM-CSF	↑	MP	19,20,35
M-CSF	↑	MP	36
IFN-α/-β	↓	MP,T	13,14,17,37–41
IFN-γ	↑↓	MP	20,42,43

[a]Induction of HIV-1 expression was observed in mature thymocytes but not in PB T cells infected in vitro and stimulated with IL-4 (23).

Upregulation of HIV production mediated by autocrine secretion or cell surface expression of TNF has been documented in vitro in acute infection of primary T cells (30) and U937 promonocytic cells (45), as well as in T lymphocytic and promonocytic cell lines persistently infected with HIV (29).

At the molecular level, the inductive effect of TNF on HIV expression has been demonstrated to be dependent on the activation of the cellular transcription factor NF-$\varkappa$B (18,28) as described earlier in cells stimulated with the phorbol ester PMA (46). The interaction of TNF with a cell surface receptor, which appears to be selecting the p55 molecule (47), leads to the physical dissociation of NF-$\varkappa$B from an inhibitory molecule known as I-$\varkappa$B. NF-$\varkappa$B, which is actually a family of related transcription factors (reviewed in Ref. 48), in its heterodimeric form of a p50/p65 complex, can then migrate to the cell nucleus and bind to two repeated consensus sequences present in the promoter/enhancer region of HIV-1, ultimately triggering or increasing viral transcription (18,28,46–48).

Several cytokines other than TNF have been described to exert inductive effects on HIV expression, although their precise mechanisms of action have not yet been identified. In addition, HIV replication in T lymphocytes can be activated by specialized cell surface receptors such as the CD3/T cell receptor complex, CD2, CD28, and other molecules (49–51). At the molecular level, several of these stimulatory pathways have been shown to activate NF-$\varkappa$B, as described for PMA and TNF, although a number of other transcription factors potentially capable of binding to other sequences on the HIV long terminal repeat (LTR) have been proposed to play a similar role in virus expression (reviewed in Ref. 52). In MPs, a number of cytokines and colony-stimulating factors (CSFs) have been shown to upregulate HIV replication (Table 1). Furthermore, in addition to transcriptional activation, evidence for cytokine-mediated post-transcriptional regulation of virus production has been described in the persistently infected promonocytic cell system U1 after stimulation with IL-6 (24). In this regard, recent studies have shown that a heterologous HIV-1 LTR linked to a reporter gene such as chloramphenicol acetyl-transferase (CAT) and transfected into U1 cells was not activated under the effect of IL-6 either alone or in synergistic combination with GC hormones, despite the fact that endogenous virus production increased up to several hundred-fold over unstimulated cells and induction of both endogenous virus and LTR activation was obtained in the same cells following stimulation with TNF-α or PMA (Poli, Kinter, and Fauci, in preparation).

Finally, evidence that certain cytokines can influence HIV production at a posttranscriptional, posttranslational level has recently been described in the case of IFN-γ. In particular, IFN-γ, in addition to inducing virus expression, also caused a significant increase in the levels of HIV particles budding and accumulating in intracellular Golgi-derived vacuoles, and a concomitant decrease in plasma-membrane-associated particles when U1 cells were stimulated by PMA (43), resembling features of intracellular virion accumulation previously described in primary macrophages infected either in vitro or in vivo (36,53).

These observations are of potential relevance not only because they provide useful tools to study the precise mechanism(s) and site of action of certain cytokines, but also because they suggest potential targets for therapeutic intervention. In this regard, a number of pharmacological agents capable of interfering with cytokine-mediated induction of HIV expression have already shown in vitro efficacy and either are being tested or are under consideration for testing in clinical protocols (54–56).

CYTOKINES SUPPRESS HIV EXPRESSION

As mentioned above, the existence of cytokines negatively acting on HIV replication was suggested by studies attempting to optimize methods of viral isolation. In particular, antibody neutralization of endogenously produced IFN-α resulted in increased virus production in mitogen-stimulated PBMC cultures (13,14,17), whereas addition of exogenous IFN-α/-β to these cells prevented infection in vitro by inhibiting the expression of HIV proteins (37,40). Later studies demonstrated that IFN-α also exerted profound suppressive effects in vitro in primary monocyte-derived macrophages (MDMs) (39) as well as in persistently infected cell lines of either T or monocytic lineage (38). Mechanistically, IFN-α (and IFN-β as well) affects multiple levels in the HIV life cycle as a function of both the cell type and the phase of virus replication. Suppression of early events, such as reverse transcription of the viral genome (41), as well as later events, such as transcription and/or translation of proviral DNA (37,39,40), have been documented in acutely infected T lymphocytic and MP cells. In addition, IFN-α has been reported to block the final phase of the virus life cycle, namely, the release of mature virions from the plasma membrane in chronically infected T and monocytic cells (38), a phenomenon known as postbudding effect, which was previously documented in cells chronically infected with animal retroviruses (reviewed in Ref. 57).

CYTOKINES WITH BIFUNCTIONAL EFFECTS
ON HIV EXPRESSION

A number of cytokines have been reported to either upregulate or suppress virus production in infected MP. The nature of these functional dichotomies still remains elusive, but is likely to be explained by both methodological differences and varying degrees of activation/differentiation of the infected MP. Transforming growth factor β (TGF-β), a potent immunosuppressive cytokine found to be expressed in PBMCs (58) as well as in macrophages and astrocytes of HIV-infected individuals (59), has been shown to inhibit viral transcription in PMA-stimulated U1 cells (25) as well as to block virus production in primary MDMs previously infected with HIV (31). However, TGF-β can also act as a potent upregulator of HIV expression during the acute infection of promonocytic U937 cells (the parental cell line of U1) or MDMs (31–33).

Interestingly, similar results have been obtained with retinoic acid, (31), a potent inducer of monocyte differentiation, suggesting the existence of common functional pathways utilized by certain cytokines and vitamins capable of exerting profound influence on HIV production. In infected primary T lymphocytes, TGF-β was found to act as an autocrine/paracrine inducer of HIV replication in PB cells stimulated with cocaine (34). However, addition of exogenous TGF-β to infected T cells in the absence of cocaine resulted in either upregulation or suppression of virus production in a concentration-dependent manner (34). Similarly, IL-4 has been described as an inducer of HIV replication in mature thymocytes (23) as well as in primary monocytes and MDMs infected in vitro (19,21,22) or in the U1 cell system in conjunction with other inductive cytokines (Poli, Kinter, and Fauci, in preparation). However, IL-4 has also been reported to suppress both constitutive and cytokine-stimulated virus production in 5-day-old infected MDMs (19). Finally, IFN-γ, an inducer of HIV expression in the U1 cell system (43), was reported earlier to exert either upregulatory, downregulatory, or no effects on HIV replication in primary MDM cultures (20).

It is likely that the apparent discordance of these findings indicates that the ability of HIV to replicate in immune cells, and particularly in MPs, is profoundly influenced by different states of cell activation and differentiation, in addition to being highly controlled by the network of virally encoded regulatory genes (52). In this regard, the recent demonstrations that *tat*-deficient viruses (60) as well as viruses profoundly mutagenized in their LTR configuration (61) could efficiently propagate in several cell types suggest a higher level of plasticity of the replicative capacity of HIV than earlier thought.

DO CYTOKINES REGULATE HIV EXPRESSION IN VIVO?

Despite the substantial body of evidence obtained in vitro, there is still no definitive proof that the mechanisms described above regulate the levels of HIV expression in infected individuals. Only manipulation of the cytokine network in either humans or relevant animal models, such as that represented by simian immunodeficiency virus (SIV) infection of macaques, will provide the ultimate answer to this important question. However, a number of observations support the hypothesis of an important role of several cytokines and/or of related mechanisms of immune activation in the pathogenesis of HIV disease.

As mentioned earlier, HIV expression in vivo occurs preferentially, if not exclusively, in tissues in which profound cell activation results as a consequence of either immunological or inflammatory stimulation (1,3–6, 59). In this context, recent evidence suggests that the B-lymphocyte system plays an important role as an in vivo regulator of virus expression from infected cells. In addition to Ab, B cells are known to produce important cytokines such as TNF-α and IL-6 after cell activation (reviewed in Ref. 62), and these cells are in a constitutively activated state in HIV-infected individuals (62,63). In vitro, B lymphocytes from HIV-infected individuals have been shown to induce HIV expression in persistently infected cell lines via release of TNF-α and IL-6, as well as to stimulate virus production when cocultured with autologous T lymphocytes obtained from infected donors (64). Furthermore, HIV gp120 envelope has been shown to further enhance the release of TNF-α and IL-6 in B lymphocytes obtained from HIV-infected individuals, as well as in B cells obtained from uninfected donors in the presence of IL-4, probably via interaction with a cell surface immunoglobulin receptor (65,66).

Finally, it is important to underscore that a large reservoir of HIV appears to reside in the germinal centers of the lymph nodes (a B-cell area) in HIV-infected individuals, where the virus is mostly found conjugated with Ab and adsorbed on the plasma membrane of follicular dendritic cells (FDCs) (3,5,65); in addition, CD4 + T lymphocytes, which infiltrate the germinal centers, are actively infected (3,4,62). It is likely that the close cell–cell contact between T and B lymphocytes and the network of FDCs that anatomically defines the germinal center of the lymph nodes plays a major role in virus expression, spreading, and, ultimately, depletion of the CD4 + T cells.

Finally, the hypothesis that cytokines may play an important role in HIV infection in vivo is supported by the evidence that several cytokines have been found elevated in the plasma and/or are spontaneously secreted by PBMCs isolated from infected individuals (Table 2). In this regard, it has recently been observed that children born from either seronegative or seropositive mothers experience a burst of cytokines such as TNF-α and IL-6 during the first weeks of life that is of even greater magnitude in infants who were vaccinated with BCG or were born from mothers infected with malaria (C. Brown, Poli, and Fauci, in preparation). Whether these "physiological" increases of cytokines can influence the more rapid course of disease that characterizes pediatric as compared to adult HIV infection remains to be established. In this regard, in parallel to very high levels of virus replication, extremely high levels of IL-6 are detectable in both the plasma and the tissues of macaques infected with the acutely lethal variant of SIV known as SIV$_{PBJ14}$ (71), which causes death in the majority of animals within a few days or weeks (72). Conversely, animal species more resistant to the acute PBJ syndrome manifest much lower levels of IL-6 in response to the infection (71). Further studies are required to elucidate the role that cytokines play in less virulent SIV infection. However, preliminary studies conducted during acute SIV infection of macaques suggest an activation of the cytokine network concomitant with the early spreading of virus in the animals (L Fox, Poli, V Hirsch, and Fauci, unpublished observations).

Table 2 Cytokines Upregulated In Vivo or Ex Vivo in HIV-Infected Individuals

Cytokine	Site/source	Producing cell	Ref.
IL-1	Plasma, PBMCs	MPs, KS	8,12
IL-6	Plasma, PBMCs, CSF[a]	MPs, B cells	
	KS, lymphomas		10–12,64–66
TNF-α	Plasma, PBMCs, CSF[a]	T, B cells, MPs	7,8,64–67
TGF-β	PBMCs, brain	MPs, astrocytes	58,59
Acid labile IFN-α	Plasma	Unknown	68
IFN-γ	Plasma	Unknown	69,70

[a]Cerebrospinal fluid.

CONCLUSIONS

There is ample evidence that the interaction of HIV with the immune system is not limited to the utilization of the cell surface CD4 molecule as a receptor for viral entry, but encompasses intimate mechanisms that control the differentiation, activation, and proliferation of T lymphocytes and MPs. The cytokine network probably plays a crucial role in determining the state of latency and expression of HIV, therefore potentially influencing the ability of the virus to spread and seed in the different cells and tissues of the organism. Delineating the mechanisms through which cytokines control HIV replication not only may provide a better understanding of the pathogenesis of this disease, but may also provide the basis for the development of more effective therapeutic strategies.

REFERENCES

1. Fauci AS, Schnittman SM, Poli G, Koenig S, Pantaleo G. Immunopathogenic mechanisms in human immunodeficiency virus (HIV) infection. Ann Intern Med 1991; 114:678-693.
2. Robey E, Axel R. CD4: collaborator in immune recognition and HIV infection. Cell 1990; 60:697-700.
3. Pantaleo G, Graziosi C, Fauci AS. New concepts in the immunopathogenesis of human immunodeficiency virus (HIV) infection. N Engl J Med 1993; 328: 327-335.
4. Pantaleo G, Graziosi C, Butini L, Pizzo PA, Schnittman SM, Kotler DP, Fauci AS. Lymphoid organs function as major reservoirs for human immunodeficiency virus. Proc Natl Acad Sci USA 1991; 88:9838-9842.
5. Fox CH, Tenner-Racz K, Racz P, Firpo A, Pizzo FA, Fauci AS. Lymphoid germinal centers are reservoirs of human immunodeficiency virus. J Infect Dis 1991; 164:1051-1057.
6. Koenig S, Gendelman HE, Orenstein JM, Dal Canto MC, Pezeshkpour GH, Yungbluth M, Janotta F, Aksamit A, Martin MA, Fauci AS. Detection of AIDS virus in macrophages in brain tissue from AIDS patients with encephalopathy. Science 1986; 233:1089-1093.
7. Reddy MM, Sorrell SJ, Lange M, Grieco MH. Tumor necrosis factor and HIV P24 antigen levels in serum of HIV-infected populations. J AIDS 1988; 1:436-440.
8. Roux-Lombard P, Modoux C, Cruchaud A, Dayer J-M. Purified blood monocytes from HIV-1 infected patients produce high levels of TNF-α and IL-1. Clin Immunol Immunopathol 1989; 50:374-384.
9. Clouse KA, Robbins PB, Fernie B, Ostrove JM, Fauci AS. Viral antigen stimulation of the production of human monokines capable of regulating HIV-1 expression. J Immunol 1989; 143:470-475.

10. Breen EC, Rezai AR, Nakajima K, Beall GN, Mitsuyasu RT, Hirano T, Kishimoto T, Martinez-Maza O. Infection with HIV is associated with elevated IL-6 levels and production. J Immunol 1990; 144:480–484.

11. Gill PS. Pathogenesis of HIV-related malignancies. Curr Opin Oncol 1991; 3:867–871.

12. Ensoli B, Barillari G, Gallo RC. Cytokines and growth factors in the pathogenesis of AIDS-associated Kaposi's sarcoma. Immunol Rev 1992; 127:147–155.

13. Barré-Sinoussi F, Chermann JC, Rey F, Nugeyre MT, Chamaret S, Gruest J, Dauguet C, Axler-Blin C, Vezinet-Brun F, Rouzioux C, Rozenbaum W, Montagnier L. Isolation of a T-lymphotropic retrovirus from a patient at risk for acquired immune deficiency syndrome (AIDS). Science 1983; 220: 868–871.

14. Gallo RC, Sarin PS, Gelmann EP, Robert-Guroff M, Richardson E, Kalyanaraman VS, Mann D, Sidhu GD, Stahl RE, Zolla-Pazner S, Leibowitch J, Popovic M. Isolation of human T-cell leukemia virus in acquired immune deficiency syndrome (AIDS). Science 1983; 220:865–867.

15. Zack JA, Arrigo SJ, Weitsman SR, Go AS, Haislip A, Chen IS. HIV-1 entry into quiescent primary lymphocytes: molecular analysis reveals a labile, latent viral structure. Cell 1990; 61:213–222.

16. Weinberg JB, Matthews TJ, Cullen BR, Malim MH. Productive human immunodeficiency virus type 1 (HIV-1) infection of nonproliferating human monocytes. J Exp Med 1991; 174:1477–1482.

17. Markham PD, Salahuddin SZ, Veren K, Orndorff SH, Gallo RC. Hydrocortisone and some other hormones enhance the expression of HTLV-III. Int J Cancer 1986; 37:67–72.

18. Osborn L, Kunkel S, Nabel GJ. Tumor necrosis factor and interleukin 1 stimulate the human immunodeficiency virus enhancer by activation of the nuclear factor kB. Proc Natl Acad Sci USA 1989; 86:2336–2340.

19. Schuitemaker H, Kootstra NA, Koppelman MHGM, Bruisten SM, Husiman HG, Tersmette M, Miedema F. Proliferation dependent HIV-1 infection of monocytes occurs during differentiation into macrophages. J Clin Invest 1992; 89:1154–1160.

20. Koyanagi Y, O'Brien WA, Zhao JQ, Golde DW, Gasson JC, Chen ISY. Cytokines alter production of HIV-1 from primary mononuclear phagocytes. Science 1988; 241:1673–1675.

21. Novak RM, Holzer TJ, Kennedy MM, Heynen CA, Dawson G. The effect of interleukin 4 (BSF-1) on infection of peripheral blood monocyte-derived macrophages with HIV-1. AIDS Res Hum Retrovird 1990; 6:973–976.

22. Kazazi F, Mathijs JM, Chang J, Malafiej P, Lopez A, Dowton D, Sorrel TC, Vadas MA, Cunningham AL. Recombinant interleukin 4 stimulates human immunodeficiency virus production by infected monocytes and macrophages. J Gen Virol 1992; 73:941–949.

23. Hays EF, Uittenbogaart CH, Brewer JC, Vollger LW, Zack JA. In vitro studies of HIV-1 expression in thymocytes from infants and children. AIDS 1992; 6:265–272.

24. Poli G, Bressler P, Kinter A, Duh E, Timmer WC, Rabson A, Justement JS, Stanley S, Fauci AS. Interleukin 6 induces human immunodeficiency virus expression in infected monocytic cells alone and in synergy with tumor necrosis factor α by transcriptional and post-transcriptional mechanisms. J Exp Med 1990; 172:151–158.

25. Poli G, Kinter AL, Justement JS, Bressler P, Kehrl JH, Fauci AS. Transforming growth factor β suppresses human immunodeficiency virus expression and replication in infected cells of the monocyte/macrophage lineage. J Exp Med 1991; 173:589–597.

26. Clouse KA, Powell D, Washington I, Poli G, Strebel K, Farrar W, Barstad P, Kovacs J, Fauci AS, Folks TM. Monokine regulation of human immunodeficiency virus-1 expression in a chronically infected human T cell clone. J Immunol 1989; 142:431–438.

27. Folks TM, Clouse KA, Justement J, Rabson A, Duh E, Kehrl JH, Fauci AS. Tumor necrosis factor alpha induces expression of human immunodeficiency virus in a chronically infected T-cell clone. Proc Natl Acad Sci USA 1989; 86:2365–2368.

28. Duh EJ, Maury WJ, Folks TM, Fauci AS, Rabson AB. Tumor necrosis factor activates human immunodeficiency virus type 1 through induction of nuclear factor binding to the NF-kB sites in the long terminal repeat. Proc Natl Acad Sci USA 1989; 86:5974–5978.

29. Poli G, Kinter A, Justement JS, Kehrl JH, Bressler P, Stanley S, Fauci AS. Tumor necrosis factor α functions in an autocrine manner in the induction of human immunodeficiency virus expression. Proc Natl Acad Sci USA 1990; 87:782–785.

30. Vyakarnam A, McKeating J, Meager A, Beverley PC. Tumour necrosis factors (α, β) induced by HIV-1 in peripheral blood mononuclear cells potentiate virus replication. AIDS 1990; 4:21–27.

31. Poli G, Kinter AL, Justement JS, Bressler P, Kehrl P, Kehrl JH, Fauci AS. Retinoic acid mimics transforming growth factor beta in the regulation of human immunodeficiency virus expression in monocytic cells. Proc Natl Acad Sci USA 1992; 89:2689–2693.

32. Lazdins JK, Klimkait T, Woods-Cook K, Walker M, Alteri E, Cox D, Cerletti N, Shipman R, Bilbe G, McMaster G. In vitro effect of transforming growth factor-β on progression of HIV-1 infection in primary mononuclear phagocytes. J Immunol 1991; 147:1201–1207.

33. Lazdins JK, Klimkait T, Woods-Cook K, Walker M, Alteri E, Cox D, Cerletti D, Shipman R, Bilbe G, McMaster G. The replicative restriction of lymphocytotropic isolates of HIV-1 in macrophages is overcome by TGF-beta. AIDS Res Hum Retrovir 1992; 8:505–511.

34. Peterson PK, Gekker G, Chao CC, Schut R, Molitor TW, Balfour HH Jr. Cocaine potentiates HIV-1 replication in human peripheral blood mononuclear cell cocultures. J Immunol 1991; 146:81–84.

35. Folks TM, Justement J, Kinter A, Dinarello CA, Fauci AS. Cytokine-induced expression of HIV-1 in a chronically infected promonocyte cell line. Science 1987; 238:800–802.

36. Gendelman HE, Orenstein JM, Martin MA, Ferrua C, Mitra R, Phipps T, Wahl LA, Lane HC, Fauci AS, Burke DS, Skillman D, Meltzer MS. Efficient isolation and propagation of human immunodeficiency virus on recombinant colony-stimulating factor 1-treated monocytes. J Exp Med 1988; 167:1428–1441.

37. Ho DD, Hartshorn KL, Rota TR, Andrews CA, Kaplan JC, Schooley RT, Hirsch MS. Recombinant human interferon alpha-A suppresses HTLV-III replication in vitro. Lancet 1985; i:602–604.

38. Poli G, Orenstein JM, Kinter A, Folks TM, Fauci AS. Interferon-α but not AZT suppresses HIV expression in chronically infected cell lines. Science 1989; 244:575–577.

39. Gendelman HE, Baca LM, Turpin J, Kalter DC, Hansen B, Orenstein JM, Dieffenbach CW, Friedman RM, Meltzer MS. Regulation of HIV replication in infected monocytes by IFN-α. J Immunol 1990; 145:2669–2676.

40. Williams GJ, Colby CB. Recombinant human interferon-beta suppresses the replication of HIV and acts synergistically with AZT. J Interferon Res 1989; 9:709–718.

41. Shirazi Y, Pitha PM. Alpha interferon inhibits early stages of the human immunodeficiency virus type 1 replication cycle. J Virol 1992; 66:1321–1328.

42. Wong GH, Krowka JF, Stites DP, Goeddel DV. In vitro anti-human immunodeficiency virus activities of tumor necrosis factor-alpha and interferon-gamma. J Immunol 1988; 140:120–124.

43. Biswas P, Poli G, Kinter AL, Justement JS, Stanley SK, Maury WJ, Bressler P, Orenstein JM, Fauci AS. Interferon-γ modulates the expression of human immunodeficiency virus in persistently infected promonocytic cells by redirecting the production of virions to intracytoplasmic vacuoles. J Exp Med 1992; 176:739–750.

44. Dinarello CA. Interleukin-1 and tumor necrosis factor: effector cytokines in autoimmune diseases. Sem Immunol 1992; 4:133–145.

45. Tadmori W, Mondal D, Tadmori I, Prakash O. Transactivation of human immunodeficiency virus type 1 long terminal repeats by cell surface tumor necrosis factor alpha. J Virol 1991; 65:6425–6429.

46. Nabel G, Baltimore D. An inducible transcription factor activates expression of human immunodeficiency virus in T cells. Nature 1987; 326:711–713.

47. Kruppa G, Thoma B, Machleidt T, Wiegmann K, Kronke M. Inhibition of tumor necrosis factor (TNF)-mediated NF-kB activation by selective blockade of the human 55-kDa TNF receptor. J Immunol 1992; 148:3152–3157.

48. Franzoso G, Bours V, Park S, Tomita-Yamaguchi T, Kelly K, Siebenlist U. The candidate oncoprotein Bcl-3 is an antagonist of p50/NF-kB-mediated inhibition. Nature 1992; 359:339–342.

49. Tong-Starksen SE, Luciw PA, Peterlin BM. Signaling through T lymphocyte surface proteins, TCR/CD3 and CD28 activate the HIV-1 long terminal repeat. J Immunol 1989; 142:702–707.

50. Perez VL, Rowe T, Justement JS, Butera ST, June CH, Folks TM. An HIV-1-infected T cell clone defective in IL-2 production and Ca^{2+} mobilization after CD3 stimulation. J Immunol 1991; 147:3145–3148.

51. Bressler P, Pantaleo G, Demaria A, Fauci AS. Anti-CD2 receptor antibodies activate the HIV long terminal repeat in T lymphocytes. J Immunol 1991; 147:2290–2294.

52. Cullen BR, Green WC. Regulatory pathways governing HIV-1 replication. Cell 1989; 58:423–426.

53. Orenstein JM, Jannotta F. Human immunodeficiency virus and papovavirus infections in acquired immunodeficiency syndrome: an ultrastructural study of three cases. Hum Pathol 1988; 19:350–361.

54. Staal FJT, Ela SW, Roederer M, Anderson MT, Herzenberg LA, Herzenberg LA. Glutathione deficiency and human immunodeficiency virus infection. Lancet 1992; 339:909–912.

55. Fazely F, Dezube BJ, Allen-Ryan J, Pardee AB, Ruprecht RM. Pentoxifylline (Trental) decreases the replication of the human immunodeficiency virus type 1 in human peripheral blood mononuclear cells and in cultured T cells. Blood 1991; 77:1653–1656.

56. Weissman D, Poli G, Bousseau A, Fauci AS. A platelet activating factor antagonist, RP 55778, inhibits cytokine dependent induction of human immunodeficiency virus expression in chronically infected promonocytic cells. Proc Natl Acad Sci USA. In press.

57. Friedman RM, Pitha PM. The effect of interferon on membrane-associated viruses. In: Friedman RM, ed. Interferon: Mechanisms of Production and Action. New York: Elsevier, 1984:319–341.

58. Kekow J, Wachsman W, McCutchan JA, Cronin M, Carson DA, Lotz M. Transforming growth factor β and noncytopathic mechanisms of immunodeficiency in human immunodeficiency virus infection. Proc Natl Acad Sci USA 1990; 87:8321–8325.

59. Wahl SM, Allen JB, McCartney-Francis N, Morganti-Kossman MC, Kossmann T, Ellingsworth L, Mai UEH, Mergenhagen SE, Orenstein JM. Macrophage- and astrocyte-derived transforming growth factor β as a mediator of central nervous system dysfunction in acquired immune deficiency syndrome. J Exp Med 1991; 173:981–991.

60. Popik W, Pitha PM. Role of tumor necrosis factor alpha in activation and replication of the tat-defective human immunodeficiency virus type 1. J Virol 1993; 67(2):1094–1099.

61. Parrott C, Seidner T, Duh E, Leonard J, Theodore TS, Buckler-White A, Martin MA, Rabson AB. Variable role of the long terminal repeal Sp1-binding sites in human immunodeficiency virus replication in T lymphocytes. J Virol 1991; 1414–1419.

62. Kehrl JH, Rieckmann P, Kozlow E, Fauci AS. Lymphokine production by B cells from normal and HIV-infected individuals. Ann NY Acad Sci 1992; 651:220–227.

63. Lane HC, Masur H, Edgar C, Whalen G, Rook AH, Fauci AS. Abnormalities of B-cell activation and immunoregulation in patients with the acquired immunodeficiency syndrome. N Engl J Med 1983; 309:453–458.

64. Rieckmann P, Poli G, Kehrl JH, Fauci AS. Activated B lymphocytes from human immunodeficiency virus-infected individuals induce virus expression in infected T cells and a promonocytic cell line, U1. J Exp Med 1991; 173: 1–5.

65. Rieckmann P, Poli G, Fox CH, Kehrl JH, Fauci AS. Recombinant gp120 specifically enhances tumor necrosis factor-alpha production and Ig secretion in B lymphocytes from HIV-infected individuals but not from seronegative donors. J Immunol 1991; 147:2922–2927.

66. Boue F, Wallon C, Goujard C, Barré-Sinoussi F, Galanaud P, Delfraissy JF. HIV induces IL-6 production by human B lymphocytes. Role of IL-4. J Immunol 1992; 148:3761–3767.

67. Grimaldi LME, Martino GV, Franciotta DM, Brustia R, Castagna A, Pristera R, Lazzarin A. Elevated alpha-tumor necrosis factor levels in spinal fluid from HIV-1 infected patients with central nervous system involvement. Ann Neurol 1991; 29:21–25.

68. Rinaldo CR, Armstrong JA, Kingsley LA, Zhou S, Ho M. Relation of alpha and gamma interferon levels to development of AIDS in homosexual men. J Exp Pathol 1990; 5:127–132.

69. Fuchs D, Hausen A, Reibnegger G, Werner ER, Werner-Felmayer G, Dierich MP, Wachter H. Interferon-γ concentrations are increased in sera from individuals infected with human immunodeficiency virus type 1. J AIDS 1989; 2:158–162.

70. Lane HC, Depper JM, Greene WC, Whalen G, Waldmann TA, Fauci AS. Qualitative analysis of immune function in patients with the acquired immunodeficiency syndrome. Evidence for a selective defect in soluble antigen recognition. N Engl J Med 1985; 313:79–84.

71. Birx DL, Lewis MG, Vahey M, Tencer K, Zack P, Jahrling P, Tosato G, Burke D, Redfield R. Association of IL-6 in the pathogenesis of acutely fatal SIV-pbj in pigtailed macaques. AIDS Res Hum Retrovir. In press.

72. Fultz PN, McClure HM, Anderson DC, Switzer WM. Identification and biologic characterization of an acutely lethal variant of simian immunodeficiency virus from sooty mangabeys (SIV/SMM). AIDS Res Hum Retrovir 1989; 5:397–409.

6

Experimental Model Systems for Studies of HIV-Associated CNS Disease

Howard E. Gendelman*

*Walter Reed Army Institute of Research
and the Henry M. Jackson Foundation
for the Advancement of Military Medicine
Rockville, Maryland*

Peter Genis*

*Walter Reed Army Institute of Research
Rockville, Maryland*

Marti Jett and Edward W. Bernton

*Walter Reed Army Institute of Research
Washington, D.C.*

**Harris A. Gelbard, Therese A. Cvetkovich, Eliot S. Lazar,
Manuel del Cerro, and Leon G. Epstein**

*University of Rochester Medical Center
Rochester, New York*

**Current affiliation:* University of Nebraska Medical Center, Omaha, Nebraska.

The opinions expressed are not necessarily those of the United States Army or Department of Defense.

INTRODUCTION

Productive HIV replication in brain tissue often, but not always, predicts neurological disease (1-5). Indeed, the CNS is a major reservoir for HIV (1-5), and virus is expressed almost exclusively in cells of macrophage lineage (brain macrophages, microglia, and multinucleated giant cells) (6-10). In affected tissue up to 15% of brain macrophages express HIV gene products (6-10). However, discrepancies between the numbers of productively infected macrophages and the severity of tissue damage were reported (4,5). These observations suggest that indirect mechanisms for tissue damage including the release of cytokines, arachidonic metabolites, and other neuronotoxic factors are mediators for tissue damage (11).

Several studies demonstrate that entry of virus into the CNS occurs early after infection, either during the acute seroconversion reaction or during subclinical infection (12-16). However, exactly how HIV enters the brain and preferentially infects macrophages are areas of intense debate. Macrophages and multinucleated giant cells were recognized early on as the major cell type harboring HIV-1 in brain tissue (17). Moreover, HIV tropism for macrophages is an essential requirement for lentiviral neuroinvasiveness (18). The virus-infected brain macrophages may originate from an expansion of latently infected monocytes that carry HIV into the brain (the "Trojan horse" hypothesis) and later produce virus (19). Alternatively, virus may penetrate the brain through a disrupted blood-brain barrier by infected T cells or as free viral particles. The role of these HIV-infected brain macrophages in disease probably revolves around metabolic, immune, and/or viral-induced secretory factors. Elucidating these events is critical to our understanding of HIV neuropathogenesis (20).

Recent reports suggest that brain dysfunction may be related to cell-encoded toxins generated from virus-infected macrophages (11,21-24). Secretory products from HIV-infected cells may alter neuronal viability, damage myelin, or stimulate neurotransmitters, resulting in neuronal dysfunction. Indeed, macrophages play important roles in steady-state immune and tissue function. Supporting this idea are recent studies demonstrating that disordered secretion of one or more cellular factors from HIV-infected macrophages or through macrophage-astrocyte interactions produces neuronal death in vitro (11,21,22). The studies suggested that HIV-infected macrophages and glial cellular interactions in brain continuously disrupt neurological function, leading to cognitive CNS dysfunction. Thus, if the macrophage plays a role in virus-induced neuropathology, it may act through cell-to-cell interactions with neurons and glia to produce CNS tissue damage (11,24). Perhaps this occurs through cytokine and/or ther neuronotoxic factor release during cell-to-cell contact. To investigate this possibility we recovered culture fluids from cell mixtures of virus-infected monocytes and astroglia. Assay of fluids after cocultivation showed high levels of arachidonic acid metabolites, cytokines, and neuronotoxic factors.

These experimental results were confirmed through studies of HIV infection in neural xenografts. Here, fetal human neural tissue was explanted into the anterior chamber of the eye of immunosuppressed adult rats (25). The neural tissue vascularized and contained all cellular brain tissue components (neurons, glia, and microglia). Moreover, the cells differentiated and formed a blood–brain barrier. Inoculation of these brain tissues with HIV-infected monocytes produced neuronal damage and glial proliferation (26).

MATERIALS AND METHODS

Isolation and Culture of Monocytes and Human Neural Cells

Monocytes were recovered from PBMCs of HIV and hepatitis B-seronegative donors after leukapheresis and purified by countercurrent centrifugal elutriation. Cell suspensions were >98% monocytes by criteria of cell morphology on Wright-stained cytosmears, by granular peroxidase, and by nonspecific esterase. Monocytes were cultured as adherent monolayers (1×10^6 cells/ml in 24-mm plastic culture wells) in DMEM (Sigma, St. Louis, MO) with recombinant human MCSF (FAP-809,Cetus Corp., Emeryville, CA) as previously described (27). Human brain tumor–derived cell lines included: U251 MG from D Bigner (28), U373 MG from B Westermark (29), and SK-N-MC (30) and H4 (HTB 148) (31) from the American Type Culture Collection (ATCC), Rockville, MD. The cells were grown as adherent monolayers in DMEM (Sigma) with 10% heat-inactivated fetal calf serum (FCS) (Sigma) and 50 μg/ml gentamicin, and characterized as to their cell of origin (32–34). Primary human astrocytes were prepared from second-trimester human fetal brain tissue obtained from elective abortions as previously described (35) and performed in full compliance with both NIH and University of Rochester guidelines. Cells were cultured as adherent monolayers in DMEM (Sigma) with 10% heat-inactivated FCS (Sigma). All culture reagents were screened and found negative for endotoxin contamination.

HIV Infection of Target Cells

Adherent monocytes cultured for 7 days were exposed at a multiplicity of infection (MOI) = 0.01 infectious virus/target cell to ADA (27,36). All viral stocks were tested and found free of mycoplasma contamination (Gen-probe II, Gen-probe Inc., San Diego, CA). Reverse transcriptase (RT) activity was determined in replicate samples of culture fluids (37).

Quantitations of Cytokine Activity

Culture fluids from control and HIV-infected monocytes were analyzed by ELISA for the human cytokines TNF-α, IL-1α, IL-1β, and IL-6 (Quantikine Immunoassay, Research and Diagnostics Systems, Minneapolis, Minnesota).

Fetal Rat and Human Brain Cortical Explant Cultures

Fetal Sprague-Dawley rat (15 days gestational age) forebrains were dissociated by tituration into a single-cell suspension and adjusted to 1×10^6 viable cells/ml. Cells were plated in poly-L-lysine treated plastic culture wells in 1:1 mixture of Eagle and Ham's F12K medium with 50 U/ml penicillin, 50 μg/ml of streptomycin, 600 μg/ml glucose, 10% horse serum, and 10% FCS) (38,39). After 5 days, cultures were treated with 10 μM cytosine arabinoside (Ara-C) (Sigma Chemical Co.) for 48 hours to deplete proliferating astrocytes, fibroblasts, and microglial cells (23). The composition of these Ara-C-treated cultures at day 10 was 70 to 85% neurons by neuron-specific enolase (NSE, Dako Corp., Carpinteria, CA), 10 to 15% microglia by latex-bead phagocytosis and rat OX-6 staining, and less than 5 to 10% astrocytes by morphology and glial fibrillary acidic protein (GFAP, Dako Corp.) staining. Cells were treated with conditioned media from cell cultures for 1 to 7 days and analyzed for neuronotoxicity.

Quantitations of Neuronal Cell Growth and Survival

The metabolic activity and number of viable cells/culture were assessed by conversion of 3-(4,5-dimethylthiazol-2yl)-2,5-diphenyl tetrazolium (MTT) bromide and color intensity measured at $OD_{490\,nm}$ (40,41). Cell morphology in neuronal cultures depleted of glial cells was examined under phase-contrast microscopy or after fixation with 80% methanol and Wright-Giemsa stain. Morphological changes in these neuron-enriched cell cultures correlated directly with MTT levels and were scored as zero (no neuritic outgrowth), + (dendritic outgrowth 2 to 4 perikaryons distance in ≥50% of cells/field), or + + (dendritic outgrowth 4 to 8 perikaryons distance in ≥50% of cells/field). Generally, 100 cells in four fields/culture were examined on successive days. In some studies, identical microscopic fields were photographed at serial intervals to decrease sampling variability.

Transplantation of Human Fetal Tissues to the Anterior Chamber of Adult Rat Eyes

Male Sprague-Dawley strain (Charles River) albino rats (100–120 days old) were maintained on cyclosporin A (Sandoz, 6.0 mg/kg/day) and housed in sterilized microisolator cages. Brain tissue from human fetuses (gestational age 11 to 17.5 weeks) was submerged in fresh human plasma at 4 °C, dissected, and minced into small (< 0.5 mm^3) fragments. The telencephalon, including both ventricular and cortical surfaces, was utilized, ensuring the presence of both neuronal and glial cellular elements (25,26). Additional human fetal tissue was stored at − 70 °C and screened for HIV infection using polymerase chain reaction (PCR) amplification techniques (26).

Preparation and HIV-1 Infection of Human Fetal Implant

Tissue fragments prepared in human plasma were combined with HIV-1 ADA-infected monocytes (see above). Replicate tissues were untreated or inoculated with uninfected monocytes. Cells were backloaded into a 50-μl Hamilton syringe. The rats were then anesthetized with ketamine (60 mg/kg), pentobarbital (20 mg/kg), and topical xylocaine (1%). Ten microliters of tissue suspension was injected through a 27-gauge needle into the anterior chamber, under direct microscope observation. The growth of the transplant and the status of the eye's anterior segment were monitored through the transparent cornea by direct ophthalmoscopy or with a stereo microscope. Seven animals received neural tissue only, seven received neural tissue and uninfected control human monocytes, and 11 animals received neural tissue and HIV-1 ADA-infected monocytes. Representative animals were sacrificed on posttransplantation days 7–14. Grafts were recovered by enucleation and prepared for histological or immunocytochemical studies as previously reported.

RESULTS

No Evidence for Neuronotoxic Activity in Culture Fluids of Uninfected or HIV-Infected Monocytes

Monocytes were infected with HIV-1 $_{ADA}$ at MOI = 0.01 for 7 days (14 days after plating). Culture fluids from the HIV-infected and control un-

infected cells were added to rat brain explants. Additions of fluids from
HIV-infected and control uninfected showed no neuronotoxicity (Figure
1 and Table 1). Fetal rat brain cells inoculated with fluids from HIV-
infected or control uninfected astroglial cells showed similar results.

Fluids from HIV-Infected Monocyte-Glial Cell Interactions Produce Neuronotoxic Factors

The absence of neuronotoxic activity from HIV-infected monocytes or
virus-infected neural cells led to assay of glial cell cocultures for neuronotoxic activities. Monocytes were infected with HIV-1_{ADA} for 7 days,
harvested from Teflon flasks, and then placed onto equal numbers of
neural cells. Fluids were harvested at 24 hours after cocultivation, then
placed on rat brain explants. In contrast to previous results, fluids from
cocultures of HIV-infected monocytes with U251 Mg, U373 Mg, HTB
148, or normal human astroglial cells were profoundly neuronotoxic (Table 1 and Figure 1). Within 2 days following the addition of fluid, neurons
were swollen and vacuolated. Calcien yellow staining showed few viable
neurons 2 days after addition of fluid (Figure 1). Dose-response analysis
of culture fluids from HIV-infected monocyte-astroglia (U251 Mg) mixtures showed significant neuronotoxicity with dilutions of $\leqslant 1/20$ of these
culture fluids. Indeed, a loss of $\geqslant 50\%$ of viable neurons per well was
evident when a 20-fold dilution of culture fluids of HIV-infected mono-
cytes-astroglia was placed onto rat fetal neurons. The toxic effects were
cell-specific. Fluids obtained from mixtures of HIV-infected monocytes
and SK-N-MC (neuroblastoma) or HIV-infected monocytes and endothelial cells showed no neuronotoxic activity. Moreover, the HIV-infected
monocyte-astroglia coculture fluids induced a marked astrogliosis in the
rat brain explant cells (Figure 2). This occurred at the same time that neuronotoxicity was observed and showed cell-specific effects for this toxicity.

Mechanisms for Neuronotoxicity from Coculture of HIV-Infected Monocytes and Astroglia

Preliminary experiments suggested that activation of the NMDA receptor
by endogenous excitatory amino acids (EAA) such as glutamate was necessary for the HIV-infected macrophage-astroglia (U251 MG) neuronotoxicity. This is of interest, as quinolinate, a weak NMDA agonist, is increased in the cerebrospinal fluid of AIDS patients and its levels correlate
with cognitive CNS dysfunction. Certain amino acids and their metabolites
(glutamate, aspartic acid, quinolinic acid) at high concentrations are

Table 1 Neuron Survival and Differentiation in Rat Brain Explants Treated for 5 Days with Culture Fluids from Uninfected and HIV-1-Infected Monocytes and Astroglia

Tissue culture medium	
Medium alone	+
Medium with M-CSF	+
Monocyte culture fluids	
Control monocytes	+ +
HIV-1$_{ADA}$-infected monocytes	+ +
HIV and its products	
HIV-1$_{HTLV-IIIB}$	+
HIV-1$_{24}$	+
HIV-1$_{ADA}$	+
HIV gp120	+
HIV-infected monocytes cocultured with	
Endothelial cells	+
SK-N-MC (neuroblastoma)	+
U251 MG (astroglia)	0
U373 MG (astroglia)	0
HTB 148 (neuroglia)	0
U251 MG astroglia cocultured with	
Uninfected monocytes	+
HIV-1$_{ADA}$	+
Freeze-thawed HIV-infected monocytes	+
Paraformaldehyde-fixed HIV-infected monocytes	+

Fetal rat brain explants were cultured for 10 days, then treated for 5 days with monocytes media, conditioned media containing 20% v/v fluids from uninfected monocytes, HIV-1$_{ADA}$ and HIV-1$_{24}$-infected monocytes, or with HIV-1$_{HTLV-IIIB}$ or HIV-1$_{ADA}$ virus stock ($>1 \times 10^8$ HIV particles/ml by grid count on transmission electron microscopy), and 500 ng/ml recombinant HIV-1$_{HTLV-IIIB}$ gp120. Conditioned media contained 20% v/v fluids from HIV-1$_{ADA}$-infected monocytes cocultured with endothelial cells, SK-N-MC (neuroblastoma), and U251 glial cells and U251 MG atroglial cells incubated with HIV-1$_{ADA}$, freeze-thawed HIV-infected monocytes, paraformaldehyde-fixed HIV-infected monocytes, and uninfected monocytes were harvested after 24 hours and assayed for neuronotoxicity. Neuron survival and extent of differentiation were estimated by cell morphology on phase contrast microscopy or on methanol-fixed, Wright-Giemsa stained slides as outlined under "Materials and Methods." Cell number was confirmed by MTT conversion as estimated by spectrophotometry at OD$_{490\,nm}$.

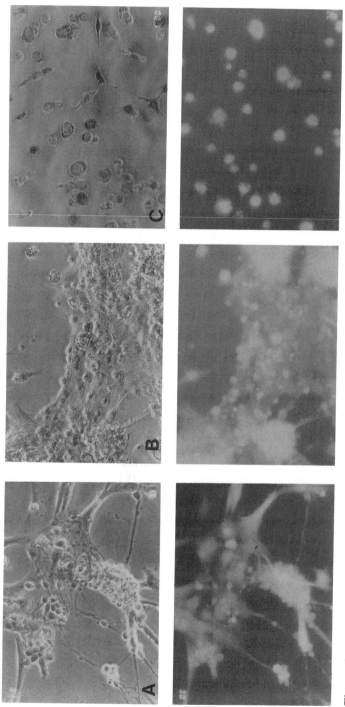

Figure 1

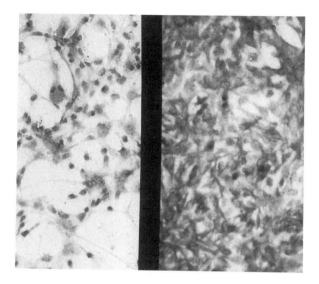

Figure 2   Astrocyte proliferation induced from culture fluids of HIV-infected monocytes and astroglia (U251 MG cells). Neuronal-enriched cell cultures at 10 days were exposed to HIV-infected monocytes (left) or culture fluids from mixtures of HIV-infected monocytes and astroglia (right). Numbers of astrocytes were determined by immunocytochemical staining using anti-GFAP antibodies ($\times$75).

Figure 1   Rat neuronal cell cultures at 10 days were exposed to a 1:10 dilution of culture fluids from monocyte-astroglial cocultures. Cultures were examined daily by phase-contrast microscopy. At day 4, cultures were stained for 90 minutes with calcein. The calcein dye is hydrolyzed by cytoplasmic esterases in living cells. (Top) phase microscopy; (bottom) identical fields under fluorescent illumination. (A) Neurons exposed to culture fluids of uninfected control monocytes show dense networks of finely branched dendrites and well-defined oval perikaria ($\times$150). (B) Neurons exposed to fluids of HIV-infected monocytes are indistinguishable from control uninfected monocyte culture fluids ($\times$150). (C) Neurons exposed to culture fluids of HIV-infected monocyte/astroglia (U251 MG) cocultures ($\times$150). Neuronal cell bodies show extensive cytoplasmic vacuolization. Dendritic outgrowths are blunted or absent. Numerous glial cells are present throughout the field. This experiment is representative of three replicate assays. Cocultivations were performed at a 1:1 cell ratio (HIV-infected monocytes/astroglia). (From J Exp Med 1992; 176:1703.)

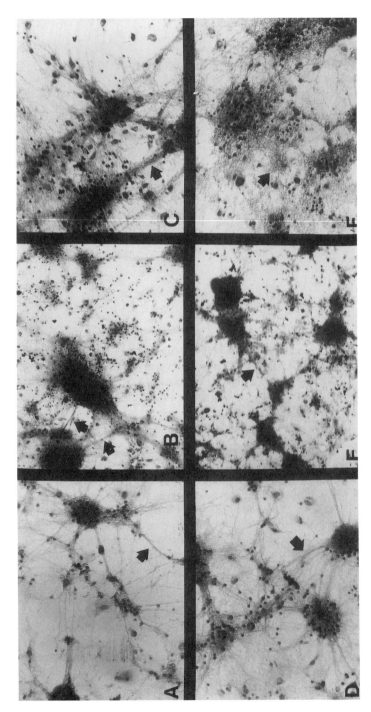

Figure 3

neuronotoxic and act through activation of NMDA receptor channel complex. NMDA antagonists can block neuronal damage for several different neurological disorders (tetanus, neurotropic viruses—for example, measles—stroke, and neurodegenerative disorders) as well as retinal ganglion cells exposed to gp120 and glutamate (23,44–48). As rat brain cells express NMDA receptors and are sensitive, in Mg^{2+}-depleted media, to the toxic effects of glutamic acid we determined whether fluids from HIV-1-infected monocytes and astroglia (U251 MG) enhanced glutamic acid neuronotoxicity. Neurons were treated for 1 hour with Mg^{2+}-free media and then inoculated with fluids of uninfected monocytes, astroglial cells (U251 MG), or cocultures of HIV-infected monocytes and 0–100 μM glutamic acid. After 1 hour, culture fluids were removed and replaced with complete neuronal media. Without glutamate, neurons treated for 18 hours with fluids from control uninfected (Figure 3A) or HIV-infected monocyte-astroglia (U251 MG) cocultures (Figure 3D) showed no evidence for neuronotoxicity. Neurons and their processes were preserved. Similar results occurred with neurons cultured with 33 μM glutamic acid with fluids from uninfected control monocytes-astroglial cells (U251 MG) (Figure 3B and C). However, neurons treated with both 33 μM glutamic acid and fluids from HIV-infected monocytes and astroglia were swollen, indicating disintegrated neuronal processes. Numerous small, pyknotic nuclei were readily identified (Figure 3E and F). These results suggested that the neuronotoxicity was NMDA-receptor mediated.

The requirements for viable HIV-infected monocytes in the neuronotoxicity were further investigated. Astroglial cells (U251 MG) were mixed with 4% paraformaldehyde-fixed or sonicated HIV-infected monocytes or HIV-1_{ADA} viral stock ($>1 \times 10^8$ total particles/ml) and fluids

---

Figure 3 Rat neuronal cell cultures at 10 days were exposed to culture fluids with or without glutamate. (A) Neurons treated with uninfected control monocytes for 18 hours. (B) Neurons exposed to 33 μm glutamate for 1 hour, then to fluids from uninfected control monocyte-astroglia (U251 MG cell) mixtures ($\times 50$). (C) High power of (B) ($\times 50$). (D) Neurons inoculated with fluids from HIV-infected monocyte-astroglia mixtures for 18 hours. (E) Neurons exposed to 33 μM glutamate for 1 hour, then treated with fluids from HIV-monocyte-astroglia mixtures ($\times 50$). (F) High power of (E) ($\times 50$). Neurons treated with glutamic acid and fluids from HIV-infected monocyte-astroglia cocultures show rounding and swelling. Complete disintegration of some neurons with perikarial swelling and loss of dendritic processes is seen.

harvested after 24 and 48 hours. Neuronotoxic activity was not observed with any of the treatments listed above, suggesting that viable cell mixtures of HIV-infected monocytes and astroglia (U251 MG) were required to produce neuronotoxicity.

Mechanisms for Neuronotoxicity Analysis of Cytokine Gene Expression During Cocultivations

A variety of cytokines may produce neurotoxicity and as such contribute to the pathogenesis of CNS disease. Two cytokines, IL-1β and TNF-α, are associated with glial proliferation, neurotoxicity, and demyelination. Interestingly, these cellular effects are all prominent features of HIV-related encephalopathy. For example, TNF, at high concentrations, is a neurotoxin (23,43,44). Human astrocytes proliferate in response to TNF-α and IL-1β (45,46), and conditioned medium from LPS-treated astrocytes stimulates HIV-1 gene expression in monocytic cells (47). These observations led us to investigate whether TNF-α and IL-1β produced the neuronotoxicity observed in supernatant fluids of HIV-infected monocytes and astroglia.

TNF-α and IL-1β protein and biological activity were seen only in coculture fluids of HIV-1-infected monocytes and astroglia (U251 MG and normal human astrocytes) (Figures 4 and 5). Maximum levels were present 12 to 48 hours following cocultivation. In a series of four replicate experiments, maximum levels of TNF-α were 1000 to 9000 pg/ml (mean of 5000), while IL-1β levels ranged from 400 to 5000 pg/ml (mean of 900) Figures 4 and 5). The underlying basis for this 10-fold difference was related to the levels of productive HIV infection. Peak cytokine levels occurred during the initial rise of RT activity, 3–5 days following virus infection, and diminished to baseline by day 10 (data not shown). TNF-α and IL-1β proteins were also detected at low levels: < 100 pg/ml in cocultures of uninfected monocytes and astroglia (U251 MG and human astrocytes). The latter results suggest that the interactions seen between HIV-infected monocytes and glia are an extension of a normal physiological rsponse. Moreover, the addition of dexamethasone, a potent inhibitor of phospholipase A, markedly reduced the cytokine response. This suggested the possible involvement of arachidonic acid metabolites in the cytokine and perhaps the neuronotoxic response. To investigate a possible temporal relationship between arachidonic acid metabolites and TNF-α we added indomethacin, a cyclooxygenase inhibitor, or nordihydroguaiaretic acid (NDGA), a lipoxygenase inhibitor, to cocultures

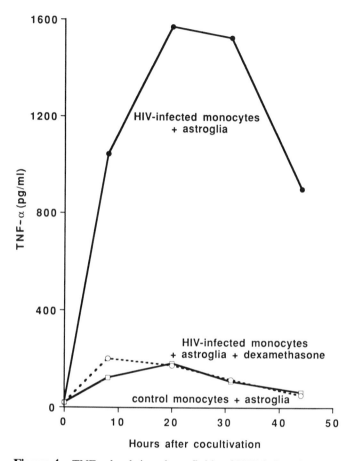

Figure 4   TNF-α levels in culture fluids of HIV-infected monocytes cocultured with astroglia (U251 MG cells). Adherent monocytes cultured for 7 days were exposed to HIV_{ADA} at a MOI $\simeq$ 0.01. Seven days after infection, HIV-infected and control uninfected monocytes were cocultured with equal numbers of astroglia. Aliquots of culture fluids were removed at various intervals and TNF-α levels measured by ELISA.

of HIV-infected monocytes and astroglia and measured TNF-α production (Table 2). The compounds were added together with equal numbers of astroglia. NDGA markedly reduced the levels of TNF-α in supernatant fluids of these cocultured cells. Interestingly, indomethacin increased TNF-α levels. This strongly suggested the involvement of arachidonates,

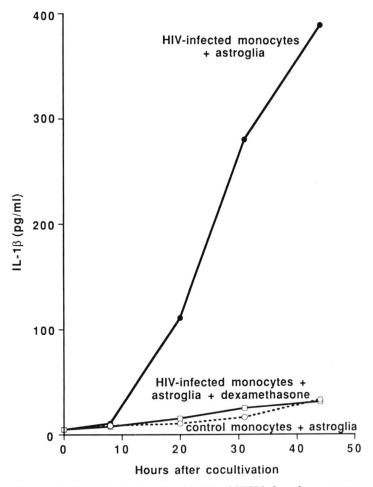

Figure 5 IL-1β levels in culture fluids of HIV-infected monocytes cocultured with astroglia (U251 MG cells). Adherent monocytes cultured for 7 days were exposed to HIV$_{ADA}$ at a MOI = 0.01. Seven days after infection, HIV-infected and control uninfected monocytes were cocultured with equal numbers of astroglia. Aliquots of culture fluids were removed at various intervals and IL-1β levels measured by ELISA.

Table 2   Effect of Arachidonic Acid Inhibitors on TNF-α Levels Following Coculture of HIV-Infected Monocytes and Astroglia

Hr after coculture	TNF-α protein (pg/ml)	
	12	48
Cell treatments		
Medium	3100	1760
Dexamethasone (10^{-5} M)	50	30
Indomethacin (0.4 μg/ml)	5030	5340
Nordihydroguaiaretic Acid (NDGA) (5 $\times$ 10^{-5} M)	602	550

Effect of arachidonic acid inhibitors on TNF production. Monocytes cultured 7 days as adherent monolayers were exposed to HIV at an MOI of 0.01. One week after infection, virus-infected monocytes were cocultured with equal numbers of U251 MG astroglial cells. At the time of coculture, the cells were incubated with medium, dexamethasone (10^{-5} M), indomethacin (0.4 μg/ml), or NDGA (5 $\times$ 10^{-5} M). TNF-α production was measured by ELISA. Data represent means of duplicate determinations for one of three experiments performed.

more exactly those of the lipoxygenase pathway, in the TNF regulatory response.

Elucidation of the Neuronotoxin: Possible Role for Arachidonic Acid Metabolites

TNF-α and/or IL-1β alone or in combination were not neuronotoxic. Recombinant human (rh-TNF-α, Amgen, Thousand Oaks, California) and rh-IL-1β (Collaborative Research, Bedford, Massachusetts), placed onto rat fetal neuronal cultures at cytokine concentrations extrapolated from coculture data (1–10 ng/ml of recombinant protein), produced no demonstrable neuronotoxicity. Moreover, vigorous screenings for mycoplasma and endotoxin contamination in cultured cells ruled out their contributory role for these effects. Viable HIV-infected monocytes are required for the generation of neuronotoxicity. Supernatant fluids from astroglial cells (U251 MG) mixed with 4% paraformaldehyde-fixed or freeze-thawed HIV-infected monocytes or HIV-1$_{ADA}$ viral stock ($>1 \times 10^8$ total particles/ml) failed to produce neuronotoxicity. These results suggested yet another component for both cytokine and neuronotoxic responses. For several reasons, arachidonic acid metabolites were thought to be this possible missing component. Arachidonic acid metabolites are

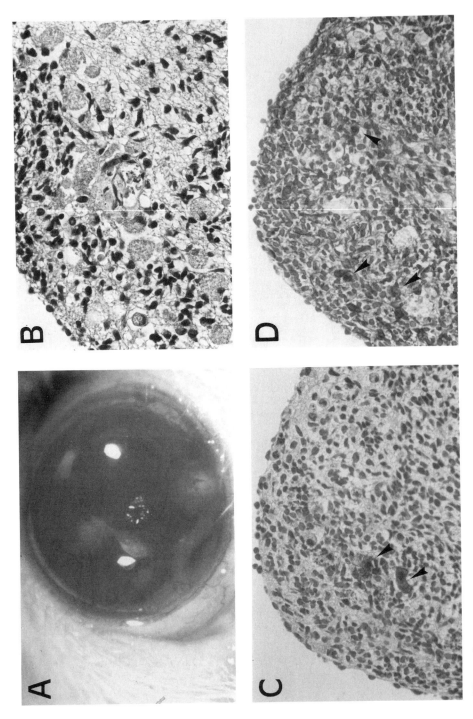

Figure 6

upregulated in monocytes after incubation with the viral envelope glyco-protein, gp120 (48). These metabolic products can regulate TNF-α and IL-1β production in macrophages and play important roles in developmental neurobiology and in certain circumstances are neuronotoxic (49–54). Furthermore, the addition of NDGA, a potent lipoxygenase inhibitor, inhibited both the cytokine and neuronotoxic responses (data not shown).

HIV Infection of Human Neural Xenografts: Relevance of the Experimental Findings to an Animal Model System

Growth of the human neural xenograft was readily observed under direct observation using a dissecting microscope (Figure 6A). Human grafts were compared among animals receiving only fetal brain tissue and those receiving brain tissue and uninfected or HIV-infected human monocytes. In all grafts, normal-appearing neuronal and glial precursors with distinct nuclei and occasional mitotic forms were readily observed. The xenografts containing HIV-1$_{ADA}$-infected monocytes showed pathological changes at 7, 10, and 14 days postinoculation (Figure 6B and D). This consisted of neuronal dropout in areas near the HIV-infected monocytes (Figure 6B) with astroglial proliferation (Figure 6D). Immunohistochemical studies using antibodies to the HIV-1 p24 (AIDS Research and Reference Reagent Program, NIAID, NIH; Dr. Kathelyn Steimer, Chiron Corporation) (55) demonstrated productive infection in the explanted monocytes (Figure 6C). Viral antigens were detected in both mononucleated and multinucleated syncytial cells' characteristics of HIV-1 encephalitis (56). Neurons in proximity to the infected monocytes were small and darkly stained with poorly defined nuclei. Immunohistochemical analysis of these tissues using anti-GFAP staining identified proliferating and reactive astrocytes

---

Figure 6 (A) Biomicroscopy of rat eye, anterior chamber, containing xenograft of 12.5-week-old human fetal brain. Several distinct, vascularized grafts are present. (B–D) Photomicrographs of anterior chamber xenograft from an animal euthanized on posttransplantation day 7 after placement of 14-week's-gestation human fetal brain and HIV-1$_{ADA}$-infected monocytes. (B) Small, triangular, pyknotic nuclei of degenerating neurons are seen surrounding a cluster of monocytes ($\times 300$). (C) HIV-1$_{ADA}$-infected monocytes (arrowheads) are identified using anti-HIV-1 p24 immunohistochemistry ($\times 250$). (D) Adjacent 5-μ section of graft in panel C demonstrating anti-GFAP immunohistochemistry. Reactive astrocytes are seen with abundant cytoplasm. Proliferating cells are shown with mitotic figures (arrowheads) ($\times 250$).

next to the virus-infected monocytes. Control uninfected human monocytes or cell-free HIV-1 infections of grafted tissues failed to replicate
these pathological findings.

DISCUSSION

We demonstrated in an experimental in vitro system and in human xenografts that interaction between HIV-infected human monocytes and astroglia produced neuronotoxicity and glial proliferation. This was associated with high levels of IL-1β and TNF-α. Although the appearance
of IL-1α and TNF-α response correlated with neuronal death, it was not
the sole neuronotoxin. The addition of TNF-α and IL-1β—separately or
in combination—to neurons at the concentrations found in HIV-infected
monocyte-astroglia culture fluids did not produce neuronotoxicity. Viable
glial cell interactions were required, as mixtures of neuronal or endothelial cells and HIV-infected monocytes failed to elicit cytokines or neuronotoxins. Moreover, HIV-infected monocyte culture fluids, sucrose-gradient
concentrated viral particles, and paraformaldehyde-fixed or freeze-thawed
HIV-infected monocyte cell membranes failed to produce cytokine or
neuronotoxic activity when placed onto astrocytes. These data, taken
together, suggested that other factor(s) were required for the observed
responses. One of these factors was identified as lipidic compounds derived from membrane phospholipids, including products of the lipoxygenase system. The large numbers of HIV-infected macrophages and the
prominent astrogliosis found in virus-infected brain tissue and neuronotoxicity in the xenograft human brain system support the biological relevance of these observations.

Pathological outcomes of HIV-1 infection in brain tissue include
neuronal loss, reactive astrogliosis, and myelin damage (56,57). Neuronal
loss (58) is strongly associated with axonal and dendritic damage in the
cortex and subcortex of affected individuals (59,60). The paucity of productively infected neurons supports indirect mechanisms for neuronal
damage seen during HIV disease (6–10). Recent reports suggest that brain
dysfunction may be related to cell-encoded toxins generated from virus-
infected macrophages (11,21,22). Secretory products from HIV-infected
cells may alter neuronal viability, damage myelin, or stimulate neurotransmitters, resulting in neuropathology.

Supporting this notion are recent studies demonstrating that disordered secretion of one or more cellular factors from HIV-infected macrophage produces neuronal death in vitro (11,21,22). In one report, HIV-
infected U937 cells, a myelomonocytic cell line, released toxic factors

that destroyed cultured chick and rat neurons (22). The monocyte-produced neurotoxin(s) were heat-stable and protease-resistant and acted by way of N-methyl-D-aspartame (NMDA) receptors. It is possible that the results described in this report represent an amplification of these previously reported findings. Indeed, HIV-infected macrophages might initiate these cellular responses, which are then amplified or modified by the astrocytes. The ultimate result is the production of cytokines and neuronotoxins. The possible role of arachidonic acid metabolites, low-molecular-weight heat-stable and protease-resistant factors, in these cytotoxic events, supports this contention. Indeed, TNF causes amplification of arachidonic acid metabolites in response to IL-1 while platelet-activating factor enhances TNF production (49–51).

An autocrine loop between arachidonic acid metabolites and cytokines, and vice versa, could explain these glial cell interactions. It is thus tempting to attribute the pathogenesis of HIV encephalopathy to secretory products produced from HIV-infected macrophages or through the interactions between HIV-1-infected macrophages and astrocytes. Perhaps interplay occurs between a number of toxic factors, including cytokines, arachidonic acid metabolites, and viral structural and/or regulatory proteins (gp120, Tat, Nef, etc). TNF and IL-1 probably contribute to the in vivo neuropathology of HIV infection. TNF regulates class I and II MHC antigens and induces proliferation of astrocytes (61). Additionally, TNF can cause meylon damage and lysis in oligodendrocytes and upregulates HIV gene expression in monocytic cells (43,44,47). Thus, TNF can facilitate the production of inflammatory infiltrates in brain parenchyma and permits the penetration of virus-infected monocytes through the blood–brain barrier. These results suggest that cytokines, viral proteins, and lipidic compounds all play roles in the neuropathogenesis of HIV disease.

There is precedent for the ability of HIV-1-infected monocytes to trigger cytokine production from astrocytes during cell-to-cell contact. The release of TGF-β, a potent chemotactic factor, is initiated from the interactions between HIV-infected macrophages and astrocytes. The production of TGF-β in brain likely permits recruitment of HIV-infected monocytes into the brain, providing a mechanism for efficient viral and disease spread (62). Although, the exact secretory factors that regulate neural injury in HIV disease probably include combinations of factors, the validity of this model system for neural injury was made from studies of human fetal brain xenografts. Here, second-trimester human brain tissue was productively infected with HIV-1$_{ADA}$-infected monocytes. These studies provide strong evidence that HIV-infected macrophages are necessary to produce neuropathology. Indeed, only xenografts containing virus-infected monocytes showed neuronal loss and reactive astrogliosis. These observations, taken together, provide strong evidence to support the hypothesis that interactions between HIV-infected monocytes and astroglia are required for the neuropathogenesis of HIV disease.

ACKNOWLEDGMENTS

We thank Ms. Victoria Hunter and Debra Joyne for excellent graphics and Christopher Welch, Victoria Lancets, and Michael Zura for excellent technical assistance. Dr. Gendelman is a Carter-Wallace Fellow. Portions of this work were supported by Public Health Service Grants AI32305 and NS28754 (L. G. E.), PAF/AMFAR grant 500258-12-PG (H. A. G.), POINS31492, and the Strong Children's Research Fund to H. A. G.

REFERENCES

1. Shaw GM, Harper ME, Hahn BE, Epstein LG, Gajdusek DC, Price RW, Navia BA, Petito CK, O'Hara CH, Groopman JE, Wong-Staal F, Gallo RC. HTLV-III infection in brains of children and adults with AIDS encephalopathy. Science (Washington, DC) 1985; 1:177.
2. Levy JA, Shimabukuro J, Hollander H, Mills J, Kaminsky L. Isolation of AIDS-associated retroviruses from cerebrospinal fluid and brain of patients with neurological symptoms. Lancet 1985; ii:586.
3. Ho DD, Rota TR, Schooley RT, Kaplan JC, Allan JD, Groopman JE, Resnick L, Felsenstein D, Andrews CA, Hirsch MS. Isolation of HTLV-III from cerebrospinal fluid and neural tissue of patients with neurologic syndrome related to the acquired immunodeficiency syndrome. N Engl J Med 1985; 313: 1493.
4. Michaels J, Sharer LR, Epstein LG. Human immunodeficiency virus type 1 (HIV-1) infection of the nervous system: a review. Immunodefic Rev 1988; 1:71.
5. Price RW, Sidtis J, Rosenblum M. The AIDS dementia complex: some current questions. Ann Neurol 1988; 23(suppl):S27.
6. Koenig S, Gendelman HE, Orenstein JM, Dal Canto MC, Pezeshkpour GM, Yungbluth M, Janotta F, Aksamit A, Martin MA, Fauci AS. Detection of AIDS virus in macrophages in brain tissue from AIDS patients with encephalopathy. Science (Washington, DC) 1986; 233:1089.
7. Wiley CA, Shrier RD, Nelson JA, Lampert PW, Oldstone MBA. Cellular localization of human immunodeficiency virus infection within the brains of

acquired immune deficiency syndrome patients. Proc Natl Acad Sci USA 1986; 83:7089.

8. Vazeux R, Brousse N, Jarry A, Henin D, Marche C, Vedrenne C, Mikol M, Wolff M, Michon C, Rozenbaum W, Bureau J-F, Montagnier L, Brahic M. AIDS subacute encephalitis: identification of HIV-1-infected cells. Am J Pathol 1987; 126:403.

9. Stoler MH, Eskin TA, Benn S, Angerer RC, Angerer LM. Human T-cell lymphotropic virus type III infection of the central nervous system—a preliminary in situ analysis. JAMA 1986; 256:2360.

10. Gabuzda DH, Ho DD, de la Monte SM, Hirsch MS, Rota TR, Sobel RA. Immunohistochemical identification of HTLV-III antigen in brains of patients with AIDS. Ann Neurol 1986; 20:289.

11. Genis P, Jett M, Bernton EW, Gelbard HA, Dzenko K, Keane R, Resnick L, Volsky DJ, Epstein LG, Gendelman HE. Cytokines and arachidonic acid metabolites produced during HIV-infected macrophage–astroglial interactions: implications for the neuropathogenesis of HIV disease. J Exp Med 1992; 176:1703.

12. Resnick L, DiMarzo-Veronese F, Schupbach J, Tourtellotte WW, Ho DD, Muller F, Shapshak P, Vogt M, Groopman JE, Markham PD, Gallo RC. Intra-blood-brain-barrier synthesis of HTLV-III specific IgG in patients with neurologic symptoms associated with AIDS or AIDS-related complex. N Engl J Med 1985; 313:1498.

13. Griffin DE, McArthur JC, Cornblath DR. Neopterin and interferon-gamma in serum and cerobrospinal fluid of patients with HIV associated neurologic disease. Neurology 1991; 4:69.

14. McArthur JC, Cohen BA, Farzedegan H, Cornblath DR, Selnes OA, Ostrow D, Johnson RT, Phair J, Polk BF. Cerebrospinal fluid abnormalities in homosexual men with and without neuropsychiatric findings. Ann Neurol 1988; 23(suppl):S34.

15. Goudsmit J, Wolters EC, Bakker M, Smit L, van der Noorda J, Hische EAH, Tutuarima JA, van der Helm HJ. Intrathecal synthesis of antibodies to HTLV-III in patients without AIDS or AIDS related complex. Br Med J 1986; 1292: 1231.

16. Cooper DA, Gold J, Maclean P, Donovan B, Finlayson R, Barnes TG, Michelmore HM, Brooke P, Penny R. Acute AIDS retrovirus infection: Definition of a clinical illness associated with seroconversion. Lancet 1985; i:537.

17. Sharer LR, Cho E-S, Epstein LG. Multinucleated giant cells and HTLV-III in the brains of AIDS encephalopathy. Hum Pathol 1985; 16:7610.

18. Sharma DP, Zink MC, Anderson M, Adams R, Clements JE, Joag SV, Narayan O. Derivation of neurotropic simian immunodeficiency virus from exclusively lymphocytotropic parental virus: Pathogenesis of infection in macaques. J Virol 1992; 66:3550.

19. Peluso R, Haase A, Stowring L, Edwards M, Ventura P. A Trojan horse mechanism for the spread of visna virus in monocytes. Virology 1985; 147:231.

20. Gendelman HE, Orenstein JM, Baca LM, Weiser B, Burger H, Kalter DC, Meltzer MS. Editorial review: the macrophage in the persistence and pathogenesis of HIV infection. AIDS (London) 1989; 3:475.

21. Pulliam L, Herndier BG, Tang NM, McGrath MS. Human immunodeficiency virus-infected macrophages produce soluble factors that cause histological and neurochemical alterations in cultured human brains. J Clin Invest 1991; 87:503.

22. Giulian D, Vaca K, Noonan CA. Secretion of neurotoxins by mononuclear phagocytes infected with HIV-1. Science (Washington, DC) 1991; 250:1593.

23. Bernton E, Bryant H, Decoster M, Orenstein JM, Ribas J, Meltzer MS, Gendelman HE. No direct neuronotoxicity by HIV-1 virions or culture fluids from HIV-1 infected T cells or monocytes. AIDS Res Hum Retrovir 1992; 8:495.

24. Tardiu M, Hery C, Peudenier S, Boespflug O, Montagnier L. Human immunodeficiency virus type 1-infected monocytic cells can destroy human neural cells after cell-to-cell adhesion. Ann Neurol 1992; 32:11.

25. Epstein LG, Cvetkovich TA, Lazar E, Dehlinger K, Dzenko K, del Cerro C, del Cerro M. Successful xenografts of second trimester human fetal brain and retinal tissue in the anterior chamber of the eye of adult immunosuppressed rats. J Neural Transplantation Plasticity 1992; 3:151–158.

26. Cvetkovich TA, Lazar E, Blumberg BM, Saito Y, Eskin TA, Reichman R, Baram DA, del Cerro C, Gendelman HE, del Cerro M, Epstein LG. Human immunodeficiency virus type 1 (HIV-1) infection of neural xenografts. Proc Natl Acad Sci USA 1992; 11:5162–5166.

27. Gendelman HE, Orenstein JM, Martin MA, Ferrua C, Mitra M, Phipps T, Wahl L, Lane HC, Fauci AS, Burke DS, Skillman D, Meltzer MS. Efficient isolation and propagation of human immunodeficiency virus on recombinant colony-stimulating factor-1-treated monocytes. J Exp Med 1988; 167:1428.

28. Bigner DD, Bigner SH, Ponten J, Westermark B, Mahaley MS, Ruoslaht E, Herschman H, Engl LF, Wikstrand CJ. Heterogeneity of genotypic and phenotypic characteristics of fifteen permanent cell lines derived from human gliomas. J Neuropathol Exp Neurol 1981; 40:201.

29. Westermark B, Ponten J, Hugosson R. Determinants for the establishment of permanent tissue culture lines from human gliomas. Acta Pathol Microbiol Scand 1973; 81:791.

30. Spengler BA, Biedler JI, Helson L, Freedman LS. Morphology and growth, tumorigenicity and cytogenetics of human neuroblastoma cells established in vitro. In Vitro 1973; 8:410.

31. Arnstein P, Taylor DOH, Nelson-Rees WA, Huebner RJ, Leanette EH. Propagation of human tumors in antithymocyte serum-treated mice. J Natl Cancer Inst 1974; 52:71.

32. Mizrachi T, Naranjo JR, Levi B-Z, Pollard HB, Lelkes PI. PC12 cells differentiate into chromaffin cell-like phenotypes in coculture with adrenal medullary endothelial cells. Proc Natl Acad Sci USA 1990; 87:6161–6165.

33. Mizrachi Y, Zeira M, Shahabuddin M, Li G, Sinangil F, Volsky DJ. Efficient binding, fusion and entry of HIV-1 into CD4⁻ negative neural cells: a mechanism for neuropathogenesis. AIDS Bull Inst Pasteur 1991; 89:81.

34. Dewhurst S, Stevenson M, McComb RD, Volsky DJ. Expression of glial fibrillary acidic protein in human glioma cell lines as detected by molecular hybridization. Acta Neuropathol (Berlin) 1987; 73:383.

35. McCarthy KD, de Vellis J. Preparation of separate astroglial and oligodendroglial cell cultures from rat cerebral tissue. J Cell Biol 1980; 85:890.

36. Gendelman HE, Baca L, Husayni H, Orenstein JM, Turpin JA, Skillman D, Kalter DC, Hoover DL, Meltzer MS. Macrophage–human immunodeficiency virus interaction: viral isolation and target cell tropism. AIDS (London) 1990; 4:221.

37. Kalter DC, Nakamura M, Turpin JA, Baca LM, Dieffenbach C, Ralph P, Gendelman HE, Meltzer MS. Enhanced HIV replication in MCSF-treated monocytes. J Immunol 1991; 146:298.

38. Choi DW, Maulucci-Gedde M, Kriegstein AR. Glutamate neurotoxicity in cortical cell culture. J Neurosci 1987; 7:357.

39. Kaufman LM, Barrett JN. Serum factor supporting long-term survival of rat central neurons in culture. Science (Washington, DC) 1983; 220:1394.

40. Manthrope M, Fagnani R, Skaper SD, Varon S. An automated colorimetric microassay for neuronotrophic factors. Dev Brain Res 1986; 25:191–198.

41. Bryant H, Burgess S, Gendelman HE, Meltzer MS, Holaday J, Bernton E. Neuronotropic activity associated with monocyte growth factors and products of stimulated monocytes. In: Frederickson RCA, McGaugh JL, Felton F, eds. Peripheral Signalling of the Brain: Role in Neural-Immune Interactions and Learning and Memory. Toronto: Hogrefe and Huber, 1991:83–99.

42. Gendelman HE, Friedman RM, Joe S, Baca LM, Turpin JA, Dveksler G, Meltzer MS, Dieffenbach C. A selective defect of interferon α production in human immunodeficiency virus–infected monocytes. J Exp Med 1990; 172:1433.

43. Robbins DS, Shirzai Y, Drysdale B, Lieberman A, Shin HS, Shin ML. Production of cytotoxic factor for oligodendrocytes by stimulated astrocytes. J Immunol 1987; 139:2593.

44. Selmaj KW, Raine CS. Tumor necrosis factor mediates myelin and oligodendrocyte damage in vitro. Ann Neurol 1988; 23:339.

45. Selmaj KN, Farooq M, Norton T, Raine CS, Brosman CF. Proliferation of astrocytes in vitro in response to cytokines. J Immunol 1990; 144:129.

46. Chung IY, Benveniste EN. Tumor necrosis factor-alpha production by astrocytes: induction by lipopolysaccharide, interferon-gamma and interleukin-1. J Immunol 1990; 144:2999.

47. Vitkovic L, Kalebic T, de Cunha A, Fauci AS. Astrocyte-conditioned medium stimulates HIV-1 expression in a chronically infected promonocyte clone. J Neuroimmunol 1990; 30:153.

48. Wahl LM, Corcoran ML, Pyle SW, Arthur LO, Harel-Bellan A, Farrar WL. Human immunodeficiency virus glycoprotein (gp120) induction of monocyte arachidonic acid metabolites and interleukin 1. Proc Natl Acad Sci USA 1989; 86:621.

49. Conti P, Reale M, Barbacane RC, Bongrazio M, Panara MR, Fiore S. The combination of interleukin 1 plus tumor necrosis factor causes greater generation of LTB_4, thromboxanes and aggregation on human macrophages than these compounds alone. In: Prostaglandins in Clinical Research: Cardiovascular System. New York: Alan R Liss, 1989.

50. Dubois C, Bissonnette E, Rola-Pleszczynski M. Platelet-activating factor (PAF) enhances tumor necrosis factor production by alveolar macrophages: Prevention by PAF receptor antagonists and lipoxygenase inhibitors. J Immunol 1989; 143:964.

51. Poubelle PE, Gingras D, Demers C, Dubois C, Harbour D, Grassi J. Rola-Pleszczynski M. Platelet-activating factor (PAF-acether) enhances the concomitant production of tumour necrosis factor-alpha and interleukin-1 by subsets of human monocytes. Immunology 1991; 72:181.

52. Lindgren JA, Hokfelt T, Dahlen S-E, Patrono C, Samuelsson B. Leukotrienes in the rat central nervous system. Proc Natl Acad Sci USA 1984; 81: 6216.

53. Shimizu T, Takusagawa Y, Izumi T, Ohishi N, Seyama Y. Enzymic synthesis of leukotriene B_4 in guinea pig brain. Int Soc Neurochem 1987; 48:1541.

54. Nicol GD, Klingberg DK, Vaska MR. Prostaglandin E_2 increases calcium conductance and stimulates release of substance P in avian sensory neurons. J Neurosci 1992; 12:1917.

55. Steimer KS, Puma JP, Power MD, Powers MA, George-Nascimento C, Stephens JC, Levy JA, Sanchez-Pescador R, Luciw PA, Barr PJ, Hallewell RA. Differential antibody responses of individuals infected with AIDS-associated retroviruses surveyed using the viral core antigen p25 gag expressed in bacteria. Virology 1986; 150:283–290.

56. Gendelman HE, Gendelman S. Neurological aspects of human immunodeficiency virus infection. In: Specter S, Bendinelli M, Friedman H, eds. Neuropathogenic Viruses and Immunity. New York: Plenum Press, 1992:229–255.

57. Navia BA, Cho ES, Petito CK, Price RW. The AIDS dementia complex. II. Neuropathology. Ann Neurol 1986; 19:525–535.

58. Ketzler S, Weis S, Haug H, Budka H. Loss of neurons in the frontal cortex in AIDS brains. Acta Neuropathol 1990; 80:92.

59. Wiley CA, Masliah E, Morey M, Lemere C, DeTeresa R, Grafe M, Hansen L, Terry R. Neocortical damage during HIV infection. Ann Neurol 1991; 29:651.

60. Everall IP, Luthert PJ, Lantos PL. Neuronal loss in the frontal cortex in HIV infection. Lancet 1991; 337:1119.

61. Mauerhoff T, PuJol-Borrell R, Mirakian R, Bottazzo GF. Differential expression and regulation of major histocompatibility complex (MHC) class I antigens on mouse astrocytes. J Neuroimmunol 1989; 18:245–255.
62. Wahl SM, Allen JB, McCarney-Francis N, Morganti-Kossmann MC, Kossmann T, Ellingsworth L, Mai UEH, Mergenhagen SE, Orenstein JM. Macrophage- and astrocyte-derived transforming growth factor β as a mediator of central nervous system dysfunction in acquired immune deficiency syndrome. J Exp Med 1991; 173:981.

7

Mycoplasma as Cofactors in AIDS

Luc Montagnier

Institut Pasteur
Paris, France

INTRODUCTION

The follow-up of cohorts of homosexuals or hemophiliacs indicates a broad variation in the so-called silent period occurring between HIV primary infection and clinical AIDS. A little more than 50% of HIV-infected individuals belonging to these various groups come down with AIDS after 10 years. Extrapolation of the curve suggests that 90–95% of them could have AIDS after 20 years.

This large variability in the duration of the silent period may be due to different factors, such as the virus strain involved, the infecting viral dose, the genetic background of the host, its immune response, and perhaps some external cofactors as well. Actually, the hypothesis that infectious cofactors could play a role in AIDS was first proposed in 1983 (1). Unlike HTLV, it was clear that HIV (LAV) has no genetic information to activate its main target cells; therefore the virus has to rely on exogeneous activation factors (antigens) to replicate on T4 lymphocytes.

This notion has since been largely confirmed, and it has been shown that the replication cycle of HIV is not completed in resting T4 lymphocytes (2). Further, the possibility has recently been raised that some superantigens may play a role in activating a large fraction of T cells (3,4). Activating factors could be multiple (bacterial, viral, fungal infections, foreign proteins) and could also play a role in the destruction of uninfected T4 lymphocytes. The binding to the CD4 receptor of viral particles, or of the viral glycoproteins, free or in immune complexes, seems to induce in human lymphocytes a signal leading to anergy (A. M. Di Rienzo, personal communication) or apoptosis (5,6) when the cell is further activated.

The fact that immune activation per se can induce significant T4 depletion has been shown by studies of anomalies of the immune system of hemophiliacs, HIV-seronegative as well as HIV-seropositive.

In a particular cohort of hemophilic children followed by A. M. Berthier in France since 1980, low number of CD4 + cells and inversion of the T4/T8 ratio were observed from the beginning of the study in some of the hemophiliacs, either seropositive or seronegative. These anomalies disappeared when the hemophiliacs were treated with highly purified fractions of factor VIII in 1988. Before 1988, they were treated in a prophylactic manner by concentrates that contained a majority of plasmatic impurities, and that were not heated until 1985. Around 50% of the hemophiliacs of this cohort had seroconverted for HIV by 1985.

Three of the hemophilic children seroconverted later, in 1986 and 1987, but it was established by PCR analysis that their lymphocytes contained HIV proviral DNA sequences before 1985 (7), therefore suggesting a late seroconversion after earlier repeated exposure to the virus. All three children showed low CD4 cell numbers even before the time of presumed infection with HIV, and the decline continued in two of them until they received purified factor VIII. These two patients have since recovered normal CD4 + cell numbers and T4/T8 ratios, although they are still HIV-seropositive.

The third child, who had a more severe depression from the beginning, continued to deteriorate even after the change to purified factor VIII and finally died of AIDS.

This example indicates that during the course of HIV infection there is a no-return point, before which suppression of immune activation is sufficient to maintain an almost normal immune status.

The irreversible phase leading to clinical AIDS could be brought about by several changes: changes in the virus (see Chapter 2) as well as changes in the host (autoimmune phenomena—see Chapter 16), or by the close association of HIV infection with another infectious agent amplifying its effects.

None of these hypotheses is exclusive of the others. The purpose of this chapter is to present the data and to discuss their interpretation concerning the role of certain species of mycoplasma in AIDS.

IN VITRO DATA

Increased Cytopathic Effect in Cells Coinfected by HIV and Mycoplasma

Our early observation (8) indicated that tetracyclines, a class of antibiotics active on mycoplasma, could greatly reduce the cytopathic effect of HIV in CEM cells. Our CEM culture were found to be heavily contaminated with *Mycoplasma arginini*, a mycoplasma often present in cell cultures.

This observation was then extended to mycoplasma strains isolated from AIDS patients or from HIV-infected individuals, found to be in coinfection with HIV-1 strains of activated peripheral blood lymphocytes, namely *M. fermentans* (9,10), *M. pirum* (11), and *M. penetrans* (12). The increased cytopathic effect includes a rapid cytolysis of single cells, besides syncytium formation directly induced by the fusiogenic activity of HIV transmembrane protein.

Since the cell lines usually utilized for growing HIV-1 or HIV-2 strains are contaminated with *M. fermentans* (MT2, MT4, H9, CEM), all the laboratory strains of HIV must be considered more or less contaminated with that mycoplasma species, and therefore their high cytopathic effect could be attributed to this contamination.

Unlike our early observations that antibiotics could reduce the cytopathic effect associated with the presence of *M. arginini*, we could not block the CPE induced by the association of a strain of *M. fermentans* with HIV-1.

In our recent experiments, a complete cytolysis of activated T4+ lymphocytes was observed 6-7 days after their infection by a mixture of HIV-1$_{LAI}$ and a *M. fermentans* strain isolated from a patient who had AIDS-like syndrome but was HIV-negative. This cytolysis was insensitive to treatment with Sparfloxacin, a fluoroquinolone, and with Tiamuline and Rovamycin (macrolide), all antibiotics endowed with a strong inhibitory effect on *M. fermentans* growth in synthetic SP4 medium and on external infection of lymphocytes. In contrast, azidothymidine added at the time of infection almost completely inhibits the CPE, indicating that the virus infection and replication were necessary for the CPE to appear.

A likely explanation, which deserves further exploration, is that virus infection will increase internalization of an intracytoplasmic form of the mycoplasma, rendering the latter resistant to antibiotics. The proliferation of this form, or the release of endolytic enzymes, will lead to the cytopathic effect observed.

Similar observations were made earlier in our laboratory with *M. pirum*, a mycoplasma species we isolated from several AIDS patients. Studies with specific antibodies against the mycoplasma proteins by immune fluorescence indicated a strong capping of the mycoplasma bodies at the surface of lymphocytes or lymphoid cells, whereas after HIV infection, intracytoplasmic fluorescence was noted.

A Complex Life Cycle
of Mycoplasma Associated with AIDS

We have observed that, under stress conditions (for instance, exhaustion of SP4 medium), the tubular structures of *M. fermentans* transform into small spherical particles, around 140–160 nm in diameter. When put into fresh medium again, these particles regenerate the plasmodial vegetative forms.

This transformation was observed earlier with other strains of mycoplasma, such as *M. hominis* (14), but was considered to correspond to degeneration. However, DNA the size of intact genome (1200–1400 kb) could be extracted from such forms (P. Carle and O. Grau, personal communication), and we believe that instead they correspond to a monogenomic form of mycoplasma. Electron microscope studies of thin sections show a thick layer of dense material (peptidoglycans?) surrounding the plasma membrane.

The same forms could be found intracellularly in lymphocytes infected with *M. fermentans*, and may constitute one of the intracellular forms. Such forms are similar to the virus-like agent (VLA) described earlier by Lo and colleagues (14) in NIH-3T3 cells transfected with DNA from a Kaposi's sarcoma tissue. VLA turned out to be a strain incognitus of *M. fermentans*.

Invasiveness of the Mycoplasmas Associated with AIDS

The mycoplasma strains isolated by Lo and coworkers (*M. fermentans, M. penetrans*) as well as the *M. pirum* and *M. fermentans* strains isolated by us from AIDS patients all have in common that they ferment glucose and hydrolyse arginine and are able to penetrate cells. Classically, mycoplasma stays at the cell surface, but clearly this is not the case for the strains mentioned above. In the case of *M. pirum* and *M. penetrans*, a differentiated "tip" or rostrum allows the mycoplasma to bind to the cell surface, and electron microscope pictures clearly show penetration of the cell membrane by the rostrum, perhaps with the help of a protease activity.

Mycoplasma bodies can be found inside the cytoplasm. An extensive replication of mycoplasma leads to the formation of vacuoles filled with mycoplasma bodies, which results in the death of the cell.

In the case of *M. fermentans*, the process of penetration seems to be different. Images of endocytosis of the dense spherical bodies can be observed with an electron microscope in thin sections of cells, and the same dense bodies can be seen inside the cytoplasm, without vacuole formation. Some of these bodies seem to be in a degenerative phase. However, larger bodies with a dense core surrounded by a translucent capsule appear inside the cytoplasm, in close association with mitochrondria.

This may result in the high replication of multiple genomic DNAs. Here, also, a lysis of cells follows. In the in vivo situation, Lo and co-workers (15) have described large numbers of bodies of *M. fermentans* in necrotic areas of the kidney or liver of AIDS patients who died of renal or hepatic failure.

This might be an extreme situation, and more moderate intracytoplasmic replication of mycoplasma can lead to more subtle alterations of the cells. It is known that mycoplasma possess several endonuclease activities (16,17). Such enzymatic activities may have a deleterious effect on cells, particularly cells of the immune system.

Enhancement of Virus Replication

Several levels of interaction between HIV and mycoplasma may exist. With a high rate of invasion by mycoplasma, cell death will rapidly occur. But in a moderate type of infection, mycoplasma may help the virus to replicate.

The first data in support of a helper effect of mycoplasma came from irradiation experiments with gamma-rays of HIV isolates. A three-log inactivation of mycoplasma growth was obtained with a dose of 500,000 rads under conditions minimizing the release of free radicals. Whereas the same inactivation of retroviruses requires several millions of rads, we observed an important inactivation of the virus infectivity on lymphocytes or lymphoid cell lines with the dose of 500,000 rads. Furthermore, partial restoration of infectivity was achieved by adding to the cell cultures an extract of *M. pirum*-soluble proteins (11).

Similarly, an antiserum raised against the binding site of the adhesine of *M. genitalium*, which has some homology with that of *M. pirum*, could

Figure 1 Homology of amino acid sequences between two mycoplasma adhesins, HLA-DR β-chain, and a constant region of HIV-1 gp120.

```
                 G  I  V  R  T  P  L  A  E  L  L  D  G  E
M.pneumoniae     G  I  V  R  T  P  L  A  E  L  L  D  G  E   1396
     1383        *     *  *  *  *  *           *  *     *

M.genitalium     G  V  V  S  T  P  L  V  N  I  N  G  Q  G  A
     1207        *     *  *  *  *  *                          1220

HLA-DR           V  V  S  T  G  L  I  Q  N  G  D  T  W  F  Q
      141        *  *     *        *  *  *                    155

HIV-1-gp120      V  V  S  T  Q  L  L  L  N  S  L  A  E  E
      254        *  *     *        *  *                       268
```

partly block infectivity of HIV-1 and HIV-2 prototypes (18). However, this experiment—which we are trying to repeat with other mycoplasma species—has two interpretations. One is that the antibody has removed a mycoplasma component (the adhesin itself) required from efficient infection of the cells by HIV.

The other interpretation is that the antibody recognizes a sequence of HIV glycoproteins essential for binding or penetration. There is indeed some homology between the binding site of the adhesin of *M. pneumoniae*, *M. genitalium*, and a conserved sequence of HIV-1 gp120. Interestingly, the same region shows also homology with the sequence of HLA-DR binding to the CD4 molecule (Figure 1).

This raises the possibility that mycoplasma surface proteins would interfere with the function of CD4-bearing lymphocytes.

Mycoplasma as Immune Activators

Several mycoplasma species have been shown to induce inflammatory cytokines (19,20). Gougeon and colleagues in our laboratory (21) has shown induction of IL-6 and TNF-α on monocytes of blood donors by *M. pirum* and *M. fermentans*. In the latter case, a protein extract of *M. fermentans* was also shown to be active.

Another possibility is that some mycoplasma protein acts as superantigens. Cole and Atkin (22) have recently shown that supernatants of *M. arthriditis* cultures contain a protein with characteristics of superantigen. This has not yet been shown for the species associated with human AIDS. However, clearly *M. pirum* and *M. fermentans* have mitogenic activity early after contact with T lymphocytes.

In summary, there are a number of ways in which mycoplasma could play a role in AIDS. Particularly attractive is the hypothesis that some mycoplasma strains form an indissociable couple with HIV strains, each partner synergizing the other: for example, HIV will help intracytoplasmic penetration of the mycoplasma, which in turn will activate expression of HIV messages and proteins. Finally, this will result in a "superactivation" of HIV, transforming a slow-growing retrovirus in a killer virus.

IN VIVO ASSOCIATION OF MYCOPLASMA WITH AIDS AND HIV INFECTION

The abovementioned data would not be meaningful for AIDS pathogenesis without the demonstration of the actual association of mycoplasma with AIDS. Such a demonstration is difficult for two main reasons.

First, unlike HIV, the isolation of mycoplasma from blood samples has proven difficult, due to the difficulty of growing in vitro the mycoplasma strains. However, we have isolated, of 150 lymphocyte cultures derived from HIV-positive patients, five strains of *M. pirum* and one strain of *M. fermentans*. These cultures were initially undertaken to isolate HIV, and the mycoplasma was isolated generally at the decline of HIV production, when the lymphocytes were dying. The supernatant of such cultures was systematically seeded in SP4 medium, a synthetic medium designed for fastidious mycoplasma.

Similarly, two strains of *M. fermentans* were isolated from two HIV-negative patients with AIDS-like syndrome. No mycoplasma could be isolated, using the same technique, from more than 100 cultures from normal healthy donors. It has been also reported, by Lo et al., that *M. fermentans* could be isolated from urine samples of HIV-positive individuals.

The second obstacle to demonstrating an association between mycoplasma and AIDS is the lack of detection of an antibody response. Due probably to the poor immunogenicity of mycoplasma proteins or to the low level of systemic infection, several studies indicate low or unspecific levels of antibodies against *M. fermentans* in HIV-positive as well as in HIV-negative patients. Similarly, using ELISA with lysat or a peptide derived from the adhesin of *M. pirum*, we could not detect a specific antibody response against this mycoplasma. However, Lo et al. (12) have recently detected antibodies against *M. penetrans* in 40% of HIV-seropositive individuals.

Indirect Evidence by PCR

DNA amplification techniques could be the methods of choice to detect mycoplasma in fresh tissues or blood cells. However, PCR requires appropriate primers for mycoplasma species, and therefore only mycoplasma in which some DNA sequences are known can be detected in this way. Moreover, only conserved genes or sequences can be utilized, due to the large genomic variability of the microorganisms.

Finally, mycoplasma-productive infection may occur in some tissues acting as a reservoir, and peripheral blood cells may be not the appropriate targets. Studies by Hawkins and colleagues (23) have found by PCR that the blood DNA of 11% of HIV-seropositive patients was positive for *M. fermentans*. This species was the only one researched.

Preliminary studies from our laboratory (O. Grau, personal communication) indicate a significant increase of positivity for *M. fermentans* as well as PCR positivity for *M. pirum* in 2 of 17 HIV-seropositive patients and in 0 of 9 seronegative healthy individuals.

Recently Lo et al. (12) isolated from HIV-positive patients a third species, *M. penetrans*, also invasive for cells. No data are yet available on the prevalence of this mycoplasma in AIDS patients.

These preliminary results suggest that not only one, but several, species of invasive, intracellular mycoplasma could be associated with HIV infection. If any of these species is an obligatory cofactor for AIDS pathogenesis, the prediction would be that in every patient at least one species should be found.

Isolation of *M. fermentans* from HIV-Negative Patients with AIDS-Like Syndrome

That *M. fermentans* per se can induce immunodepression is further suggested by our isolation of a peculiar strain from a patient who was HIV-negative by all criteria but had AIDS. The patient had repetitive episodes of cryptococcal meningitis and was highly lymphopenic, with almost no CD4+ lymphocytes.

The mycoplasma was isolated from a 1-month culture of its activated lymphocytes (mostly NK cells) and was also detected by PCR in fresh, uncultured, bone marrow cells (bone marrow of the patient showed extensive aplasia). Fresh peripheral blood leukocytes were negative by PCR. The patient had no antibodies against his own mycoplasma.

The mycoplasma could be grown to high titers (10^{11}) in SP4 medium. It was cytopathic for activated T4 lymphocytes, showing a high degree of intracellular invasiveness.

We suspect that the mycoplasma was at the origin of the bone marrow aplasia, and possibly of the severe immune depression.

Other patients are now the subjects of similar research. The situation of these patients may just represent an extreme case, whereas in HIV-positive patients, the mycoplasma is only the "helper" of the virus.

At any rate, such results encourage us to continue a thorough investigation of the role of mycoplasma in AIDS.

ACKNOWLEDGMENTS

We thank Drs. A. Blanchard, O. Grau, and M.-L. Gougeon for their helpful comments.

REFERENCES

1. Montagnier L, Chermann JC, Barré-Sinoussi F, et al. A new human T-lymphocytic retrovirus: characterization and possible role in lymphadenopathy and acquired immune deficiency syndromes. In: Gallo RC, Essex ME, Gross L, eds. Cold Spring Harbor, NY: Cold Spring Harbor Laboratory Press, 1984: 363-379.
2. Zack JA, Arrigo SJ, Weitsman SR, Haislip ASG, Chen LSY. HIV-1 entry into quiescent primary lymphocytes: molecular analysis reveals a labile, latent viral structure. Cell 1990; 61:213-222.
3. Marrack P, Kappler J. The staphylococcal enterotoxins and their relatives. Science 1990; 248:705-711.
4. Groux H, Torpier G, Monté D, Mouton Y, Capron A, Ameisen JC. Activation-induced death by apoptosis of CD4 lymphocytes from immunodeficiency virus-infected asymptomatic individuals. J Exp Med 1992; 175:331-340.
5. Ameisen JC, Capron A. Cell dysfunction and depletion in AIDS: the programmed cell death hypothesis. Immunol Today 1991; 12:102-105.
6. Banda NM, Bernier J, Kurahara DK, et al. Cross-linking by HIV gp120 primes T cells for activation-induced apoptosis. J Exp Med 1992; 176:1099-1106.
7. Moncany M, Berthier A, Markoulatos P, Montagnier L. Late seroconversion in three multitransfused young haemophiliacs confirmed by HIV PCR analysis. In press.
8. Lemaître L, Guétard D, Hénin Y, Montagnier L, Zerial A. Protective activity of tetracycline analogs against the cytopathic effect of the human immunodeficiency viruses in CEM cells. Res Virol 1990; 141:5-16.
9. Lo SC, Tsai S, Benish JR, Shih JW, Wear DJ, Wong DM. Enhancement of HIV-1 cytocidal effects in CD4 + lymphocytes by the AIDS-associated mycoplasma. Science 1991; 251:1074-1076.
10. Lemaître M, Hénin Y, Destouesse F, Ferrieux C, Montagnier L, Blanchard A. Role of mycoplasma infection in the cytopathic effect induced by human immunodeficiency virus type 1 in infected cell lines. Infect Immun 1992; 60: 742-748.
11. Montagnier L, Blanchard A, Guétard D, et al. A possible role of mycoplasmas as co-factors in AIDS. In: Girard M, Valette L, eds. Retroviruses of Human AIDS and Related Animal Diseases: Proceedings of the Colloque des Cent Gardes. Lyon, France: Fondation M. Mérieux, 1991;9-17.
12. Wang RYH, Shih JWK, Grandinetti T, Pierce PF, Hayes MM, Wear DJ, Alter H, Lo SC. High frequency of antibodies to *Mycoplasma penetrans* in HIV-infected patients. Lancet 1992; 340:1312-1316.
13. Freundt EA and Razin S. The mycoplasma. In: Krieg NR, Holt JG, eds. Bergey's Manual of Systematic Bacteriology, Vol. 1, Baltimore: Williams and Wilkins, 742-770.
14. Saillard C, Carle P, Bové JM, Bébéar C, Lo SC, Shih JWK, Wang RYH, Rose DL, Tully JG. Genetic and serologic relatedness between *Mycoplasma fer-*

mentans strains and a mycoplasma recently identified in tissues of AIDS and non-AIDS patients. Res Virol 1990; 141:385–395.

15. Bauer FA, Wear DJ, Angritt P, Lo SC. Mycoplasma fermentans (incognitus strain) infection in the kidneys of patients with acquired immunodeficiency syndrome and associated nephropathy: a light microscopic, immunohisto- chemical, and ultrastructural study. Hum Pathol 1991; 22:63–69.

16. Halden N, Wolf JB, Leonard WJ. Identification of a novel site specific pro- duced by Mycoplasma fermentans: discovery while characterizing DNA bind- ing proteins in T lymphocyte cell lines. Nucl Acid Res 1989; 17:3491–3494.

17. Marcus PI, Yoshida I. Mycoplasmas produce double-stranded ribonuclease. J Cell Physiol 1990; 143:416–419.

18. Montagnier L, Berneman D, Guetard D, Blanchard A, et al. Inhibition de l'infectiosité de souches prototypes du VIH par des anticorps dirigés contre une séquence peptidique du mycoplasme. CR Acad Sci Paris 311:425–430.

19. Mühlradt PF, Quentmeier H, Schmitt E. Involvement of interleukin-1 (IL-1), IL-6, IL-2, and IL-4 in generation of cytolytic T cells from thymocytes stim- ulated by a Mycoplasma fermentans-derived product. Infect Immun 1991; 59:3962–3968.

20. Mühlradt PF, Schade U. MDHM, a macrophage-stimulatory product of Mycoplasma fermentans, leads to in vitro interleukin-1 (IL-1), IL-6, tumor necrosis factor, and prostaglandin production and is pyrogenic in rabbits. Infect Immun 1991; 59:3969–3974.

21. Montagnier L, Gougeon ML, Olivier R, et al. Factors and mechanisms of AIDS pathogenesis. In: Rossi GB, Beth-Giraldo E, Chieco-Bianchi L, Dian- zani F, Giraldo G, Verani P, eds. Science Challenging AIDS. Basel: Karger.

22. Cole BC, Atkin CL. The Mycoplasma arthritidis T-cell mitogen, MAM: a model superantigen. Immunol Today 1991; 12:271–276.

23. Hawkins RE, Rickman LS, Vermund SH, Carl M. Association of mycoplasma and human immunodeficiency virus infection: detection of amplified Myco- plasma fermentans DNA in blood. J Infect Dis 1992; 165:581–585.

8

Effects of HIV on Signal Transduction Mechanisms

Anthony J. Pinching and Keith E. Nye

The Medical College of Saint Bartholomew's Hospital
London, England

INTRODUCTION

On reviewing the pathogenetic mechanisms underlying HIV-induced immunodeficiency and AIDS, it is clear that the virus has pervasive effects on many of the key players in the cellular immune system. Some of these effects are mediated directly by viral infection of cells (CD4 lymphocytes and antigen-presenting cells) and immune responses directed toward them; other effects are mediated by viral proteins, most notably the gp120 envelope glycoprotein, affecting the function of T lymphocytes, antigen-presenting cells, and B lymphocytes. Other effects on these and other cells are consequent upon these primary changes, and are largely mediated by alterations in the quantity and type of cytokine signals deriving from cells directly infected or affected by HIV.

There is a natural inclination to seek a single unifying mechanism for these diverse effects, but one should avoid the temptation to seek the conceptual "magic bullet," a singular mechanism that explains everything, attractive though that be. It is far more likely that the effects of HIV on the immune system—and indeed on other systems, such as the nervous system—may be a mix of several mechanisms. The exact mix may vary between individuals and virus strains, and even within one individual over time. This clearly applies to the many mechanisms proposed to explain how CD4 cells become depleted.

In this chapter, we are primarily concerned with exploring the cellular mechanisms underlying HIV-induced CD4-cell dysfunction. Our data suggest that similar mechanisms may apply to macrophages and other antigen-presenting cells. They may provide useful leads in the exploration of neuropathogenetic mechanisms and may also provide links with some of the mechanisms proposed for CD4-cell depletion, but we recognize that many other factors and mechanisms are likely to apply.

INTRACELLULAR SIGNALING CHANGES

HIV-Infected Cells In Vitro

We have shown (1) that chronically HIV-infected H9 lymphoblastoid cells have increased baseline intracellular calcium levels in comparison with uninfected H9 cells. When stimulated with phytohemagglutinin (PHA) or anti-CD3 monoclonal antibody, the uninfected cells show a substantial rise in intracellular calcium, reaching a peak within 100 seconds; these changes closely resemble the pattern seen in freshly isolated normal human lymphocytes. HIV-infected H9 cells, whose baseline calcium levels are at or a little above the plateau seen in PHA- or anti-CD3-stimulated cells, show only a very small increment in calcium levels with either stimulus.

The major mechanism controlling intracellular calcium levels in response to such stimuli is the inositol polyphosphate second messenger pathway, specifically the production of inositol trisphosphate—Ins $(1,4,5)P_3$, which releases calcium from intracellular stores—and inositol tetrakisphosphate—Ins $(1,3,4,5)P_4$, which may modulate this response and/or open plasma membrane calcium channels. Whereas resting uninfected H9 cells had low levels of $InsP_3$ and undetectable $InsP_4$, HIV-infected H9 cells had raised levels of both (1). PHA or anti-CD3 stimulation of uninfected cells produced a rise in $InsP_3$ and, to a lesser extent, in $InsP_4$, while HIV-infected H9 cells showed a slight fall in $InsP_3$ but a further rise in $InsP_4$. These are likely to be responsible for the altered intracellular calcium at baseline and after stimulation.

Thus, HIV infection induces a state of chronic activation of CD4 lymphoblastoid cells that renders them refractory to further CD3-mediated signals, providing a mechanism to explain the suppression of such responses.

Cells from HIV-Infected Patients

We went on to show (2) that lymphocytes from patients with HIV infection showed identical changes in intracellular calcium, with elevated baseline values and blunted response to CD3-mediated stimuli. Similarly, freshly isolated lymphocytes from these patients showed increased $InsP_3$ and markedly increased $InsP_4$.

On stimulation with PHA or anti-CD3, control lymphocytes showed a prompt and marked rise in $InsP_3$, followed by a lesser rise in $InsP_4$ (2); a gradual increase in the inactive metabolite $Ins(1,3,4)P_3$, reflected the metabolism of $Ins(1,3,4,5)$ by a 5'-phosphatase. By contrast, the lymphocytes from HIV-infected patients showed virtually no change in $Ins(1,4,5)$ P_3 on stimulation, but there was a rise from an increased baseline of Ins $(1,3,4,5)P_4$; there was a delayed and very small rise in $Ins(1,3,4)P_3$, suggesting an inhibition of the 5'-phosphatase. Some of the fall in $InsP_4$ was due to action of a 3'-phosphatase converting it back to $Ins(1,4,5)P_3$. These changes were more pronounced in patients with more advanced HIV diseases; patients with AIDS showed not only complete inhibition of the 5'-phosphatase but also a marked inhibition of the 3'-phosphatase. Further studies (see "Mechanism of Intracellular Signaling Changes" below) have been performed to elucidate the mechanism of the inhibition of these enzymes.

Cells from Patients Receiving Zidovudine Treatment

Having shown a progressively more marked inhibition of the controlling phosphatases of this pathway with the evolving natural history of HIV infection, it was logical to assess the impact of antiretroviral therapy on this marker of lymphocyte dysfunction. First, it could indicate whether the changes were reversible by inhibiting viral replication. Second, it could provide a tool with which one could monitor improvement in immune dysfunction with such therapy; it could serve as an additional "surrogate" marker of benefit to the evidently imprecise and temporally dissociated CD4 rise that occurs transiently after starting zidovudine.

To provide a simpler quantitative assay for these longitudinal studies, we studied phosphatase activity by examining the effect of patient lymphocyte lysates on the metabolism of labeled Ins(1,3,4,5)P$_4$, analyzing the metabolites by HPLC. We confirmed, using this technique, that patients with AIDS showed marked inhibition of the 3'-phosphatase and complete inhibition of the 5'-phosphatase before treatment. There was progressive improvement in the activity of both enzymes at 4, 6, 8, and 12 weeks to levels more typical of untreated asymptomatic seropositive subjects (2). Improved levels were maintained for up to 14 months in the six patients studied for this duration, although transient deterioration was seen just before and in association with intercurrent opportunistic infections. Asymptomatic or mildly symptomatic patients started with less impairment but improved to normal or near-normal values over a similar time course.

These changes closely paralleled the improvement in PHA-induced proliferation and interferon-γ production in the same patients, and some occurred despite the fact that there was no significant change in the number or percentage of CD4 cells at these time points. Moreover, the changes correlated well with the temporal improvements in patients' clinical state in response to zidovudine therapy, in contrast to the CD4 "blip." These results show the reversibility of the signaling defects and show that zidovudine-induced immunological benefit, at least in terms of reversal of lymphocyte dysfunction, lasts for well over a year. Simplified assays of this type may well provide a valuable additional marker for evaluating and monitoring the immunological effects of antiretroviral agents.

Signal Transduction Changes in Alveolar Macrophages

We have also studied intracellular calcium levels and inositol polyphosphate metabolism in alveolar macrophages obtained by bronchoalveolar lavage of HIV-infected patients (3). In essence, these cells show changes very similar to those seen in lymphocytes with elevated intracellular calcium and inositol polyphosphate second messengers.

MECHANISM OF INTRACELLULAR SIGNALING CHANGES

Inhibitory Effect of HIV-Infected Patient Cell Lysates

Using the lysate system to assess InsP$_4$ metabolism, we showed that lysates from HIV-infected patients were able to inhibit almost completely the 5'-phosphatase activity present in control lysates (4). This confirmed the idea that the activity was being inhibited by a cytosolic factor. We also showed that red cell lysates from AIDS patients showed normal activity, confirming that this was not a global cellular defect.

Effect of rgp120 on Normal Lymphocytes

Lysates of control lymphocytes preincubated with recombinant HIV gp120 (Celltech) showed effects similar to those induced by patient lysates, confirming the data of Kornfeld et al. (5). The role of cross-linking—for example, by antibody—has been thought to be important in this effect (6), although we have shown that it is not essential in our system. Nef protein had no effect.

Inhibition of 5'-Phosphatase by ATP

One possible mechanism for the inhibition of 5'- and 3'-phosphatases would be elevated intracellular ATP levels, which preferentially inhibit the 5'-phosphatase, while having some effect on the 3'-phosphatase. We have shown in separate experiments that patient cells have raised ATP levels of about 7 mM (7). We assayed $InsP_4$ metabolism with normal and patient cell lysates in the presence of added ATP between 2 and 10 mM (4). Phosphatase activity in control cells could be partially but not completely inhibited by 5 and 10 mM, the levels being about the same as those found in asymptomatic HIV-infected subjects. The latter could be very slightly further inhibited, but not totally. Patients with AIDS had no activity detectable at any level of ATP. These data suggest that while the raised ATP levels found in patient cels can account for a part of the inhibition of 5'- and 3'-phosphatases, they cannot be wholly responsible as ATP cannot produce the complete inhibition seen in AIDS patients.

Possible Role of Higher Inositol Polyphosphates

It has been shown that $Ins(1,3,4,5,6)P_5$ can inhibit the 5'- and 3'-phosphatases (SB Shears, personal communication), with a preferential effect on the latter. We have consistently observed a small peak of $Ins(3,4,5,6)P_4$ in patient cells although we have yet to quantitate levels of $InsP_5$ and $InsP_6$ to determine whether they are sufficient alone, or together with raised ATP, to account for the observations (8).

Possible Role of Tyrosine Kinase Mediated—Regulation

The question of how HIV affects the behavior of predominantly uninfected cells present in patients' peripheral blood, whether mediated by gp120 alone or by other means, remains to be fully explained. It is likely that the activity of these phosphatases is physiologically regulated and we have evidence for an associated regulatory protein in cytosol (8); this appears to need phosphorylation to be activated. A likely pathway for its phosphorylation would be by the CD4-associated p56lck in its activated form. The tyrosine kinase activity of p56lck may be switched on by p56fyn. Ligation of CD4 leads to the phosphorylation of Y394 and Y505 on p56lck; phosphorylation of y394 is essential for tyrosine kinase activity, but this activity is regulated by Y505 phosphorylation. CD45, a tyrosine phosphatase, removes the phosphate group from Y505, thus activating P56lck. Alternatively, activation may be effected by CD2 and/or CD28. The association of CD3 and CD4 with these other transmembrane proteins offers a possible means whereby gp120, either through CD4 or through CD4 and other gp120-binding ligands, could ihhibit the 5'-phosphatase and 3'-phosphatase—essentially by the enhanced activity of a normal physiological regulator.

DISCUSSION

Our data, together with those of others (5,6,9–11), have shown that HIV infection in vitro and in vivo—and at least in part through the action of gp120—causes chronic activation of CD4 lymphocytes and macrophages. This causes the cells to be refractory to further stimulation and hance to appear biologically suppressed in functions that require additional CD3-mediated signals. This results from inhibition of the regulatory phosphatases of the inositol polyphosphate pathway, which itself probably results from changes in other intracellular mediators, including ATP, $InsP_5$, and tyrosine kinase–mediated regulation.

We have previously reviewed the possible role of these mechanisms in the immunopathogenesis of HIV disease in relation to other observations in the literature (12). They provide a unifying explanation for much of the cellular dysfunction attributable to CD4 cells and macrophages, and we have preliminary data suggesting that dendritic cell dysfunction (13) may also have similar origins. It has not escaped our attention that such activation could, through raised intracellular calcium levels, for example, lead to apoptosis and thus provide one of a number of possible mechanisms for CD4-cell depletion. It is also possible that altered intracellular signaling underlies the neuronal dysfunction—and even depletion—seen in HIV encephalopathy, whether these be provoked by viral products such as gp120 or by macrophage-derived mediators.

Our studies provide a means for explaining many of the cellular changes seen in HIV infection. They also indicate ways in which natural history and, in particular, response to antiretroviral and other therapies may be monitored and evaluated from the immunological perspective.

Furthermore, the unusual changes induced by HIV have provided novel insights into the regulation and relationships of the inositol polyphosphate pathway of signal transduction.

ACKNOWLEDGMENTS

This work was supported by the Medical Research Council. We are most grateful to Professor R. Michell, Dr. R. F. Irvine, and Dr. S. B. Shears for their help and advice in the development of our work and ideas.

REFERENCES

1. Nye KE, Pinching AJ. HIV infection of H9 lymphoblastoid cells chronically activates the inositol polyphosphate pathway. AIDS 1990; 4:41–45.
2. Nye KE, Knox KA, Pinching AJ. Lymphocytes from HIV-infected individuals show aberrant inositol polyphosphate metabolism which reverses after zidovudine therapy. AIDS 1991; 5:413–417.
3. Nye KE, Moss F, Pinching AJ. Alveolar macrophages from HIV-infected patients show chronic activation via the inositol polyphosphate pathway. In preparation.
4. Nye KE, Riley GA, Pinching AJ. The defect seen in the phosphatidylinositol hydrolysis pathway in HIV-infected lymphocytes and lymphobastoid cells is due to inhibition of the inositol 1,4,5-trisphosphate/1,3,4,5-tetrakisphosphate 5-phosphomonoesterase. Clin Exp Immunol 1992; 89:89–93.
5. Kornfeld H, Cruickshank WW, Pyle SW, Berman JS, Center DM. Lymphocyte activation by HIV-1 envelope glycoprotein. Nature 1988; 335:445–448.
6. Mittler RS, Hoffman MK. Synergism between HIV gp120 and gp120-specific antibody in blocking human T-cell activation. Science 1989; 245:1380–1382.
7. Nye KE, Laurence NJ, Pinching AJ. ATP levels in lymphocytes from HIV-infected patients. Unpublished observations.
8. Nye KE, Pinching AJ. Studies on the mechanisms underlying inhibition of the inositol 1,4,5-trisphosphate/1,3,4,5-tetrakisphosphate 5-phosphomonoesterase by HIV. Unpublished observations.
9. Gupta S, Vayuvegula B. Human immunodeficiency virus associated changes in signal transduction. J Clin Immunol 1987; 7:486–489.
10. Linette GP, Hartzman RJ, Ledbetter JA, June C. HIV-1 infected T-cells show a selective signalling defect after perturbation of CD3/antigen receptor. Science 1988; 241:573–576.
11. Cefai D, Debre P, Kaczorek M, Idziorek T, Autrun B, Bismuth G. Human immunodeficiency virus-1 glycoproteins gp120 and gp160 specifically inhibit the CD3/T-cell-antigen receptor phosphoinositide transduction pathway. J Clin Invest 1990; 86:2117–2124.

12. Pinching AJ, Nye KE. Defective signal transduction—a common pathway for cellular dysfunction in HIV infection? Immunology Today 1990; 11:256–259.
13. Macatonia SE, Lau R, Patterson S, Pinching AJ, Knight SC. Dendritic cell depletion and dysfunction in HIV infection. Immunology 1990; 71:38–44.

9

Programmed Cell Death (Apoptosis) and AIDS

Jean Claude Ameisen

Unité INSERM U167-CNRS 624
Institut Pasteur
Lille, France

INTRODUCTION

Human immunodeficiency virus (HIV) infection leads in around 10 years to immune incompetence and to cell loss and tissue atrophy in several organs, including the brain and the bone marrow. The major pathological feature of AIDS is the progressive collapse of the two most complex regulatory networks of the human body, the immune system and the central nervous system (1). In each of these organs, AIDS induces the loss of a selective cell population: CD4+ T-cell depletion in the immune system, leading to immune deficiency; and neuronal loss in the brain, leading to brain atrophy and dementia (1,2). An intriguing feature of AIDS, to which little attention has been paid, is that cell loss is not associated with detectable necrosis, or significant inflammation, in particular in the brain and the bone marrow. Another intriguing feature, which has received much attention, is that before cell loss can be detected, cell dysfunction is observed. Most functional studies in HIV-infected people have focused on cells from the immune system. It has been found that CD4+ T-helper cells present early functional defects that precede any significant decrease in this cell population, and are detected only a few weeks or months after seroconversion. These functional defects are characterized in vivo by a failure of CD4+ T cells to mediate delayed-type hypersensitivity reactions to self–major histocompatibility complex (MHC)-class II-restricted recall antigens, and in vitro by a selective loss of the ability of T cells to proliferate to these recall antigens, as well as to defined polyclonal activators such as pokeweed mitogen (3–8).

The pathogenesis of AIDS was initially viewed as being related solely to direct virus-mediated cell destruction of defined target-cell populations. However, this concept has been challenged in recent years by the following series of observations. First, CD4+ T-cell dysfunction is observed at a time when very few peripheral blood CD4+ T cells are infected (9,10). Second, neuronal loss is observed in the brain (2), while neurons, in contrast to CD4+ T cells, do not seem to be targets for HIV infection, HIV in the central nervous system being expressed almost exclusively in cells of the macrophage lineage (11,12). Finally, chimpanzees, the only primate model that can be productively and chronically infected with HIV-1, seem not to develop any AIDS-related disease.

The pathogenesis of immune and nervous cell loss has become a major problem in AIDS research, with obvious potential therapeutic implications. Cell depletion, cell dysfunction, and tissue atrophy, as well as the paradoxical observation of B-cell and CD8+ T-cell hyperactivation, in spite of the apparent complete lack of CD4+ T-helper-cell function, have been related to various distinct and sometimes contradictory mechanisms (reviewed in Ref. 13). Two sets of questions have been raised in recent years: the first one concerns the identification of the viral or host-mediated effectors that may induce cell dysfunction or cell killing; the second question is the topic of this chapter, and concerns the mechanisms whereby cells die in HIV-infected people, and our proposal that cell dysfunction and cell loss may represent two aspects of a single unique mechanism, the inappropriate induction of a physiological cell-suicide process, termed programmed cell death (PCD) (13).

THE PROGRAMMED CELL DEATH HYPOTHESIS
OF AIDS PATHOGENESIS

Cells have two known major ways to die (14,15). The first one, necrosis, always associated with disease, is a spectacular consequence of cell aggression by several agents, including infectious pathogens, complement, antibodies plus complement, toxins, or hypoxemia. During necrosis, cell swelling and rupture of the cell membrane lead to the release of proteases and other intracellular toxic enzymes, causing the death of bystander cells, an inflammatory reaction, and a scarring process that will disorganize the architecture of the tissue or the organ in which necrosis is occurring.

Identified several decades ago as an important feature in embryonic development (16), but only recently the focus of an increasing number of studies, PCD—apoptosis, or activation-induced cell death—represents a physiological form of cell deletion that radically differs from necrosis (14,15). It is involved in physiological processes in which cell deletion is part of homeostasis, such as the shaping of organs and tissues during embryogenesis (14,15), and also tissue turnover in adult life, including endocrine-dependent tissue atrophy and hemopoietic stem-cell-number regulation (15,17).

During development, PCD has been shown to play an essential role in the shaping and maturation of the immune system and the brain. In the brain, PCD leads to the deletion of around 50% of neurons that fail to establish appropriate synaptic connections (18). In the thymus, PCD leads to the deletion of around 90% of normal immature thymocytes (19). In this cell population, PCD is a physiological response to T-cell-receptor (TcR) stimulation, and is involved in the negative selection of the T-cell repertoire, the clonal deletion of autoreactive thymocytes, and the establishment of self-tolerance (19).

There are several morphological and biochemical differences between apoptosis and necrosis: the best-known characteristics of apoptosis are the regular fragmentation of the entire cellular DNA, due to the activation of an endogenous endonuclease, into regular multiples of an oligonucleosome-length unit of 180 base pairs; the condensation of nuclear chromatin; the maintenance of cell-membrane integrity; and the segmentation of the cytoplasm into multiple bubbles that are ingested by neighboring epithelial or monocytic cells of the microenvironment. In contrast to necrosis, PCD does not induce bystander-cell death or inflammation, or tissue disorganization, and therefore remains most often undetected if not thoroughly investigated (14,15,17).

The most important difference between PCD and necrosis, however, is of a functional nature. In most instances, PCD is an active cell-suicide process that requires activation signals, signal transduction, gene expression, and protein synthesis in the dying cell (15,17,20,21). Therefore, PCD is regulated by signals provided by the local environment. Unlike cell degeneration or necrosis, PCD can be induced or suppressed in most cell populations by the withdrawal or addition of defined activation signals (15,17,20,21). In other terms, whatever is triggering cell death, when a cell dies by necrosis, the only way to prevent it is to remove the aggressing agent; when cells undergo PCD, cell death can be prevented, in most cases, by the sole modulation of cell signaling.

In a paper first submitted in May 1990, we proposed a theoretical model of AIDS pathogenesis that related most features of the disease to a single putative mechanism: programmed cell death dysregulation (13). We postulated that most immunological and nonimmunological defects leading to AIDS, including brain atrophy and dementia, may be related to the abnormal induction of PCD in several cell populations, including CD4+ T cells and neurons, as a consequence of indirect interference of HIV with inter- and intracellular signaling, leading to PCD in response to activation signals that normally lead to cell differentiation or proliferation. We proposed that such a mechanism could account for the two major CD4+ T-cell defects in HIV-infected people: their early in vitro dysfunction and their progressive and late in vivo depletion, leading to AIDS. In this model, the reason that these cells do not proliferate in vitro to stimuli, including recall antigens, would be that these stimuli induce cell suicide. In vivo, T-cell suicide after activation would be an ongoing process that would progressively overwhelm the renewal capacity of the immune system and lead to the progressive disappearance of this cell population, independently of any HIV-mediated cytopathogenic effect. In contrast with the normal generation and maintenance of immune memory, stimulation of both naive and memory mature CD4+ T cells would lead in HIV-infected people to a form of inappropriate and continuous negative selection of the repertoire in response to non-self antigens expressed by various pathogens and the environment.

The hypothesis also provided a possible explanation for two paradoxical features in HIV-infected people. The first is the existence and persistence of B-cell and CD8+ T-cell hyperactivation; PCD, an active process associated with early lymphokine secretion (22) and with release of nucleosomes that can activate B cells (23), could account for a truncated and inappropriate form of helper function provided by dying CD4+ T cells. The second paradox is the persistence of a very low percentage of HIV-infected CD4+ T cells until the last stages of the disease (9,10). Since HIV proviral integration and expression requires CD4+ T-cell activation, a rapid CD4+ T-cell-suicide process in response to activation may allow infection only of rare activated bystander cells. This would be consistent with a previous hypothesis on a general role for apoptosis induced by cyto-toxic lymphocytes and natural killer cells in limiting certain viral infections (24), and with the recent observation that apoptosis of insect cells prevent the spread of baculovirus infection (25).

Our model also questioned the validity of two prevailing concepts that reached beyond the scope of AIDS pathogenesis. The first one was that TcR stimulation could lead in mature T cells to either proliferation or clonal anergy, but not, as in immature thymocytes, to clonal deletion (19). Our hypothesis of AIDS pathogenesis implied, however, that a cell-death program could remain functional in mature CD4 + T cells, and be expressed in certain circumstances, such as incomplete or inappropriate T-cell activation. The second prevailing concept, at that time, was that pathological and deleterious cell death is due to cell aggression by necrosis, accumulation of toxic metabolites, or cytopathic effects of infectious agents, and that programmed cell death represents a beneficial and physio-logical form of cell death, including the form of PCD that is induced by effector cytotoxic lymphocytes and natural killer cells in target cells in-fected by intracellular pathogens (21,24). Our model implied, however, that in the absence of any effector cells, cell suicide in response to inap-propriate activation signals could lead to disease. Programmed cell death, and cell proliferation, are physiological processes that are highly active during embryogenesis, and become tightly regulated during adult life. Oncoviruses cause cancer by dysregulating the expression of genes in-volved in the control of cell proliferation. Our hypothesis proposed that lentiviruses cause cell dysfunction and cell loss by a converse capacity to dysregulate, through indirect mechanisms, the expression of genes involved in the control of physiological death programs.

Based on previous findings on normal PCD in thymocyte develop-ment, the hypothesis made several experimentally testable predictions that could allow one to assess its validity or serve to falsify it (13). We made the following proposals:

1. The failure of T cells to proliferate in vitro to polyclonal stimuli may be related to detectable activation-induced CD4 + T-cell death, with characteristic features of apoptosis, including regular cellular DNA fragmentation and ultrastructural aspects of chrom-atin condensation.
2. As in immature thymocytes (20), T-cell death may be prevented either by inhibitors of gene expression or signal transduction such as cyclosporin A or by addition of activation cosignals that may also restore CD4 + T-cell proliferation to stimuli.

3. Investigation of the nature of the in vitro response of memory CD4+ T cells to recall antigens raised two potential problems: first, it is impossible to know whether failure of proliferation to recall antigens is related to abnormal in vitro T-cell response or to the fact that the antigen-specific memory CD4+ T cells have already been deleted in vivo (26,27); second, since memory CD4+ T cells specific for any given antigen are rare (around 1/10,000) and since apoptosis is a process that spares bystander cells, memory CD4+ T-cell death in response to self-MHC-II-dependent recall antigens could not be expected to be detectable.

4. Therefore, in order to investigate whether T-cell death occurs in response to TcR mobilization by self-MHC-II-dependent ligands, we proposed the use of bacterial superantigens (28), which previously had never been tested in T cells from HIV-infected individuals. Superantigenss mimic in an enhanced way CD4+ T-cell response to recall antigens by binding to MHC-II molecules and interacting with defined $V\beta$ TcR molecules expressed by up to 30% of human T cells, inducing in vitro proliferation in both memory and naive normal mature human CD4+ T cells and PCD in normal human immature thymocytes (28,29). We predicted that in CD4+ T cells from HIV-infected people, superantigens may induce PCD in a percentage of cells (20–30%) high enough to allow detection.

5. Activation cosignals that may prevent CD4+ T-cell apoptosis and restore proliferation to polyclonal activators may also restore proliferation to specific recall antigens of memory CD4+ T cells that have not already been deleted in vivo. If true, this would allow one to assess the extent of the CD4+ T-cell repertoire remaining in vivo, at any given time, in an HIV-infected individual.

6. Finally, if CD4+ T-cell PCD were to represent a crucial event in the pathogenesis of AIDS, we postulated that it should not be detectable in the HIV-infected chimpanzee that does not develop any AIDS-related disease (13).

EXPERIMENTAL FINDINGS

Programmed Cell Death of Mature Murine T Cells

After our hypothesis was first submitted for publication, a series of experimental observations from murine models was published that indicated that TcR stimulation can lead to PCD in mature CD4+ or CD8+ T cells in several circumstances, either in vitro or in vivo. Mature murine T-cell PCD was detected in vitro when TcR stimulation is performed 1) in resting T cells in the presence of particular cosignals such as the antibody-mediated ligation of CD4 (30) or the binding to the T-cell MHC-I molecule of a CD8 molecule expressed by a bystander CD8 + T cell (31) (the *veto* phenomenon) or 2) in preactivated T cells that have received a prior stimulation by IL-2 alone (32), that are restimulated in the absence of accessory cells (33), or in which consecutive TcR stimulation is performed under different conditions (34). Together, these findings suggested that a death program might be functional in mature T cells and that its expression might have a physiological role in both the maintenance of extrathymic self-tolerance and the ending of a normal immune response to non-self-antigens. In the latter case, it is tempting to speculate that PCD may occur in low-affinity or bystander-activated T cells as well as terminally differentiated effector T cells, and spare memory T cells, leading to a relative increase in the antigen-specific memory T-cell repertoire and participating in the expansion of immune memory. In the context of our hypothesis, these findings had at least two implications: on the one hand, they provided support to the possibility that induction of PCD in the mature CD4 + T cells might be achieved by a virus that 1) interacts with the CD4 molecule and 2) may interfere with CD4 + T-cell activation and accessory-cell function; on the other hand, they also suggested that induction of mature T-cell PCD may not necessarily lead to pathology unless it interferes with the generation or maintenance of T-cell memory.

Our hypothesis postulated that the entire CD4 + T-cell population from HIV-infected people was primed in vivo for suicide upon further TcR stimulation by self-MHC-II-dependent ligands. In this context, bacterial superantigens were proposed as tools allowing one to reveal the existence of this priming in in vitro assays, and as factors that may induce in vivo broad deletions in CD4 + T cells from HIV-infected people (13). Surprisingly, a series of subsequent papers revealed three unsuspected features of superantigens: 1) in vivo, after an initial phase of spectacular T-cell proliferation and expansion that lasts several days, superantigens —in contrast to antigens—lead to the depletion of the peripheral T cells expressing the corresponding Vβ molecules, a deletion process that has been shown to involve PCD (35), and 2) two different murine retroviruses that induce deletions of mature peripheral T cells expressing defined Vβ molecules—murine mammary tumor virus (MMTV) and murine leukemia virus (MuLV)—were shown to encode superantigens (36,37). These findings have led Janeway (38) to propose the hypothesis that superantigens encoded by HIV might contribute to AIDS pathogenesis. In this context, the priming for and the induction of PCD would be due to a single factor, the viral superantigen. In line with this model, Primi and colleagues (39; Chapter 12) have reported that AIDS-patient T cells present losses in the $V\beta$ T-cell repertoire that may be due to a deletion process involving superantigens. However, it should be noted that both MMTV and MuLV are oncoviruses, not lentiviruses as HIV is, and that no superantigen encoded by HIV has been detected to date.

Programmed Cell Death, HIV Infection, and AIDS

Since publication of our hypothesis (13), reports from six laboratories, including ours, have indicated a possible relationship among HIV infection, AIDS, and T-cell PCD, by showing that 1) CD4 + and CD8 + T cells from HIV-infected people are abnormally programmed to undergo PCD; 2) the cytopathic effect of HIV in CD4 + T cells is related to PCD induction; and 3) CD4 cross-linking by HIV envelope and antienvelope antibodies is able to prime normal human CD4 + T cells for PCD after TcR stimulation.

In our laboratory, Groux et al. (40–42) confirmed the hypothesis that in vitro activation of CD4 + T cells from HIV-infected people with pokeweed mitogen or bacterial superantigens leads to cell death by apoptosis, and that cell death can be prevented either by the T-cell signal transduction inhibitor, cyclosporin A, or by the addition of T-cell activation cosignals. Gougeon et al. (44; Chapter 10) reported that the accelerated in vitro death of CD4 + and CD8 + T cells from HIV-infected people, which Montagnier et al. (43) had previously observed in serum-free medium in the absence of any stimulation, is due to apoptosis, and that in vitro activation of both CD4 + and CD8 + T cells with ionomycin, or of CD4 + T cells with superantigens, significantly increases the percentage of cells undergoing PCD (44). Miedema et al. (45; Chapter 11) presented evidence showing that the previous finding in his laboratory of a failure of T cells from HIV-infected people to proliferate in vitro to a CD3 MAb (27) was related to the induction of PCD in CD4 + and CD8 + T cells. During the same period, the in vitro cytopathic effect of HIV was shown by Carson's group (46) and Hovanessian's laboratory (47) to be due to PCD induction, a finding that provided an explanation for the previous observation by Hovanessian's group (48) that in vitro death of CD4 + T cells after HIV infection is preceded by the accumulation of histones, a consequence of internucleosome cleavage during PCD.

Recent findings suggest a role for the interaction of the HIV envelope with the CD4 molecule in the programming of CD4 + T cells for death by apoptosis. First, PCD induction in vitro in HIV-infected CD4 + T-cell cultures could be prevented by an anti-HIV envelope antibody, added after infection, that interferes with CD4–HIV envelope interaction and allows productive HIV infection to proceed in vitro in the absence of CD4 + T-cell death (46). Second, Cohen et al. (49) reported that CD4 + T-cell death consecutive to CD4–HIV envelope interaction between uninfected and infected cells (syncytia formation) is an active process that can be prevented by selective inhibitors of T-cell activation. Hovanessian et al. (Chapter 3) have presented evidence indicating that such cell death is due to apoptosis, and that apoptosis can be selectively blocked by CD4 antibodies that do not prevent binding of HIV envelope to the CD4 molecule. Third, and finally, extending the findings by Newell et al. (30) in murine CD4 + T cells, Finkel et al. reported at the Keystone Symposium (March 1992) that cross-linking of the CD4 molecule by gp120 plus anti-gp120 antibodies primes normal human CD4 + T cells for PCD in response to subsequent TcR stimulation (50).

Together, these findings suggest that the HIV envelope protein and the immune response to it may help induce CD4 + T-cell apoptosis in AIDS by at least two distinct means: in uninfected CD4 + T cells that are in close vicinity to HIV-infected cells—a situation that is likely to occur in the lymph nodes, in particular through contacts between CD4 + T cells and HIV-infected accessory cells—but also in uninfected CD4 + T cells that are at a distance from any HIV-infected cell, through the binding to the CD4 molecule of HIV envelope–antienvelope immune complexes. An essential question that remains to be addressed is whether PCD, in all these instances, can be prevented by the sole modulation of cell signaling.

Additional Potential Induction Mechanisms and In Vivo Relevance of PCD

Although the HIV envelope protein is a tempting candidate for PCD induction in CD4 + T cells, additional potential mechanisms that are not mutually exclusive may be involved in the priming of both CD4 + and CD8 + T cells for apoptosis in HIV-infected people. Potential candidate mechanisms—such as putative HIV-encoded superantigens; molecular mimicry between viral proteins and the self; cross-reactive autoantibodies directed against T-cell surface molecules, including MHC-II, Apo1, or Fas; and inappropriate cosignaling provided by accessory cells—are discussed elsewhere in the context of PCD induction (51). The two-signal model of T-cell activation, a paradigm in cellular immunology for almost 20 years, implies that T-cell proliferation requires both TcR stimulation by antigen and appropriate cosignaling provided by antigen-presenting accessory cells, such as monocytes, macrophages, B cells, follicular dendritic cells, or Langerhans cells (52–54). It has been known for several years that TcR stimulation in the absence of appropriate cosignaling leads to T-cell anergy (53). During the last 2 years, however, it has been reported, as mentioned above, that TcR stimulation in the presence of inappropriate cosignaling can also lead to T-cell death by apoptosis. Therefore, a virus that has the capacity to infect not only CD4 + T cells but also antigen-presenting accessory cells may have several ways to interfere with intercellular signaling and to prime T cells for apoptosis. It is important to note that during the first years following seroconversion (the clinical latent phase of HIV infection), most of the virus in HIV-infected people seems to be trapped in the lymph nodes, and to be associated with the accessory cells (55,56). Therefore, the abnormal in vitro behavior of T cells from the peripheral blood (which represent, at any given time, only around 2% of the T-cell pool in the body) may be an indirect consequence, in HIV-infected people, of a priming of T cells for PCD occurring in the lymph nodes, through defective interaction between T cells and accessory cells.

Finally, it remains to be investigated whether cell loss that occurs in nonimmunological organs from HIV-infected people, such as neuronal loss (2), may also be related to inappropriate induction of PCD (13). In this context, it is interesting to note that the infected cells in the brain are of macrophage lineage, accessory cells to the neurons, and that findings presented by Gendelman et al. (57; Chapter 6) show that infected monocytes are able to induce neuronal cell death.

A paradoxical but central question in AIDS pathogenesis is whether death of mature CD4 + T cells may be enough to account for CD4 + T-cell depletion in vivo, or if impairment of renewal of CD4 + T cells is also involved. The finding that CD8 + T cells from HIV-infected individuals also undergo PCD in vitro (44,45) adds relevance to this question. An interesting result was presented by McCune at the Keystone Symposium in March 1992: in immunodeficient SCIDhu mice reconstituted with human fetal thymus, HIV infection leads to thymus involution and CD4 + thymocyte loss, and thymocyte apoptosis can be detected in vivo. This is the first identification of apoptosis in vivo related to HIV infection, and it is consistent with the idea that any mechanism that will induce abnormal apoptosis in mature T cells may be at least as effective in interfering with T-cell renewal.

PCD induction may not lead to disease as long as it does not prevent generation or renewal of effector cells or maintenance of memory cells. Our model of AIDS pathogenesis postulated that inappropriate induction of T-cell PCD may not be unique to AIDS. We proposed that, in contrast to chronic PCD induction, transient T-cell PCD may even have a beneficial role in the control of acute lymphotropic viral infections, such as measles (13). This hypothesis, although not yet tested in measles, is supported by recent findings showing that acute benign Epstein-Barr virus (EBV)-induced infectious mononucleosis in children is associated with transient in vitro PCD of a large proportion of CD4 + and CD8 + T cells (58).

In a chronic infection such as HIV infection, is ongoing T-cell PCD a mere anecdotal consequence of an ongoing ineffective stimulation of the immune system, or does T-cell PCD play a central role in the pathogenesis of AIDS? Such questions have remained unresolved issues for most abnormal features that have been identified so far in HIV-infected people and proposed as potential pathogenic mechanisms. Animal models, however, provide relevant models that allow one to discriminate between pathogenic and nonpathogenic chronic retroviral infections. It has recently been shown that feline leukemia virus strains that induce lymphopenia and disease in vivo also induce lymphocyte PCD in vitro, whereas strains that do not lead to disease in vivo do not lead to lymphocyte PCD in vitro (59). We have addressed this question in simian models of lentiviral infections, which are more closely related to AIDS. In a collaborative study performed in our laboratory by Groux et al., and in collaboration with M. Girard, E. Muchmore, A. Venet, J. P. Lévy, D. Dormont, A. M. Aubertin, and F. Barré-Sinoussi, it was observed that T cells from chimpanzees experimentally infected with HIV-1 (which do not develop disease) are not programmed to undergo PCD in vitro, and that T cells from macaques experimentally infected with SIV (which develop a disease closely resembling AIDS) are abnormally programmed to undergo in vitro PCD in response to stimulation (60). Similar findings have been presented by Gougeon et al. (Chapter 10) and were reported by Julio Lavergne's group at the VIII International Congress of Immunology, Budapest (August 1992). Together, these findings support the hypothesis that inappropriate and chronic induction of T-cell PCD may be closely related to AIDS pathogenesis, and is not the sole consequence of the ability of a given lentivirus to infect CD4 + T cells, or of an ongoing stimulation of the immune system. They also suggest that simian models of AIDS-related diseases may be important in exploring the possible consequences of therapeutic strategies aimed at the prevention of T-cell PCD.

PCD DYSREGULATION, CELL DEPLETION, AND CELL IMMORTALIZATION

Genes that are involved in coordinate regulation of physiological PCD during development have been characterized in the nematode *Caenorhabditis elegans* (61). In mammals, three genes involved in the control of PCD have recently been identified: two, Bcl-2 and c-myc, are oncogenes; one, p53, is an antioncogene, a tumor suppressor gene. Physiological expression of the Bcl-2 gene prevents PCD induction in myeloid precursors and also in B lymphocytes, in which case it participates in the development and maintenance of immune memory. Abnormal consitutive expression of Bcl-2 leads to B-cell immortalization, and the development of tumors, such as in human follicular B-cell lymphoma, EBV-infected B cells, and transgenic mice in which additional activation is provided, for example, constitutive c-myc expression (reviewed in Ref. 62). Surprisingly, expression of the sole c-myc, a potent oncogene, has been shown to induce PCD (63), an effect that is prevented when the Bcl-2 gene is coexpressed (64). Thus, the development of tumors—in some cell populations, at least —requires the coordinated expression of oncogenes that may exert opposite regulatory effects on PCD. This model is consistent with the finding that inactivation, through mutation, of the tumor suppressor gene p53 may be involved in cancer development by abrogating the physiological cell dependence on growth factors for the prevention of PCD (65).

Together, these findings suggest that inappropriate expression of genes involved in the physiological control of PCD may lead to disease, either by inducing excessive cell loss and preventing cell renewal or by inducing cell immortalization, leading to oncogenesis.

There is now evidence that a cell-suicide program is functional in various normal mature cell populations including T cells, and may participate in cell renewal, regulation of cell function, control of viral dissemination, and prevention of cell immortalization. This death program can be triggered by a wide range of mechanisms, including the deprivation of growth factors, incomplete or defective activation, or, alternatively, excessive and prolonged activation, which may be involved in superantigen-mediated T-cell death and neurotransmitter-mediated "excitotoxicity" of neurons.

This raises several important questions, with potential therapeutic implications. The first is that in vitro observations of PCD might, like in vitro observations of cell proliferation, raise complex problems of correlation with the in vivo fate of the cells. Another question is that in vivo modulation of PCD might not be devoid of deleterious effects. In particular, therapeutic strategies effective in preventing T-cell PCD and restoring T-cell proliferation in HIV-infected people could induce an increase in viral production and the number of infected cells and, besides any effect on the viral infection, the breaking of self-tolerance, the dysregulation of the immune response, or the development of tumors. For all these reasons, animal models of AIDS-related diseases will be required to further investigate the possible role of PCD in the pathogenesis of the disease and the possible consequences of in vivo treatment designed to prevent PCD. A third question in such a context is whether tumors, such as Kaposi's sarcoma and B-cell lymphoma, that are frequent in HIV-infected people are the sole consequence of a progressive immunodeficiency. AIDS-Kaposi's sarcoma cells represent an intriguing model, since they appear to depend on growth factors released by other cells in order to become transformed (66). It is therefore possible that PCD dysregulation may be a broad target of HIV-mediated interference with cell signaling that leads, depending on the cell types, either to excessive PCD and cell loss or to cell immortalization.

The main implication of our hypothesis was that the possible involvement of PCD in the pathogenesis of immunodeficiency and neurological disorders in HIV-infected people may represent the basis for the development of new therapeutic strategies that may have relevance to disease beyond the scope of AIDS (13). Interdisciplinary studies will be required to assess whether PCD dysregulation is central to AIDS pathogenesis, to further characterize the molecular control of cell survival and cell death, to identify the viral and host genes that may be involved in PCD dysregulation, and to explore to what extent in vivo control of PCD can be achieved.

REFERENCES

1. Fauci AS. The human immunodeficiency virus: infectivity and mechanisms of pathogenesis. Science 1988; 239:617–622.
2. Everall IP, Luthert PJ, Lantos PL. Neuronal loss in the frontal cortex in HIV-infection. Lancet 1991; 337:1119–1121.
3. Lane HC, Depper JM, Greene WC, Whalen G, Waldmann TA, Fauci AS. Quantitative analysis of immune function in patients with AIDS: evidence for a selective defect in soluble antigen recognition. N Engl J Med 1985; 313:79.
4. Shearer GM, Bernstein DC, Tung KSK, Via CS, Redfield R, Salahuddin SJ, Gallo RC. A model for the selective loss of MHC self-restricted T-cell immune responses during the development of AIDS. J Immunol 1986; 137:2514.
5. Hofmann B, Jakobsen KD, Odum N, Dickmeiss E, Platz P, Ryder LP, Pedersen C, Mathiesen L, Bygbjerg I, Faber V, Svejgaard A. HIV-induced immuno-

deficiency: Relatively preserved PHA as opposed to decreased PWM responses may be due to possibly preserved responses via CD2/PHA pathway. J Immunol 1989; 142:1874.

6. Miedema F, Petit AJC, Terpestra FG, Eeftinck Schattenkerk JKM, DeWolf F, Al BJM, Roos M, Lange JMA, Danner SA, Goudsmit J, Schellekens PTA. Immunological abnormalities in HIV-infected asymptomatic homosexual men. J Clin Invest 1988; 82:1908.

7. Clerici M, Stocks NI, Zajac RA, Boswell RN, Lucey DR, Via CS, Shearer GM. Detection of three distinct patterns of helper cell dysfunction in asymptomatic HIV-seropositive patients: independence of CD4+ cell numbers and clinical staging. J Clin Invest 1989; 84:1892.

8. Clerici M, Stocks NI, Zajac RA, Boswell RN, Bernstein DC, Mann DL, Shearer GM, Berzofsky JA. Il-2 production used to detect antigenic peptide recognition by T-helper lymphocytes from asymptomatic HIV-seropositive individuals. Nature 1989; 339:383.

9. Schnittman SM, Psallidopoulos MC, Lane HC, Thompson L, Baseler M, Massari F, Fox CH, Salzman NP, Fauci AS. The reservoir for HIV-1 in human peripheral blood is a cell that maintains expression of CD4. Science 1989; 245:305.

10. Brinchmann JE, Albert J, Vartdal F. Few infected CD4+ T cells but a high proportion of replication-competent provirus copies in asymptomatic HIV-1 infection. J Virol 1991; 65:2019.

11. Koenig S, Gendelman H, Orenstein J, Dal Canto M, Pezeshkpour G, Yungbluth M, Janotta F, Aksamit A, Martin M, Fauci A. Detection of AIDS virus in macrophages in brain tissue from AIDS patients with encephalopathy. Science 1986; 233:1089.

12. Michaels J, Sharer LR, Epstein LG. HIV-1 infection of the nervous system: a review. Immunodefic Rev 1988; 1:71.

13. Ameisen JC, Capron A. Cell dysfunction and depletion in AIDS: the programmed cell death hypothesis. Immunol Today 1991; 4:102–105.

14. Duvall E, Wyllie AH. Death and the cell. Immunol Today 1986; 7:115–119.

15. Tomei LD, Cope FO, eds. Apoptosis: the molecular basis of cell death. Current Communications in Cell and Molecular Biology. Cold Spring Harbor, NY: Cold Spring Harbor Laboratory Press, 1991.

16. Glucksman A. Cell deaths in normal vertebrate ontogeny. Biol Rev 1951; 26: 59–86.

17. Raff M. Social controls on cell survival and cell death. Nature 1992; 356: 397–400.

18. Oppenheim RW. Cell death during development of the nervous system. Annu Rev Neurosci 1991; 14:453–501.

19. Blackman M, Kappler J, Marrack P. The role of the TcR in positive and negative selection of developing T cells. Science 1990; 248:1335–1341.

20. McConkey DJ, Orrenius S, Jondal M. Cellular signaling in programmed cell death (apoptosis). Immunol Today 1990; 11:120–121.

21. Golstein P, Ojcius DM, Young JDE. Cell death mechanisms and the immune system. Immunol Reviews 1991; 121:29–65.
22. Odaka C, Kisaki H, Tadakuma T. T-cell receptor-mediated DNA fragmentation and cell death in T-cell hybridoma. J Immunol 1990; 144:2096–2101.
23. Bell DA, Morrison B, Vandenbygaart P. Immunogenic DNA-related factors: Nucleosomes spontaneously released from normal murine lymphoid cells stimulate proliferation and immunoglobulin synthesis of normal mouse lymphocytes. J Clin Invest 1990; 85:1437–1496.
24. Clouston WM, Kerr JFR. Apoptosis, lymphocytotoxicity and the containment of viral infections. Med Hypothesis 1985; 18:399–404.
25. Clem RJ, Fechheimer M, Miller LK. Prevention of apoptosis by a baculovirus gene during infection of insect cells. Science 1991; 254:1388–1390.
26. Schnittman SM, Lane HC, Greenhouse J, Justement JJ, Baseler M, Fauci AS. Preferential infection of CD4+ memory T cells by HIV-1: Evidence for a role in the selective T-cell functional defects observed in infected individuals. Proc Natl Acad Sci USA 1990; 87:6058–6062.
27. Van Noesel CJM, Gruters RA, Terpstra FG, Schellekens PTA, van Lier RAW, Miedema F. Functional and phenotypic evidence for a selective loss of memory T cells in asymptomatic HIV-infected men. J Clin Invest 1990; 86:293–299.
28. Marrack P, Kappler J. The staphylococcal enterotoxins and their relatives. Science 1990; 248:705–711.
29. Jenkinson EJ, Kingston R, Smith CA, Williams GT, Owen JJT. Antigen-induced apoptosis in developing T cells: a mechanism for negative selection of the TCR repertoire. Eur J Immunol 1989; 19:2175–2177.
30. Newell MK, Haughn LJ, Maroun CR, Julius MH. Death of mature T cells by separate ligation of CD4 and the TCR for antigen. Nature 1990; 347:286–289.
31. Sambhara S, Miller R. Programmed cell death of T cells signaled by the T cell receptor and the α_3 domain of class I MHC. Science 1991; 252:1424–1427.
32. Lenardo MJ. Interleukin 2 programs mouse $\alpha\beta$ T-lymphocytes for apoptosis. Nature 1991; 353:858–861.
33. Liu Y, Janeway CA Jr. INFγ plays a critical role in induced cell death of effector T cell: a possible third mechanism of self-tolerance. J Exp Med 1990; 172:1735–1739.
34. Russel JH, White CL, Loh DY, Meleedy-Rey P. Receptor-stimulated death pathway is opened by antigen in mature T cells. Proc Natl Acad Sci USA 1991; 88:2151–2155.
35. Kawabe Y, Oshi A. Programmed cell death and extrathymic reduction of Vβ8+ CD4+ T cells in mice tolerant to *Staphylococcus aureus* enterotoxin B. Nature 1991; 349:245–247.
36. Choi YW, Kappler JW, Marrack P. A superantigen encoded in the open reading frame of the 3' long terminal repeat of mouse mammary tumor virus. Nature 1991; 350:203–207.

37. Hügin AW, Vacchio M, Morse HC. A virus-encoded superantigen in a retrovirus-induced immunodeficiency syndrome of mice. Science 1991; 252:425–427.

38. Janeway CA Jr. MLS: makes a little sense. Nature 1991; 349:459–461.

39. Imberti L, Sottini A, Bettinardi A, Puoti M, Primi D. Selective depletion in HIV infection of T cells that bear specific T cell receptor Vβ sequences. Science 1991; 254:860–862.

40. Ameisen JC, Groux H, Torpier G, Mouton Y, Capron A. Programmed T cell death (apoptosis) and AIDS pathogenesis. VII International Conference on AIDS, Florence, June 16–21, 1991. Abstr WA 1235.

41. Groux H, Monté D, Bourrez JM, Capron A, Ameisen JC. L'activation des lymphocytes T CD4$^+$ de sujets asymptomatiques infectés par le VIH entraîne le déclenchement d'un programme de mort lymphocytaire par apoptose. CR Acad Sci Paris (Série III) 1991; 312:599–606.

42. Groux H, Torpier G, Monté D, Mouton Y, Capron A, Ameisen JC. Activation-induced death by apoptosis in CD4$^+$ T cells from HIV-infected asymptomatic individuals. J Exp Med 1992; 175:331–340.

43. Montagnier L, Guétard D, Rame V, Olivier R, Adams M. Viral and immunological factors of AIDS pathogenesis. In Girard M, Valette L, eds. Retroviruses of Human AIDS and Related Animal Diseases. IV Colloque des Cent Gardes 1989. Lyon, France: Fondation M Mérieux, 1990:11–17.

44. Gougeon ML, Olivier R, Garcia S, Guétard D, Dragic T, Dauguet C, Montagnier L. Mise en évidence d'un processus d'engagement vers la mort cellulaire par apoptose dans les lymphocytes de patients infectés par le VIH. CR Acad Sci Paris (Série III) 1991; 312:529–537.

45. Meyaard L, Otto SA, Jonker RR, Mijnster M, Keet R, Miedema F. Programmed death of T cells in HIV-1 infection. Science 1992; 257:217–219.

46. Terai C, Kornbluth R, Pauza C, Richman D, Carson D. Apoptosis as a mechanism of cell death in cultured T lymphoblasts acutely infected with HIV-1. J Clin Invest 1991; 87:1710–1715.

47. Laurent-Crawford AG, Krust B, Muller S, Rivière Y, Rey-Cuillé MA, Béchet JM, Montagnier L, Hovanessian A. The cytopathic effect of HIV is associated with apoptosis. Virology 1991; 185:829–839.

48. Krust B, Laurent A, Cointe D, Rey MA, Meurs E, Marié I, Hovanessian AG. Some cellular and viral parameters implicated in the pathogenesis of HIV infection. In: Girard M, Valette L, eds. Retroviruses of Human AIDS and Related Animal Diseases. V Colloque des Cent Gardes 1990. Lyon, France: Fondation M Mérieux, 1991:41–45.

49. Cohen DI, Tani Y, Tian H, Boone E, Samelson L, Lane HC. Participation of tyrosine phosphorylation in the cytopathic effect of HIV-1. Science 1992; 256:542–545.

50. Banda NK, Bernier J, Kurahara D, Kurrle R, Haigwood N, Sekaly R, Finkel TH. Crosslinking CD4 by HIV gp120 primes T cells for activation-induced apoptosis. J Exp Med 1992; 176:1099–1106.

51. Ameisen JC. Programmed cell death and AIDS: from hypothesis to experiment. Immunol Today 1992; 13:388–391.

52. Bretscher P, Cohn M. A theory of self-nonself discrimination. Science 1970; 169:1042–1049.

53. Jenkins M. The role of cell division in the induction of clonal anergy. Immunol Today 1992; 13:69–73.

54. Janeway CA Jr. The immune system evolved to discriminate infectious nonself from noninfectious self. Immunol Today 1992; 13:11–16.

55. Pantaleo G, Graziosi C, Butini L, et al. Lymphoid organs function as major reservoirs for HIV. Proc Natl Acad Sci 1991; 88:9838–9842.

56. Fox CH, Tenner-Racz K, Racz P, Firpo A, Rizzo PA, Fauci AS. Lymphoid germinal centers are reservoirs of HIV-1 RNA. J Infect Dis 1991; 164:1051–1057.

57. Genis P, Jett M, Bernton W, Boyle T, Gelbard H, Dzenko K, Keane R, Resnick L, Mizrachi Y, Volsky D, Epstein L, Gendelman HE. Cytokines and arachidonic metabolites produced during HIV-infected macrophage-astroglia interactions: implications for the neuropathogenesis of HIV disease. J Exp Med 1992; 176:1703–1718.

58. Uehara T, Miyawaki T, Ohta K, Tamaru Y, Yokoi T, Nakamura S, Taniguchi N. Apoptotic cell death of primed CD45RO⁺T lymphocytes in EBV-induced infectious mononucleosis. Blood 1992; 80:452–458.

59. Rojko JL, Fulton RM, Rezanka LJ, et al. Lymphocytotoxic strains of feline leukemia virus induce apoptosis in feline T4-thymic lymphoma cells. Lab Invest 1992; 66:418–426.

60. Ameisen JC, Groux H, Plouvier B, Torpier G, Mouton Y, Capron A. Programmed cell death (apoptosis) and AIDS pathogenesis: theory and experimental approach. In: Girard M, Valette L, eds. Retroviruses of Human AIDS and Related Animal Diseases. VI Colloque des Cent Gardes 1991. Lyon, France: Fondation M Mérieux, 1992:19–24.

61. Hengartner M, Ellis R, Horvitz H. *Caenorhabditis elegans* gene *ced-9* protects cells from programmed cell death. Nature 1992; 356:494–499.

62. Korsmeyer S. Bcl-2: a repressor of lymphocyte death. Immunol Today 1992; 13:285–288.

63. Evan GI, Wyllie AH, Gilbert CS, Littlewood TD, Land H, Brooks M, Waters CM, Penn LZ, Hancock DC. Induction of apoptosis in fibroblasts by c-myc protein. Cell 1992; 69:119.

64. Bissonnette R, Echeverry F, Mahboubi A, Greene DR. Apoptotic cell death induced by c-myc is inhibited by Bcl-2. Nature 1992; 359:552–554.

65. Yonish-Rouach E, Resnitzky D, Lotem J, Sachs L, Kimchi A, Oren M. Wilde-type p53 induces apoptosis of myeloid leukaemic cells that is inhibited by IL-6. Nature 1991; 352:345–347.

66. Nair BC, De Vico AL, Nakamura S, Copeland TD, Chen Y, Patel A, O'Neil T, Oroszlan S, Gallo RC, Sarngadharan MG. Identification of a major growth factor for AIDS-Kaposi's sarcoma cells as oncostatin M. Science 1992; 255:1430–1432.

10

Programmed Cell Death in HIV Infection and Correlation with AIDS Pathogenesis

Marie-Lise Gougeon, Sylvie Garcia, and Luc Montagnier

Institut Pasteur
Paris, France

Jonathan Heeney

Laboratory of Viral Pathogenesis
Rijswijk, The Netherlands

INTRODUCTION

One of the difficulties in understanding the complex pathology of human immunodeficiency virus (HIV) infection is explaining the progressive depletion, and finally the complete disappearance, of the CD4+ helper-T-cell population, which leads to the destruction of the immune system. Functional defects of helper T cells are observed very early after HIV infection and are characterized by the impairment of in vitro T-cell receptor (TcR)-dependent activation in response to major histocompatibility complex (MHC)-restricted recall antigens (1) or to anti-CD3 monoclonal antibodies (2). The functional defects of helper T cells are followed by the progressive disappearance of CD4 lymphocytes during disease progression. Although the loss of CD4 + cells appears to result primarily from their destruction following infection—whether by viral cytopathic effect, host-mediated cytotoxicity, or both (3)—the magnitude of immunological defects observed in infected individuals during the asymptomatic phase of HIV infection is disproportionately high in comparison to the level of infectious virus and to the number of CD4 + -infected cells (4-6), suggesting that factors other than virus-induced cytopathogenicity may be involved. Some indirect mechanisms have to be considered in which the effect of the virus must be amplified by its interaction with the functional network of the immune system.

Recently, we and others (7-12) suggested that the loss of CD4 + cells in asymptomatic HIV-infected individuals is associated with lymphocyte activation. Activation, however, does not result in cell proliferation, but rather in cell depletion, through a mechanism known as programmed cell death (PCD) (13-17).

The morphological characteristics of PCD have been called *apoptosis,* as opposed to *necrosis*, the morphology of accidental cell death. In general, the cell undergoing apoptosis is submitted to profound structural changes. One of these is an apparent modification of the cytoskeleton so that the plasma membrane undergoes a process of rapid blebbing. The nuclear collapse is another feature of apoptosis: chromatin becomes extremely condensed and tends to marginate in crescents around the nuclear envelope. The nucelar collapse, visible by light or electron microscopy, indicates extensive damage to chromatin, which is degraded into single and multiple oligonucleosomes. Because nucleosomes are spaced regularly at approximately 180-200 base-pair (bp) intervals along eukaryotic chromatin, an electrophoretic separation of DNA reveals a "ladder" pattern of bands averaging about 200 bp, 400 bp, 600 bp, and so on. The DNA is cleaved in the internucleosomal linker region, where it is relatively weakly associated with histone H1 (16,17). This fragmentation of DNA is enzymatic and generally occurs after activation of a calcium-dependent endogenous endonuclease (17).

Apoptosis is an active cell-suicide mechanism that is involved, for instance, in the negative intrathymic selection of the T-cell repertoire, which leads to the clonal deletion of autoreactive T cells, and to the establishment of self-tolerance (18). Immature thymocytes undergo apoptosis in response to glucocorticoids, hormones, calcium ionophores, and antibodies to the CD3 TcR (19-21). Mature T lymphocytes appear to be resistant to apoptosis. However, in some circumstances, antigen-receptor signaling may lead to the re-emergence of a cell-death program in mature T cells (22–25).

An interesting question raised by our observations concerns the reasons for the inappropriate re-emergence of a cell-death program in mature T cells from HIV-infected patients. In this chapter we present and discuss our recent observations that in HIV infection PCD may contribute in vivo to the depletion of reactive T cells after antigenic stimulation. Furthermore, these observations are strengthened by experiments performed on HIV-infected chimpanzees and SIV-infected macaques, showing a correlation between the emergence of a cell-depletion program and AIDS pathogenesis.

PCD IN PERIPHERAL LYMPHOCYTES
FROM HIV-INFECTED INDIVIDUALS

Our earlier studies (26) indicated that when peripheral blood lymphocytes (PBLs) separated on Ficoll gradient were cultured in medium in the absence of exogenous stimulation, there was a significant difference in daily loss of viability between lymphocytes from healthy HIV-negative individuals and those from HIV-infected individuals. This in vitro-induced premature cell death of patients' lymphocytes did not represent the death of infected cells, and it was observed early in the asymptomatic phase of the disease and was more pronounced in the AIDS stage (Figure 1).

A preliminary analysis of the phenomenon was carried out with a two-color cytofluorometry assay consisting of double-staining of cultured lymphocytes with two nucleic acid dyes, ethidium bromide and orange acridine. Subsequent analysis by flow cytometry of the stained cells in cultures of patients' PBLs revealed the early occurrence of a living population, not stained by ethidium bromide and weakly stained with orange acridine (10,26). This population was absent in cultures from seronegative donors. We made the hypothesis that the weak staining with orange acridine of cultured lymphocytes was the consequence of chromatin condensation in the nuclei of these cells, and this feature represents one of the structural changes occurring during the process of cell death by apoptosis.

We have confirmed that, under these conditions, patients' lymphocytes were dying of apoptosis. Apoptosis was monitored by the presence of oligonucleosomal DNA fragments in the nuclei of cultured lymphocytes: when analyzed by electrophoresis on an agarose gel, the DNA is

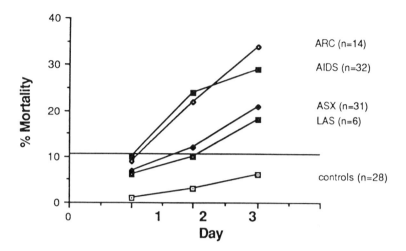

Figure 1 In vitro loss of viability of lymphocytes from HIV-infected patients as compared to seronegative donors. PBLs from HIV-infected individuals and from controls were cultured during 1 to 3 days at 10^6 cells/ml in culture medium composed of RPMI-1640, 1 mM glutamine, 10 mM hepes, 1% penicillin/strepto-mycin, 10% FCS. Cell death was assessed by trypan blue permeability. Each point represents the mean of percent mortality in lymphocyte cultures from several donors. Patients were staged according to CDC surveillance definitions: stage II (ASX), stage III (LAS), stage IVA (ARC), stage IVC/IVD (AIDS), and controls.

resolved in discrete bands, the size of a nucleosomal DNA unit (200 bp) or a multiple of this size, if the digestion is not complete (Figure 2). Thus, a significant fraction of lymphocytes from HIV-infected individuals undergoes apoptosis after a short culture time, so the total DNA shows the characteristic oligonucleosomal bands.

Figure 2 Triggering by ionomycin of the apoptosis process in peripheral lymphocytes from HIV-infected individuals. (A) Peripheral lymphocytes from two seronegative donors (lanes 1–4) and two asymptomatic HIV-infected individuals (CDC stage IIB, no treatment) (lanes 5–8) were stimulated for 24 hours with ionomycin (Calbiochem) 1 μM (lanes 1, 2, 5, 6) or unstimulated (lanes 3, 4, 7, and 8). At the end of the culture, 2×10^6 cells were collected and DNA fragmentation was analyzed as reported (10,12). (B) Electron micrograph of ultrathin sections (uranyl acetate staining) from HIV-positive patients' lymphocytes cultured for 4 hours as described above in the presence of ionomycin 1 μM. (a) Normal lymphocyte; (b) lymphocyte with condensed chromatin; (c) apoptotic lymphocyte.

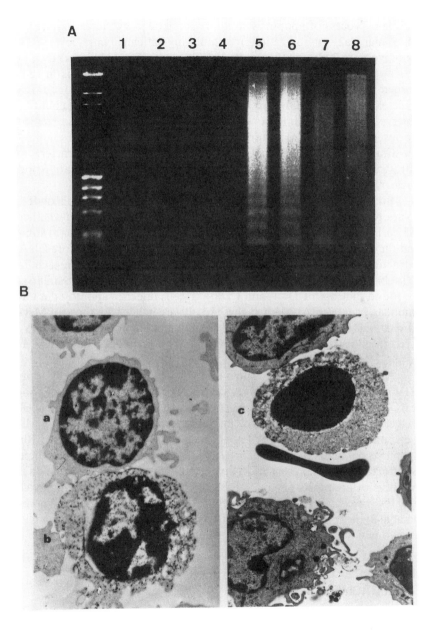

This process of apoptosis could be accelerated by increasing the intracellular Ca2 + mobilization by stimulating patients' lymphocytes with ionomycin for 24 hours (Figure 2), the Ca2 + ionophore being known to activate the endogenous endonuclease and to induce apoptosis in cells primed for this cell death, such as immature thymocytes (21). Under the same experimental conditions, no oligonucleosomal fragments could be observed in cultures from seronegative donors. Confirmation was obtained by observing with the electron microscope ultrathin sections of ionomycin-stimulated patients' lymphocytes. These cells display characteristic ultrastructural changes of apoptosis such as chromatin condensation and nuclear shrinkage (Figure 2).

Both CD4 + and CD8 + cells from HIV-infected individuals undergo apoptosis upon activation with ionomycin: this was observed whether the purification of CD4 + and CD8 + T cells was carried out prior to stimulation with ionomycin or was done at the end of the culture before DNA extraction (12). This suggests that the triggering of apoptosis in each T-cell subpopulation does not depend on the presence of the other. Similarly, we found that both CD4 + and CD8 + T cells undergo apoptosis in unstimulated cultures. Altogether, these results are in line with those of Meyaard et al. (11), who recently showed that stimulation of T cells from HIV-infected patients with cross-linked CD3 antibodies induces apoptosis in both CD4 + and CD8 + T cells.

Altogether, these results show that CD4 + and CD8 + T cells from HIV-infected patients are primed in vivo for a suicide process by apoptosis. They also suggest that a fraction of these cells have already been triggered in vivo for apoptosis by unknown stimuli and consequently will die spontaneously in vitro. Another fraction has been programmed for apoptosis but needs further in vitro activation to undergo apoptosis. These two fractions may represent cells in two distinct stages of PCD (see below). Analysis of apoptosis ex vivo on freshly isolated lymphocytes indicates very low percentages of apoptotic cells in HIV-infected patients and comparable to the control values (Table 1). This is probably related to the rapid in vivo elimination of these cells by macrophages.

INFLUENCE OF INHIBITORS ON IONOMYCIN-INDUCED DNA FRAGMENTATION

Apoptosis depends on the intracellular availability of certain key proteins, including a calcium-magnesium-dependent endonuclease (16,17). We thus analyzed, with various inhibitors, the requirements of apoptosis in pa-

Table 1 Apoptosis in Freshly Isolated PBLs from Asymptomatic HIV-Infected Individuals (% apoptotic nuclei in PBLs ex vivo)

	1	2	3	4	5	6	7	8	9	10	11	12
Controls	2	3	2	<1	1	1	3	2	<1	1	2	1
Patients	<1	<1	3	5	2	1	2	1	1	<1	1	3

Apoptosis was tested in freshly isolated PBLs from asymptomatic HIV-infected individuals and from seronegative donors by staining the nuclei of the cells with propidium iodide, as described in the text.

tients' lymphocytes to explore whether new macromolecular synthesis was necessary. We reported that, as shown for mouse thymocytes (15,21,27), induction of apoptosis by ionomycin in peripheral lymphocytes is an active mechanism that requires protein synthesis and involves functional endogenous endonuclease (12). Similar results were reported by Groux et al. (8) in PWM and staphylococcal enterotoxin (SEB)-induced apoptosis, and Meyaard et al. (11) in anti-CD3-induced cell death. On the other hand, apoptosis observed when the cells were cultured in the presence only of medium was not sensitive to inhibitors such as actinomycin-D or cycloheximide, indicating that new macromolecular synthesis was not necessary for death to occur. In addition, Zn^{2+} ions, known to inhibit the activity of the endonuclease, did not affect spontaneous apoptosis, a situation also observed in thymocytes (27).

These results suggest that, according to Arends and Wyllie (15), at least two lymphocyte T-cell subpopulations can be distinguished in HIV-infected patients, as a function of their stages with regard to apoptosis. The first one has been primed in vivo for apoptosis, presumably in response to cell-type-specific signals. Apoptosis is initiated upon culture in such primed cells, through activation of effector molecules, by triggering mechanisms. These triggering mechanisms include the controlled influx of calcium into the cell by nonspecific stimuli such as calcium ionophores or specific stimuli such as anti-TcR stimulation or superantigen activation. The second T-cell subpopulation, which shows a spontaneous apoptosis, has already been triggered for apoptosis by in vivo signals and will proceed into apoptosis in vitro, without the need for additional activation signals. The insensitivity to the inhibitors may indicate that these cells, primed for apoptosis, already contain the complete machinery for death and that a mild cellular injury, such as that induced by in vitro culture, will trigger the apoptosis process in these cells.

INFLUENCE OF BACTERIAL SUPERANTIGENS ON ACTIVATION-INDUCED APOPTOSIS

Physiological activators of T lymphocytes are antigens that are recognized, in the context of MHC molecules, through their interaction with the variable V portions of the TcR α and β chains (28). However, T cells recognize another category of ligands—the superantigens—on the basis of the expressed Vβ alone, independently of the other variable TcR segments. The superantigens bind to MHC proteins and this complex, by engaging Vβ, can stimulate many T cells. Toxins produced by different types of bacteria, including staphylococci, streptococci, and mycoplasmas, act as superantigens and cause toxic and septic shock, triggering overstimulation of the immune system (29).

Normal immature thymocytes respond to activation by undergoing apoptosis, and we and others (8–12) have shown that such a cell-death program exists in peripheral T cells from HIV-infected patients. We thus addressed the possibility, as recently proposed (7), that in HIV-infected patients, T cells primed for apoptosis will die instead of being activated when stimulated through their TcR. This process would induce in vivo the progressive depletion of antigen-reactive mature T cells.

Since, owing to the large repertoire of T-cell specificities, it would be difficult to detect in vitro induction of apoptosis in response to classic antigens, we investigated whether the suicide program in lymphocytes from HIV-infected patients could be triggered by a superantigenic stimulation. Several superantigens were used: SEB, streptococcal erythrogenic toxin A (ETA), and mycoplasma arthritidis mitogen (MAM). The study was realized on lymphocytes from clinically asymptomatic HIV-infected patients (12). Quantification of apoptosis was performed using a recently described flow-cytometry method (30) than quantifies the percentage of apoptotic nuclei in a cell suspension after propidium iodide staining in hypotonic buffer. As shown in Figure 3, superantigenic activation by staphylococcal enterotoxins triggers the apoptotic program in patients' lymphocytes, not in control lymphocytes, and this process occurs very quickly—during the first 48 hours of stimulation. The rapidity of the activation-induced apoptosis is compatible with an abnormal stimulation of programmed T cells that causes their death instead of their activation.

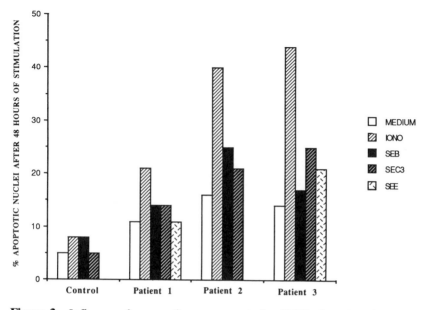

Figure 3 Influence of superantigens on apoptosis of PBLs from HIV-infected patients. PBLs from asymptomatic HIV-infected patients or from a seronegative control were stimulated for 24 hours with ionomycin (1 μg/ml) or staphylococcal enterotoxins (1 μg/ml). The percentage of apoptotic nuclei in the cultures was determined as described (30). Results are the mean of duplicate cultures, and SDs (not shown) were < 10% of the mean. Results of one representative experiment are shown.

The pattern of apoptotic response to the superantigens varies among patients. This may be related to variable proportions, from one patient to another, of programmed T cells expressing the matching Vβ molecules, or it may reflect a refractory state correlated with the in vivo depletion of the corresponding T-cell clones. Such a deleterious process is suggested by a recent report (31) that shows the selective elimination in vivo in HIV-infected patients at the AIDS stage of T cells that express a defined set of Vβ sequences.

While both CD4 + and CD8 + T cells seem to be programmed for apoptosis, CD4 + cells died preferentially consequent to the stimulation with the superantigen SEB, which is probably due to the CD4 + T-cell tropism of this antigen. This observation suggests that the T-cell tropism of the activator used to induce apoptosis in patients' lymphocytes will determine which subpopulation will die: ionomycin (10,12) and anti-CD3 antibodies (11) will activate the death of both CD4+ and CD8+ T cells, while SEB will induce selectively the death of CD4+ T cells (8,12).

PREVENTION OF APOPTOSIS: INFLUENCE OF CYTOKINES

In preliminary studies we observed that a crude preparation of cytokines secreted by PHA-activated human T lymphocytes (TCGF) restored the in vitro viability of patients' lymphocytes (10,26): addition of TCGF (10% v/v) at the initiation of the culture prevented the apparition of the population weakly stained by orange acridine in a nonstimulated 3-day culture (10,26) and in parallel prevented the ionomycin-induced apoptosis (10,12).

Although cytosolic Ca^{2+} increase has been shown to be at the origin of cell death in thymocytes in response to specific stimuli (13,19,32), it also mediates proliferation in mature T lymphocytes provided that other independent signals delivered by accessory cells and including protein kinase C (PKC) activation are delivered (33). Moreover, agents that activate PKC block endonuclease activation in thymocytes (21,27,34,35). Since TCGF was able to prevent activation-induced apoptosis as well as spontaneous apoptosis, we tested whether interleukin-1 (IL-1), a known activator of PKC that is present in TCGF, was responsible for this protection.

Indeed, a mixture of IL-1α and IL-2 was sufficient to prevent spontaneous and ionomycin-induced apoptosis (12). It is worth noting that IL-2 alone had no effect on apoptosis. Furthermore, these cytokines not only prevented apoptosis but, in some patients, also restored in vitro superantigenic T-cell stimulation. The importance of a cosignal delivery in prevention of apoptosis has also been reported by Groux et al. (8), who showed that the cosignal given through the CD28 molecule was able to restore the proliferative response of T cells from HIV-infected individuals to SEB, PWM, and tetanus antigen.

RELEVANCE OF THESE DATA TO AIDS PATHOGENESIS

We asked whether the phenomenon of priming for PCD was unique to HIV-1-infected humans developing AIDS or could also be observed in another primate species susceptible to AIDS, the rhesus macaques experimentally infected with SIV_{sm}-derived strains. These animals develop a chronic persistent lentivirus infection that results in T-helper-cell loss and

Table 2 Correlation Between Priming for PCD and AIDS Pathogenesis

	Apoptosis	Antihistone antibodies[a]	AIDS
HIV-1-infected humans	+	+	+
HIV-1-infected chimpanzees	−	−	−
SIV-infected macaques	+	+	+

[a]See the text.

the development of AIDS, with the same pattern of disease progression and opportunistic infections as observed in HIV-infected humans.

We have studied the state of spontaneous and ionomycin-induced apoptosis in peripheral cells of SIV-infected macaques (Table 2). We found a stronger spontaneous apoptosis in infected macaques than in controls, and, as found in lymphocytes from HIV-infected humans, ionomycin induced a great enhancement of apoptosis (12). As a corollary, chimpanzees represent a species that can be productively infected by HIV-1 but does not develop disease. We reported that their peripheral lymphocytes do not seem to be abnormally programmed for apoptosis since the values of spontaneous and ionomycin-induced apoptosis were very low and similar to those found in uninfected chimpanzees (12). The HIV-positive chimpanzees did not show any sign of immune depression, particularly CD4 + T-cell depletion, although they actively replicated HIV-1. Therefore, our results suggest that, in HIV-infected humans and SIV-infected macaques, priming for PCD is correlated with AIDS pathogenesis, particularly CD4 cell depletion.

The occurrence of apoptosis in vivo, even in asymptomatic HIV-infected patients, is suggested by the presence of high-affinity antihistones and anti-RNP antibodies in the majority of 150 sera or plasma from HIV-infected individuals (36). Such antibodies are likely to appear upon release of nucleosomal histones in the circulation, after cell death by apoptosis. Furthermore, in SIV-infected macaques, the development of anti-H2B antibodies has been correlated with the development of disease (37). In conclusion, there is a correlation among the abnormal re-emergence in peripheral lymphocytes of a priming for PCD, the presence in patients' sera of autoantibodies and antihistones, and AIDS pathogenesis (Table 2).

CONCLUSION

One of the common characteristics of HIV infection is the gradual depletion of T4 lymphocytes during the development of AIDS. Apoptotic mechanisms—induced as a direct consequence of HIV replication (38,39) or as an indirect effect of HIV infection (8–12)—are possibly the major contributors of T4-cell depletion. The mechanism by which T lymphocytes become primed in vivo is not yet clear. The events leading to apoptosis in both direct and indirect mechanisms are probably different, since cycloheximide and cyclosporin A suppress induction of apoptosis in the indirect but not in the direct mechanism.

The re-emergence of a cell-depletion program in mature T cells from HIV-infected humans could proceed from different mechanisms, and several hypotheses have been proposed. The first one is that, during HIV infection, apoptosis can be induced by inappropriate delivery of activating signals. Recent observations in the murine model (25) showed that, when preceded by ligation of CD4, signaling of mature T cells through TcR-$\alpha\beta$ results in T-cell unresponsiveness due to the induction of activation-dependent cell death by apoptosis. In HIV-infected patients, the priming of CD4+ T cells for apoptosis following activation could be induced either by the HIV-gp120 or gp120–anti gp120 complexes, or by anti-CD4 autoantibodies, as suggested by Ameisen and Capron (7).

However, other mechanisms should be envisaged for the priming of CD8+, since the re-emergence of a cell-depletion program in HIV-infected patients concerns both CD4+ and CD8+ T cells. This default could be the consequence, as proposed for thymocytes (35), of a lack of adequate second signaling by antigen-presenting cells, due to a defective antigen-presenting cell function related to their infection by HIV (2). Indeed, as discussed above, cosignaling with IL-1α or CD28 MAb restores the activation of patients' T cells. Alternatively, the priming for death could occur intrathymically in the immature CD4+CD8+ thymocytes, whose maturation will lead to peripheral CD4+ and CD8+ T cells abnormally programmed for activation-induced cell death.

Another hypothesis was recently formulated after the discovery that superantigens are encoded by a murine retrovirus (mammary tumor virus) (40). This theory proposes that HIV might cause, in conjunction with class II genes, cell anergy and depletion of uninfected CD4+ T cells by encoding a superantigen. Progression of CD4 T-cell depletion would require cycles of mutation in the retroviral superantigen gene, resulting in the elimination of CD4 T cells bearing different Vβs over time. The main difference between this hypothesis and the hypothesis that priming for PCD would occur through gp120-CD4 recognition is that the second one implies that the loss of CD4+ T cells in AIDS patients is a random phenomenon occurring during antigenic or superantigenic activation, while the first one assumes that T-cell depletion is a strictly Vβ-selective process. Results obtained in several laboratories are compatible with either hypothesis (31,41), and we have recently found a Vβ-specific anergy in T lymphocytes from 50% of asymptomatic HIV-infected individuals (G. Dadaglio, S. Garcia, and M. L. Gougeon, submitted). We are currently analyzing the potential role of the virus itself in the induction of this Vβ-specific anergy.

Thus, a combination of several hypotheses may be envisaged to account for the regular and complete CD4 depletion occurring during HIV infection.

ACKNOWLEDGMENTS

This work was supported by grants from the ANRS, the CNRS, and the Pasteur Institute. We would like to acknowledge Drs. A.M. Berthier, B. Dupont, G. Gonzales, M. Kierstetter, G. Pialloux, and R. Roué, for their collaboration in the clinical aspects of this work (Hôpital Bégin, Centre Médical Rey-Leroux).

REFERENCES

1. Shearer GM, Clerici M. Early T helper cell defects in HIV infection. AIDS 1991; 5:245–253.
2. Miedema F, Petit AJC, Terpstra FG, et al. Immunological abnormalities in human immunodeficiency virus (HIV) infected asymptomatic homosexual men: HIV affects the immune system before CD4 + T helper cell depletion. J Clin Invest 1989; 82:1908–1913.
3. Fauci AS. The human immunodeficiency virus: infectivity and mechanisms of pathogenesis. Science (Washington, DC) 1988; 239:617–622.
4. Ho DD, Mougdil MS, Alam M. Quantification of human immunodeficiency virus type 1 in the blood of infected persons. N Engl J Med 1989; 321:1621–1625.
5. Schnittman SM, Psallidopoulos MC, Lane HC, et al. The reservoir for HIV-1 in human peripheral blood is a T cell that maintains expression of CD4. Science 1989; 245:305–308.
6. Bagasra O, Hauptman SP, Lischner HW, Sachs M, Pomerantz RJ. Detection of human immunodeficiency virus type 1 provirus in mononuclear cells by in situ polymerase chain reaction. N Engl J Med 1992; 326:1385–1391.
7. Ameisen JC, Capron A. Cell dysfunction and depletion in AIDS: The programmed cell death hypothesis. Immunol Today 1991; 12:102–105.

8. Groux H, Torpier G, Monté D, Mouton Y, Capron A, Ameisen JC. Activation-induced death by apoptosis from human immunodeficiency virus-infected asymptomatic individuals. J Exp Med 1992; 175:331–340.

9. Gougeon ML, Olivier R, Garcia S, Guétard D, Dragic T, Dauguet C, Montagnier L. Evidence for an engagement process toward apoptosis in lymphocytes of HIV-infected patients. CR Acad Sci Paris 1991; 312:529–537.

10. Gougeon ML, Garcia S, Guétard D, Olivier R, Dauguet C, Montagnier L. Apoptosis as a mechanism of cell death in peripheral lymphocytes from HIV1-infected individuals. In: Janossy G, Autran B, Miedema F, eds. Immunology of HIV Infection. Basel: Karger, 1992:115–126.

11. Meyaard L, Otto SA, Jonker RR, Mijnster MJ, Keet R, Miedema F. Programmed death of T cells in HIV-1 infection. Science 1992; 257:217–219.

12. Gougeon ML, Garcia S, Heeney J, Tschopp R, Lecoeur H, Guétard D, Rame V, Dauguet C, Montagnier L. Programmed cell death in AIDS-related HIV and SIV infections. AIDS Res Hum Retrovir. In press.

13. Duvall E, Wyllie AH. Death and the cell. Immunol Today 1986; 7:115–119.

14. Cohen JJ, Duke RC. Apoptosis and programmed cell death in immunity. Annu Rev Immunol 1992; 10:267–293.

15. Arends MJ, Wyllie AH. Apoptosis: mechanisms and roles in pathology. Int Rev Exp Pathol 1991; 32:223–254.

16. Wyllie AH, Morris RG, Smith AL, Dunlop D. Chromatin cleavage in apoptosis: association with condensed chromatin morphology and dependence on macromolecular synthesis. J Pathol 1991; 142:67–77.

17. Arends MJ, Morris RG, Wyllie AH. Apoptosis: The role of the endonuclease. Am J Pathol 1990; 136:593–608.

18. Blackman M, Kappler J, Marrack P. The role of the TCR in positive and negative selection of developing T cells. Science (Washington, DC) 1990; 248:1335–1338.

19. Smith CA, Williams GT, Kingston R, Jenkinson EJ, Owen JJT. Antibodies to CD3/T cell receptor complex induce death by apoptosis in immature T cells in thymic cultures. Nature 1989; 337:181–184.

20. Shi Y, Sahai BM, Green DR. Cyclosporin A inhibits activation-induced cell death in T cell hybridomas and thymocytes. Nature 1989; 339:625–628.

21. McConkey DJ, Hartzell P, Amador-Perez JF, Orrenius S, Jondal M. C++ dependent killing of immature thymocytes by stimulation via the CD3/TCR complex. J Immunol 1989; 143:1801–1806.

22. Russel JH, White CL, Loh DY, Meleedy-Rey P. Receptor-stimulated death pathway is opened by antigen in mature T cells. Proc Natl Acad Sci USA 1991; 88:2151–2159.

23. Janssen O, Wesselborg S, Heckl-Ostreicher B, et al. T-cell receptor signaling induces death by apoptosis in human T-cell receptor gamma delta+ T cells. J Immunol 1991; 146:35–41.

24. Lucas M, Solano F, Sanz A. Induction of programmed cell death (apoptosis) in mature lymphocytes. FEBS Lett 1991; 279:19–21.
25. Newell MK, Haughn LJ, Maroun CR, Julius MH. Death of mature T-cells by separate ligation of CD4 and the T cell receptor for antigen. Nature 1990; 347:286–288.
26. Montagnier L, Guétard D, Rame V, Olivier R, Adams M. Virological and immunological factors of AIDS pathogenesis. In: Girard M, Valette L, eds. Retroviruses of Human AIDS and Related Animal Diseases. France: Pasteur Mérieux, 1989:11–17.
27. Kizaki H, Tadakuma T, Okada C, Muramatsu J, Ishimura C. Activation of a suicide process of thymocytes through DNA fragmentation by calcium ionophores and phorbol esters. J Immunol 1989; 43:1790–1794.
28. Davis MM, Bjorkman PJ. T cell antigen receptor genes and T cell recognition. Nature 1988; 334:395–402.
29. Marrack P, Kappler J. The staphylococcal enterotoxins and their relatives. Science (Washington, DC) 1990; 248:705–712.
30. Nicoletti I, Migliorati G, Grignani F, Riccardi C. A rapid and simple method for measuring apoptosis by propidium iodide staining and flow cytometry. J Immunol Methods 1991; 139:271–279.
31. Imberti L, Sottini A, Bettinardi A, Puoti M, Primi D. Selective depletion in HIV infection of T cells that bear specific T cell receptor Vβ sequences. Science 1991; 254:860–862.
32. Jenkinson EJ, Kingston CA, Smith CA, Williams GT, Owen JJT. Antigen-induced apoptosis in developing T cells: a mechanism for negative selection of the TCR repertoire. Eur J Immunol 1989; 19:2175–2180.
33. Crabtree GR. Contingent genetic regulatory events in T lymphocyte activation. Science 1989; 243:355–361.
34. Lorentz RG, Allen PM. Thymic epithelial cells lack full capacity for antigen presentation. Nature 1989; 340:557–559.
35. McConkey DJ, Orrenius S, Jondal M. Cellular signaling in programmed cell death (apoptosis). Immunol Today 1990; 11:120–121.
36. Muller S, Richalet P, Laurent-Crawford A, Karakat S, Rivière Y, Porrot F, Chamaret S, Briand JP, Montagnier L, Hovanessian A. Presence in HIV-seropositive patients of autoantibodies typically found in non-organ specific autoimmune diseases. AIDS 1992; 6:933–942.
37. Fultz PN, Stricker RB, McClure HM, Anderson DC, Switzer WM, Horaist C. Humoral response to SIV/SMN infection in macaque and Mangabey monkeys. AIDS 1990; 3:319–329.
38. Laurent-Crawford AG, Krust B, Muller S, Riviè Y, Rey-Cuillé MA, Béchet JM, Montagnier L, Hovanessian A. The cytopathic effect of HIV is associated with apoptosis. Virology 1991; 185:829–839.

39. Terai C, Kornbluth, RS, Pauza CD, Richman DD, Carson DA. Apoptosis as a mechanism of cell death in cultured T lymphoblasts acutely infected with HIV-1. J Clin Invest 1991; 87:1710–1715.

40. Choi Y, Kappler JW, Marrack P. A superantigen encoding in the open reading frame of the 3' long terminal repeat of mouse mammary tumour virus. Nature 1991; 350:203–207.

41. Banda NK, Bernier J, Kurahara DK, Kurrle R, Haigwood N, Sekamy RP, Finkel TH. Crosslinking CD4 by human immunodeficiency virus gp120 primes T cells for activation-induced apoptosis. J Exp Med 1992; 176:1099–1106.

11

Immunological and Virological Mechanisms of CD4+ T-Cell Depletion

Frank Miedema, Linde Meyaard, Marijke Roos, Sigrid Otto, Thijs Tersmette, and Peter Schellekens

Central Laboratory of the Netherlands Red Cross Blood Transfusion Service and University of Amsterdam Amsterdam, The Netherlands

INTRODUCTION

There is ample evidence that in HIV-1-infected individuals the number of CD4+ lymphocytes in peripheral blood is the best prognostic marker for progression to AIDS (for review see Ref. 1). While clear cytopathic effects of HIV on CD4+ cells are observed in vitro, it is still not understood how HIV infection may result in massive CD4+ T-cell depletion in vivo. Direct cytopathic effects cannot account for CD4 depletion since only relatively few cells are productively infected. Therefore, research has concentrated on systemic effects of HIV infection through immunological mechanisms that may explain CD4-cell loss. In addition, it has been noted that CD4+ T-cell depletion may not in all cases be a slow, continuous, rather linear process, but may vary according to the type of HIV variant that is present in vivo, which is suggestive for a virus-induced mechanism of CD4 depletion. This chapter presents evidence for new im-munological (2) and virological mechanisms (3), and their possible con-tribution to CD4 depletion and immune dysfunction are discussed.

PROGRAMMED DEATH OF T CELLS IN HIV INFECTION

Programmed cell death (PCD), also known as apoptosis or activation-induced cell death, is a physiological mechanism of cell deletion that dif-fers morphologically and biochemically from necrosis. PCD has been de-scribed as playing a role in a wide variety of immunological regulatory processes. The process is characterized by a typical cellular morphology and degradation of the chromatin into discrete fragments that are multi-ples of about 190 base pairs of DNA.

Early in HIV infection, in clinically stable asymptomatic individuals, immunological abnormalities can already be demonstrated. HIV infection affects both CD4 + and CD8 + T-cell function, such as interleukin-2 pro-duction, and proliferation after stimulation with recall antigens and CD3 antibodies before CD4 + T-cell numbers are decreased (4,5). Early in in-fection, this T-cell nonresponsiveness is caused by a selective deletion of T-memory cells (6), which cannot be explained by direct HIV infection, since only 1 in 10,000 to 1 in 1000 T cells are infected (7). In addition to deletion of T-memory cells, in long-term infected persons an intrinsic non-responsiveness in both CD4 + and CD8 + cells is observed. We have pre-viously demonstrated that this defect is not at the level of induction of early activation events such as increased intracellular calcium concentra-tion and activation of protein kinase C (6).

PCD in PBMCs from HIV-Infected Individuals

We tested the hypothesis that T-cell nonresponsiveness in HIV infection is caused by PCD. We studied peripheral blood mononuclear cells (PBMCs) from 29 asymptomatic HIV-1-infected persons (CDC class II or III) selected for having normal CD4 + T-cell counts (mean 540/mm^3, range 320–880) but who had impaired reactivity to TCR/CD3-mediated stimulation (data not shown). After overnight culture transmission, elec-tron microscopy revealed extensive peripheral chromatin condensation and dilation of the endoplasmatic reticulum under the cell membrane but preservation of mitochondrial structures as features of PCD in PBMCs from an HIV-infected individual (Figure 1). Moreover, the DNA-cleavage pattern typical for PCD was observed in cultured PBMCs from HIV-in-

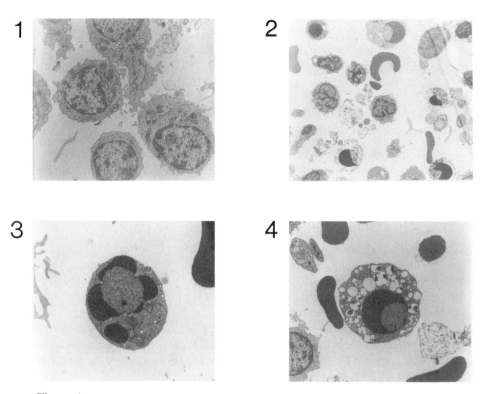

Figure 1 Transmission electron microscopy analysis of the typical morphological changes in cells undergoing PCD. PBMCs from a seronegative control (1) and PBMCs from an HIV-infected individual (2-4) were cultured overnight in the presence of CD3 antibodies.

fected individuals. The extent of DNA fragmentation was determined by a modification of the method of Sellins (8). High- and low-molecular-weight fractions from lysed cells were separated and the low-molecular-weight fraction, containing fragmented DNA, was subjected to gel electrophoresis. DNA fragments corresponding to 1-7 nucleosomes were identified by gel electrophoresis, but longer fragments were also detected, forming a smear in the gel near the origin of migration. In unstimulated cultures, DNA fragmentation was observed in none of the seronegative controls and in 15 of 29 of the HIV-infected men. After stimulation with anti-CD3 MAbs, PBMCs from all HIV-infected persons showed DNA fragmentation, compared with 14 of 37 seronegative controls. PBMCs from homosexual controls ($n = 8$) showed essentially the same pattern as those from heterosexual subjects. Zn^{2+}, known to inhibit endonucleases and DNA fragmentation in PCD, prevented the DNA fragmentation (data not shown), supporting the fact that the cells died due to PCD.

PCD Is Enhanced by CD3-Mediated Stimulation and Occurs in Both CD4+ and CD8+ Cells

Cells undergoing PCD can be labeled in in situ nick translation. Biotin-labeled nucleotides can be incorporated into the DNA of cells with DNA-strand breaks. This provides a specific and accurate method to determine the percentages of apoptotic cells (9). The results obtained from PBMCs from 34 asymptomatic HIV-infected individuals from the Amsterdam cohort, with CD4+ T-cell numbers ranging from 70 to 950/mm³, and 17 seronegative controls are shown in Figure 2. On culturing, PBMCs from HIV-infected individuals die in significantly higher percentages than PBMCs from seronegative controls. Up to 25% of the cells were apoptotic after stimulation with anti-CD3, which supports the data obtained by analysis of DNA fragmentation.

DNA fragmentation was observed in cell fractions highly enriched for either CD4+ or CD8+ cells (Figure 3). PCD therefore does not seem to be restricted to CD4+ cells, in agreement with reported nonresponsiveness in both CD4+ and CD8+ T cells.

HIV infection induces immune abnormalities, already at the asymptomatic stage. Here we demonstrate PCD-mediated T-cell depletion upon short term in vitro culture of PBMCs from asymptomatic HIV-infected men. Moreover, FACS analysis revealed that this cell death could be enhanced by in vitro polyclonal T-cell stimulation. These results suggest that the apparent T-cell nonresponsiveness in these persons may be explained, at least in part, by in vitro deletion of reactive cells by PCD, reflecting a process already induced in vivo.

With respect to the underlying mechanism by which T cells in HIV-infected men are nonresponsive to normal CD3/TCR activation signals, several alternatives may be envisaged. Because only a few cells are infected, a systemic effect of HIV proteins or disturbances of cytokine regulatory networks rather than direct viral infection are likely to be involved. Recently, it has been proposed that in HIV infection interaction of soluble gp120 with CD4, previously shown to lead to impaired lymphocyte function, would prime CD4+ T cells for PCD (10). This hypothesis is sup-

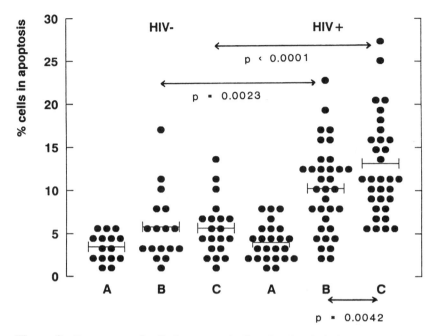

Figure 2 Percentage of cells in apoptosis directly after isolation (A) or after overnight culture in the absence (B) or presence (C) of CD3 antibodies. In PBMCs from 34 HIV-1-seropositive and 17 seronegative controls, percentages of apoptotic cells were determined by in situ nick translation (9). Percentages of apoptotic cells in HIV-infected individuals were significantly higher compared to those in controls as determined in the Mann-Whitney U-test. The increase by polyclonal stimulation of apoptosis in HIV-infected individuals was significant as determined by the Wilcoxon Matched-Pairs Signed-Ranks Test.

ported by results obtained with mature murine lymphocytes, which die of PCD after stimulation via TCR/CD3 when CD4 was previously cross-linked by anti-CD4 antibodies (11). CD4-gp120 ligation, however, is not likely to be the only mechanism to account for PCD in HIV infection, because it does not explain PCD observed in CD8 + cells. The CD8 + T-cell subset in HIV-infected individuals contains increased percentages of cells with phenotypes associated with activation, which are severely defective in their proliferative response to polyclonal activators and are reported to die in culture (12).

In our studies we observe apoptosis after stimulation with reagents that induce normal proliferative responses in lymphocytes from infected

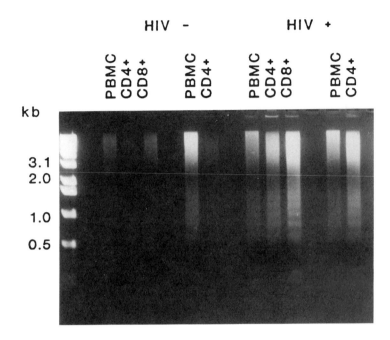

Figure 3   PCD of cells of HIV-1-infected individuals occurs in both the CD4 + and the CD8 + subset after overnight culture in the absence or presence of anti-CD3 antibodies.

men. This strongly indicates that low responsiveness to low-dose CD3 or to PWM is not simply caused by induction of PCD under those conditions and hence PCD is not the main cause of decreased T-cell function in vitro, as has been postulated by Ameisen and Capron (10).

In HIV infection, encountering antigen may cause a continuous PCD-mediated depletion of T cells in vivo. Compared to loss of memory cells due to direct HIV infection, which affects only small percentages of cells, PCD may be the principal mechanism for deletion of reactive T cells. In the early phase of infection, rapid-memory T-cell turnover initially is compensated for by increased T-cell renewal, reflected by phenotypic changes but relatively stable CD4 + numbers. Gradual deletion of immune regulatory T cells by PCD may contribute to the attenuation of the immune system, leading to emergence and high-rate replication of virulent HIV variants associated with rapid CD4 + cell decline and progression to AIDS (13).

BIPHASIC DECLINE OF CD4 + T CELLS DURING PROGRESSION TO AIDS CORRELATES WITH HIV PHENOTYPE

Longitudinal data on the rate of decline of CD4 + lymphocyte numbers in individuals who remained asymptomatic and who progressed to AIDS are relatively sparse (1,14,15). These studies show a low and constant rate of decline of CD4 + cells in groups of asymptomatic HIV-infected persons and a constant but more rapid loss of CD4 + cells in groups of persons who finally progress to AIDS. Phillips et al. (15) therefore concluded that differences in rate of decline of CD4 + lymphocytes, together with differences in CD4 + cell numbers at the time of infection, may account for the variation observed in the duration of the asymptomatic period. However, in a preliminary study we obtained evidence for differential rates of CD4 + cell decline associated with the presence of certain HIV biological variants (13). In particular, rapid CD4 + cell decline was observed in individuals with syncytium-inducing (SI), T-cell-line tropic HIV isolates. Since in general these isolates are not present from seroconversion on, but emerge in the course of HIV infection (16), one would predict a change in the rate of CD4 + cell decline that correlates with the appearance of SI variants.

To address this point, we prospectively followed the rate of CD4 + cell decline in 187 HIV-1-infected homosexual men over a period of 5 years, with emphasis on the period just before the diagnosis of AIDS. In 43 individuals of this cohort, the relationship between the rate of CD4 + cell decline and the phenotype of HIV-1 isolates was investigated. From October 1984 to March 1986, 961 homosexual men were enrolled into a prospective longitudinal study on risk factors for HIV infection and AIDS as previously described. In 238 men, antibodies to HIV-1 were present at the onset of the study. A series of at least three CD4 + lymphocyte counts was available for 198 of these 238 men. By January 1, 1990, AIDS had developed in 56 of the 198 men with at least three CD4 + cell counts. Patients with Kaposi's sarcoma, which may manifest at higher CD4 + lymphocyte counts than other AIDS-defining conditions ($n = 11$), were totally excluded from the analysis, leaving in the study 187 HIV-infected men, 45 of whom had developed AIDS. The phenotype of HIV-1 isolates was determined in 43 men—23 men aselectively chosen from the group who were still asymptomatic at the end of the study and 20 aselectively from the group who progressed to AIDS. As controls, 44 HIV-1-seronegative homosexual men were followed longitudinally during the same observation period.

At 3-monthly intervals, PBMCs were isolated from heparinized venous blood by density gradient centrifugation on Ficoll-Paque. Absolute numbers of CD4+ lymphocytes were determined by flow cytofluorometry. HIV-1 was recovered from cryopreserved, sequentially sampled, PBMCs as described before (17). Briefly, patient cells were repeatedly cocultivated with phytohemagglutinin (PHA)-prestimulated PBMCs from seronegative individuals in the presence of polybrene and IL-2, and cultures were screened for syncytium formation. Virus replication was detected by the testing of culture supernatants for HIV-1 p24 core antigen in a capture assay (17).

According to the in vitro properties, the isolates could be divided into three groups: first, SI isolates with high replication rates (detection of replication after 4–7 days of culture) that could be transmitted to the H9 T-cell line (SI); second, high-replicating non-SI isolates that could not be transmitted to the H9 cell line (Fast-NSI); and third, low-replicating (detection of replication after 9–28 days of culture) non-SI isolates that were not transmissible to the H9 cell line (Slow-NSI). When an SI variant was cultured, phenotyping was extended to samples obtained 1 and 2 years before the final sample.

CD4 Depletion Kinetics

The kinetics of CD4+ cell decline was analyzed in nonprogressors and progressors to AIDS during a 5-year follow-up. In nonprogressors during the follow-up period a continuous and steady decline of the mean number of CD4+ cells occurred, from a mean of $0.7 \times 10^9/L$ at 9 months to $0.4 \times 10^9/L$ at 54 months. In the same observation period, the CD4+ cell numbers in HIV-1-seronegative controls remained relatively stable. In progressors, until 18 months before AIDS diagnosis, the decline of CD4+ lymphocytes was slow and steady; however, from 18 months onward, when mean CD4+ cell numbers were about $0.4 \times 10^9/L$, the decline was much faster. At the time of diagnosis of AIDS, mean CD4+ cell numbers were $0.14 \times 10^9/L$ (10th–90th percentiles: 0.03×10^9–$0.31 \times 10^9/L$). To determine the rate of CD4+ lymphocyte decline, linear trend regression analysis was performed. Figure 4 shows the CD4 cell counts of progressors and nonprogressors with linear trend lines fitted through the data points of the nonprogressors, and through those of the progressors divided into periods before and after the 18-month time point preceding AIDS. The regression coefficients of these trend lines show that

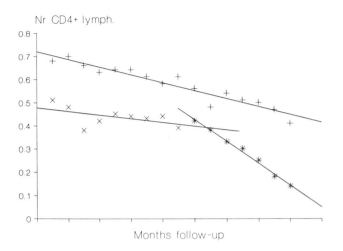

Figure 4   Linear trend lines of CD4 + cell decline in HIV-1-infected homosexual men. (Top) nonprogressors (+). (Bottom) progressors divided into two periods: (*) more than 18 months preceding AIDS diagnosis and (×) 18 months or less before diagnosis.

nonprogressors lose their CD4 + cells at a rate between 4.9 × 10⁶ and 6.9 × 10⁶/L/month. CD4 + cell decline in the progressors more than 18 months before diagnosis of AIDS is even slightly less (3.3 × 10⁶/L/month). However, in the last 18 months preceding diagnosis, the decline is 5 times faster (15.7 × 10⁶/L/month).

The regression coefficients of each single person in the three groups defined in Figure 4., i.e., nonprogressors and progressors before and after the 18-month time point, were determined. The rates of CD4 + cell loss in nonprogressors and progressors more than 18 months before AIDS diagnosis were similar. The median of CD4 + cell decline in nonprogressors was 5 × 10⁶/L/month. Progressors in the period more than 18 months preceding diagnosis lost 4 × 10⁶ CD4 + cells/L/month and in the period less than 18 months before diagnosis 17 × 10⁶ CD4 + cells/L/month. As expected, these cell losses differ only slightly from those calculated on the lines fitted to the means of the CD4 + cells per group. Apparently, as reflected in positive regression coefficients, CD4 + cell numbers remained stable in about 15–20% of the nonprogressors. In approximately 25% of the progressors, CD4 + cell decline in the period less than 18 months before diagnosis was similar to that in the asymptomatic group and in the progressor group more than 18 months preceding diagnosis. Less than 10% of the progressors did not show a decline in the period less

than 18 months preceding AIDS diagnosis; however, these men had significantly lower CD4 + cell numbers compared to those men who showed
declining cell numbers from 18 months onward (data not shown).

Association of CD4 + Cell Decline and HIV-1 Subtypes

Figure 5 shows box plots of the rates of CD4 + lymphocyte decline per
individual divided into groups according to HIV-1 biological phenotypes.
The median and range in the SI group was much lower than in the Fast-
NSI or Slow-NSI group ($p < 0.0005$). It appeared that the median and
range of CD4 + cell loss in individuals with SI variants were almost identical to those in progressors in the 18-month period before diagnosis.
The median of the Fast-NSI and Slow-NSI groups was in the range of
nonprogressors and of the progressors more than 18 months before diag-

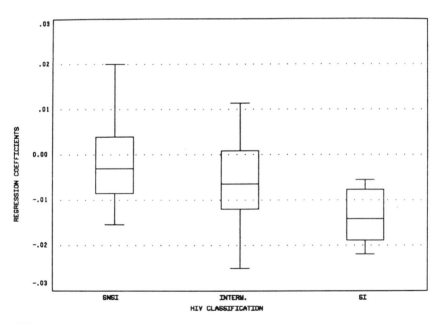

Figure 5 Box plots of regression coefficients of the linear trend lines fitted
through the CD4 + cell numbers of each individual, in which the time periods
were classified according to the presence of different HIV isolates. SNSI: time
period during which slow-growing non-SI isolates were present ($n = 16$). INTERM.:
time period during which fast-growing non-SI isolates were present ($n = 21$). SI:
time period during which SI isolates were present ($n = 14$).

nosis. When an SI type was present, there was always a loss of CD4+ cells, while a substantial part of individuals with Slow-NSI and Fast-NSI types did not lose these cells during the observation period.

Thus, over a period of 4.5 years, we observed in nonprogressing individuals a constant decline of 4.9×10^6 CD4+ lymphocytes/L/month, about the same magnitude as reported in the literature (15). However, when analyzing CD4+ cell depletion in persons who progressed to AIDS, at about 18 months before AIDS a "critical event" seems to occur, leading to a 3–5 times more rapid decline of CD4+ lymphocytes. Because around this point of time neither a change in the clinical condition of the individuals was observed nor indications were present for the occurrence of infections other than HIV-1, we hypothesized that a change in the behavior of HIV-1 might be responsible. This hypothesis was substantiated by the finding of a significant correlation between the fast decline of CD4+ cells and the presence of more virulent HIV-1 subtypes. These results, obtained in a large cohort of infected people, are compatible with a role for HIV biological variants in AIDS pathogenesis postulated before on a relatively small number of observations (13).

Our results demonstrate that, next to absolute numbers of CD4+ cells, the rate of CD4+ cell decline is a powerful prognostic marker for progression to AIDS. Therefore, fast-declining CD4+ cell numbers might be considered an additional treatment criterion for early therapy. However, a considerable overlap exists between the rate of decline in the group that will progress to AIDS in less than 18 months and that in both groups of nonprogressors and progressors more than 18 months before AIDS diagnosis. It appeared that, using CD4+ cell decline, progressors and nonprogressors can be distinguished only within 18 months before diagnosis of AIDS. To accurately assess the rate of decline, at least three time points over 6 months should be used. Calculation of decline over such a short period will result in even more overlap of rates of decline between groups of progressors and nonprogressors than in the current study. Besides, the period of time preceding AIDS will be reduced to a mere 9–12 months, which may prove to be late for the installation of antiretroviral treatment, e.g., with zidovudine.

This study confirms the importance of CD4+ cell numbers as a parameter for the immune status of HIV-infected individuals and as a short-term predictor for the progression to AIDS. However, it also emphasizes the need for addition, longer-term prognostic markers as criteria for early therapy. Next to such parameters as beta-2 microglobulin (18) and T-cell reactivity (19), biological phenotyping of HIV isolates may prove to be useful in this respect.

REFERENCES

1. Lange JMA, De Wolf F, Goudsmit J. Markers for progression in HIV infection. AIDS 1990; 3(suppl 1):153-160.
2. Meyaard L, Otto SA, Jonker R, Mijnster MJ, Keet RPM, Miedema F. Programmed death of T cells in HIV-1 infection. Science 1992; 257:217-219.
3. Schellekens PThA, Tersmette M, Roos M, et al. Biphasic rate of CD4+ cell decline during progression to AIDS correlates with HIV-1 phenotype. AIDS 1992; 6:665-669.
4. Miedema F, Petit AJC, Terpstra FG, et al. Immunological abnormalities in human immunodeficiency virus (HIV)-infected asymptomatic homosexual men. HIV affects the immune system before CD4+ T helper cell depletion occurs. J Clin Invest 1988; 82:1908-1914.
5. Gruters RA, Terpstra FG, De Jong R, Van Noesel CJM, Van Lier RAW, Miedema F. Selective loss of T-cell functions in different stages of HIV infection. Eur J Immunol 1990; 20:1039-1044.
6. Van Noesel CJM, Gruters RA, Terpstra FG, Schellekens PTA, Van Lier RAW, Miedema F. Functional and phenotypic evidence for a selective loss of memory T cells in asymptomatic HIV-infected men. J Clin Invest 1990; 86:293-299.
7. Schnittman SM, Psallidopoulos MC, Lane HC, et al. The reservoir for HIV-1 in human peripheral blood is a T cell that maintains expression of CD4. Science 1989; 245:305-308.
8. Sellins KS, Cohen JJ. Gene induction by γ-irradiation leads to DNA fragmentation in lymphocytes. J Immunol 1987; 139:3199-3206.
9. Jonker RR, et al. Detection of apoptosis using fluorescent *in situ* nick translation. In preparation.
10. Ameisen JC, Capron A. Cell dysfunction and depletion in AIDS: the programmed cell death hypothesis. Immunol Today 1991; 12:102-105.
11. Newell MK, Haughn LJ, Maroun CR, Julius MH. Death of mature T cells by separate ligation of CD4 and the T-cell receptor for antigen. Nature 1990; 347:286-288.
12. Prince HE, Jensen ER. HIV-related alterations in CD8 cell subsets defined by in vitro survival characteristics. Cell Immunol 1991; 134:276-286.
13. Tersmette M, Lange JMA, De Goede REY, et al. Association between biological properties of human immunodeficiency virus variants and risk for AIDS and AIDS mortality. Lancet 1989; i:983-985.
14. Eyster ME, Gail MH, Ballard JO, Al-Mondiry H, Goedert JJ. Natural history of human immunodeficiency virus infections in hemophiliacs: Effects of T-cell subsets, platelet counts, and age. Ann Intern Med 1987; 107:1-6.
15. Phillips AN, Lee CA, Elford J, et al. Serial CD4 lymphocyte counts and development of AIDS. Lancet 1991; 337:389-392.

16. Tersmette M, Gruters RA, De Wolf F, et al. Evidence for a role of virulent HIV variants in the pathogenesis of AIDS obtained from studies on a panel of sequential HIV isolates. J Virol 1989; 63:2118–2125.

17. Tersmette M, De Goede REY, Al BJM, et al. Differential syncytium-inducing capacity of human immunodeficiency virus isolates: frequent detection of syncytium-inducing isolates in patients with acquired immunodeficiency syndrome (AIDS) and AIDS-related complex. J Virol 1988; 62:2026–2032.

18. Fahey JL, Taylor JM, Detels R. The prognostic value of cellular and serologic markers in infection with human immunodeficiency virus type 1. N Engl J Med 1990; 322:166–172.

19. Schellekens PTA, Roos MTL, De Wolf F, Lange JMA, Miedema F. Low T-cell responsiveness to activation via CD3/TCR is a prognostic marker for AIDS in HIV-1 infected men. J Clin Immunol 1990; 10:121–127.

12

T-Cell-Receptor Repertoire in AIDS: New Insights Into the Pathogenesis of the Disease

Luisa Imberti, Alessandra Sottini, Alessandra Bettinardi, Cinzia Mazza, and Daniele Primi

Consiglio Nazionale delle Ricerche (CNR)
Institute of Chemistry
School of Medicine
University of Brescia
Brescia, Italy

INTRODUCTION

The enormous progress achieved in recent years toward understanding HIV's complex molecular biology has not been a determinant condition for resolving the central enigma of AIDS: the mechanism by which the infection leads to the almost complete elimination of CD4 + T cells. The interaction between gp120, the external envelope glycoprotein of HIV, and the CD4 molecule is a crucial event for T-cell infection, but it is indubitable that the progressive loss of CD4 lymphocytes during disease progression cannot be accounted for solely by the direct cytopathicity of HIV, since only a minority of these cells harbors the infecting virus (1,2).

Furthermore, the cytopathic effect of HIV described in in vitro studies does not fully explain the long time of virus latency (3,4), the fact that infected chimpanzees do not develop AIDS (5), and the reason that herpes virus HHV-6, which also infects and kills CD4 + cells in vitro (6), does not induce AIDS symptoms in vivo.

Several other mechanisms have been proposed over the years to explain CD4 + cell depletion, including immunosuppression (7), clonal deletion (7), syncyzia formation between infected and uninfected cells, and, last, selective infection and destruction of memory T cells (8). Cell dysfunction and depletion have thus been related to a wide range of different, and often contradictory, mechanisms. Recent developments in this area of research have provided new evidence suggesting, for instance, that cross-reaction between viral proteins and self-components may result in autoimmune processes triggered by HIV (9–11).

A different view of the immunodepletion occurring in AIDS has recently emerged following the observation that the loss of CD4 + cells in HIV-infected patients is associated with lymphocyte activation. Activation, however, does not result in cell proliferation but rather in cell death, through a mechanism known as programmed cell death, or apoptosis (12, 13). This is clearly a very important finding that opens new lines of research. It is known that apoptosis is the result of complex molecular physiological and pathological mechanisms, but the nature of the triggering signals starting the cascade of molecular events that eventually lead to cell death during HIV infection is still unclear.

Here we describe our current views on the mechanisms by which HIV may induce apoptosis in uninfected cells.

T-CELL DEPLETION IN AIDS IS
NOT A RANDOM PHENOMENON

There are currently two hypotheses accounting for a role of apoptosis in the pathogenesis of AIDS. The first one states that, during HIV infection, apoptosis can be induced by inappropriate delivery of activating signals (12). The gp120, gp120-antibody anti-gp120 immune complexes or anti-CD4 autoantibodies can all interact with CD4, and this interaction, in the absence of costimulatory signals, may result in active cell suicide processes of widespread biological importance. Thus, the rate of in vivo cell depletion would depend on the level of circulating CD4 ligands rather than on the number of infected lymphocytes.

The second hypothesis was formulated after the discovery that endogenous superantigens are encoded by the open reading frame within the 3' long terminal repeat of mouse mammary tumor viruses (MMTV) (14–19). Superantigens differ from conventional antigens in that they selectively interact with MHC class II and Vβ polypeptide chains of the T-cell receptor (TcR) (20–23). Thus, each superantigen has a characteristic affinity for a set of Vβ elements and stimulates virtually all T cells bearing those elements, regardless of their antigenic specificity. Following an initial proliferation, superantigen-driven T cells paradoxically become anergic and eventually die (24–28). It has been proposed that HIV might cause, in conjunction with class II genes, cell anergy and depletion of uninfected CD4+ T cells, by encoding a superantigen expressed on activated infected cells (29). The hypothesis also states that the progression of CD4+ T-cell depletion requires cycles of mutation in the retroviral superantigen gene(s), resulting in the elimination of CD4+ T cells bearing different Vβs over time. A variation of this latter theory is that molecules with superantigenic properties may be carried by opportunistic bacteria, including mycoplasma that appear to be a cofactor for AIDS.

The main difference between the two postulates is that the first one implies that the loss of CD4 in AIDS patients is a random phenomenon, while the second one suggests that T-cell depletion is strictly a Vβ-selective process.

Results recently obtained in our laboratory (30) are rather compatible with the latter hypothesis. The analysis of TcR-variable regions revealed that the Vα repertoire expressed by six AIDS patients was similar to that of normal healthy individuals, suggesting that Vα segments are not specifically involved in the phenomena leading to cell elimination. The Vβ repertoire of the same cells, on the other hand, was characterized by the lack of expression of several Vβ-family-specific genes and by the random absence of other Vβ elements. In the same study we observed that patients with long history of HIV infection but without signs of opportunistic infections also displayed important alterations in their TcR Vβ repertoire.

This latter observation suggests that the abnormalities of the T-cell repertoire are related to HIV itself and not to the secondary effects of opportunistic infection. The data also indicate that, in the course of HIV infection, CD4+ cells are not randomly deleted and that the nature of the TcR Vβ gene expressed on the surface of a given cell may strongly influence its final fate. A corollary of this finding is that the delivery of signals through the T-cell receptor is a determinant event for cell death in

AIDS. Thus, an understanding of the nature of these signals is essential for full comprehension of the pathogenesis of this disease.

IS AN HIV-ENCODED SUPERANTIGEN RESPONSIBLE FOR CELL DELETION IN AIDS?

In considering the possible mechanisms responsible for alteration of the TcR Vβ repertoire, our first selection was the action of a superantigen. This choice was almost inevitable because of the current knowledge of the genetic and biological effects of these substances. Given the implication of this possibility for understanding the pathogenesis of the disease, it is essential to consider which of the HIV genes might encode for such a putative superantigen. It is difficult to predict the biological property of a protein on the sole basis of structural information and, therefore, the eventual characterization of a putative HIV-encoded superantigen will be achieved only by directly testing the biological properties of all HIV-encoded proteins. Theoretical considerations, however, may help to restrict the field of the most likely candidates.

Recently, Haase et al. (31) proposed that the product of the *nef* gene has several characteristics that make it the HIV-encoded protein most likely to behave as a superantigen. This gene has been believed to encode for a regulatory negative factor, but later studies cast doubts on this hypothesis. *nef* is strikingly reminiscent of the mammary tumor virus superantigen, which is encoded by a gene—also located at the 3′ end of the viral genome—called *naf* (for negative acting factor of transcription). Both genes display a modest effect on transcription in vitro, but *naf* clearly acts as a superantigen. This may be an important evolutionary function for a gene whose role in the life cycle of the mammary tumor virus has been controversial.

As pointed out by Haase et al. (31), *nef* is not necessary for viral growth in vitro, but it is essential for maintaining high virus loads and for the development of AIDS in the simian model. Simian immunodeficiency virus (SIV), derived from molecular clones in which *nef* cannot be transcribed, is virtually indistinguishable in vitro, but only SIV with a transcriptional open reading frame in *nef* replicates in vivo, and it is fully pathogenic. Moreover, monkeys inoculated with SIV derived from clones in which *nef* was deleted remain healthy.

The *nef* gene has an additional property required for a putative superantigen-encoding gene. It is one of the lentivirus genes that evolves largely by mutation at extraordinarily rapid rates. This hypervariability in *nef* could spawn the many different *nef* mutants required to eliminate helper T cells with different Vβ specificities. It is also important to underline that only the primate lentiviruses (HIV and SIV) have a *nef* gene, and these lentiviruses are also the only ones that clearly, by themselves, cause immunodeficiency. Other animal lentiviruses, such as visna, that have similar genomes but lack *nef*, cause infections that resemble those caused by primate lentiviruses in every respect, except that immune function remains intact.

On the basis of all the abovementioned evidence, Haase et al. (31) have proposed that *nef* is the most likely candidate, among the HIV-encoded proteins, to behave as a superantigen. This hypothesis clearly provides an interesting model that apparently should be easy to verify experimentally. It may turn out, however, that direct evidence for an HIV-encoded superantigen may not be so easy to obtain, because of alterations of the secondary structures of recombinant proteins that may modify their natural biological activity. Thus, the idea that an HIV-encoded superantigen plays a major role in the pathogenesis of HIV remains, for the moment, an interesting hypothesis that still requires direct experimental support.

It is important to emphasize that our results do not exclude the possibility that exogenous superantigens may also play a key role in the progression of the disease. This hypothesis has recently received experimental support from the finding that gp120, HLA class I (32), and some exogenous superantigens share a very short sequence motif that encodes an epitope recognized by a monoclonal antibody (L31). Interestingly, the L31 monoclonal antibody was obtained by immunizing a BALB/c mouse with recombinant gp120 protein (32).

Direct binding experiments demonstrated that the L31 monoclonal antibody recognizes not only gp120, but also the superantigen *Staphylococcus* enterotoxin B (SEB). Furthermore, we could also demonstrate that the simultaneous incubation of peripheral blood mononuclear cells (PBMCs) obtained from healthy donors with 100 ng/ml of SEB (which in soluble form does not display a stimulatory activity) and L31 resulted in vigorous cell proliferation, similar to that obtained with cultures triggered by insolubilized SEB. The selective involvement of TcR in the activation mediated by L31 was clearly demonstrated by cytofluorimetric analysis with anti-TcR Vβ monoclonal antibodies. The T-cell population triggered by insolubilized SEB was strongly enriched in Vβ12 molecules as compared to the population of resting cells. The same type of enrichment was also obtained with T cells triggered by the combined effect of soluble SEB and L31, suggesting that the monoclonal antibody acts by enhancing the triggering potential of SEB, probably by cross-linking it on the T-cell surface.

Although these experiments concerned only one superantigen (SEB), they raise the intriguing possibility that the immune response directed against HIV proteins may potentiate the effect of exogenous superantigens that may be normally circulating in the body at physiological concentrations.

INTERACTIONS OF gp120 WITH T-CELL SURFACE MOLECULES

Although the evidence that HIV-infected patients have profound alterations in the TcR Vβ repertoire can be easily explained by the action of a superantigen, we also considered alternative mechanisms that may explain equally well the biased Vβ repertoire observed in HIV-infected patients.

In 1990 Newell et al. (33) demonstrated that signaling through the variable regions of the TcR complex results in T-cell death by apoptosis if preceded by ligation of CD4. This experimental model may reflect the conditions that occur in vivo in the course of HIV infection. The high affinity of gp120 for CD4 is well documented, while the nature of the ligand for TcR Vβ segments is only speculative. We considered the possibility that gp120 can, besides binding to CD4 with high affinity, interact, perhaps with lower affinity, with some TcR Vβ segments. The CD4 cells expressing those particular Vβ genes will therefore die by apoptosis through a mechanism similar to the one described by Newell et al., as a direct consequence of the double engagement of their CD4 and TcR molecules (Figure 1).

To prove the validity of this hypothesis, it was necessary to demonstrate that gp120 can bind to particular Vβ elements. We therefore designed an in vitro experiment that directly addressed this problem. First, PBMCs from healthy individuals were activated with the superantigens SEE, SEB, and SEC2, which selectively expand those cells bearing Vβ regions for which specific monoclonal antibodies are available. After 3 days of culturing, the activated cells were washed and incubated overnight with or without various doses of insolubilized gp120. Flow cytometric analysis with fluorescein-labeled antibodies specific for Vβ5, Vβ6, Vβ8, and Vβ12 revealed that preincubation with gp120 resulted in membrane downmodulation of some, but not all, Vβ segments and that the phenomenon was dependent strictly on the concentration of gp120 added to the cultures. Interestingly, different Vβ segments were modulated in cell samples deriving from different donors, suggesting that polymorphic structures may be involved in this interaction.

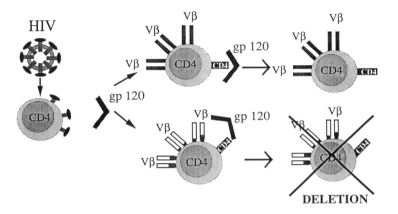

Figure 1   Putative model of interaction between gp120 and Vβ elements. The double engagement of gp120 with particular Vβ chains and CD4 molecules may result in apoptosis, while the interaction of gp120 with CD4 only is not sufficient to provoke programmed cell suicide.

In a second series of experiments, PBMCs were first incubated overnight with or without gp120 and, after being washed, were recultured for 5 days in the presence of SEE, SEB, and SEC2. Flow cytometric analysis using fluoresceined anti-Vβ antibodies revealed that, in some samples, preincubation with gp120 favored the expansion of those cells bearing Vβ6 and Vβ8 but not of those bearing Vβ5 and Vβ12.

Taken together, these observations raise the intriguing possibility that some Vβ segments may act as a coreceptor for gp120. The existence of a second receptor for HIV has been inferred from several instances of indirect evidence but, up to now, the biochemical characterization of such a receptor has been very elusive. If some Vβ segments turn out to be natural low-affinity ligands for gp120, then this second receptor will be easily characterized, first by its selective clonal distribution—in contrast to CD4, which is polyclonally expressed—and second by the low affinity of its interaction with gp120. Most important, if the interaction of Vβ segments with the HIV envelope protein is demonstrated by other experimental data, many still-obscure aspects of the pathogenetic effects of HIV infections will become much more understandable. In particular, it will be possible not only to gain new knowledge about the pathogenetic mechanisms of HIV, but also to design more efficient strategies for immunointervention and vaccines.

AUTOIMMUNITY AND TcR

Any theory accounting for depletion of self-components cannot ignore a possible involvement of autoimmune events. Autoimmunity against CD4 (34–36) and MHC (9,32,37) products in the course of HIV infection is a well-documented phenomenon that may account for some of the pathogenic effects of AIDS. The presence of autoantibodies reacting with non-clonally distributed molecules, however, cannot easily explain the restricted T-cell repertoire alterations observed in AIDS patients. We therefore considered the possibility that the immune response against HIV proteins may induce cross-reactive antibodies capable of interacting with particular Vβ elements. The production of such autoantibodies will lead to death by apoptosis of those CD4 cells that express the relevant Vβ genes and have already been in contact with gp120 (Figure 2).

A comparison of the amino acid sequences of gp120 and the known human TcR segments recently carried out in our laboratory has revealed that gp120 shares common motifs with some Vβ genes. Interestingly,

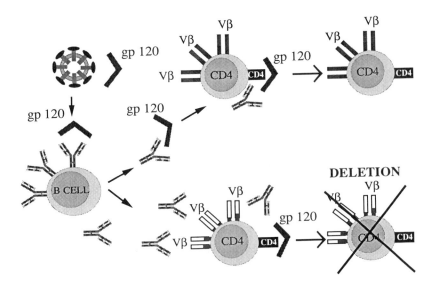

Figure 2 Putative mechanism of cell death induced by anti-TcR Vβ antibodies. The binding of anti-Vβ cross-reactive antibodies with cells that have already been in contact with gp120 may lead to apoptosis.

some of these motifs map in the most potentially antigenic region of the relevant Vβ segments. On the basis of this evidence, we constructed a first series of peptides corresponding to the putative immunogenic regions of Vβ4, Vβ19, and Vβ20, and we combined them with sera obtained from normal donors and from HIV-infected patients. Immunoreactivity against these peptides was preferentially found in several sera of AIDS patients, and the specificity of these reactions was verified by inhibition experiments with the homologous peptides.

Furthermore, we have recently obtained a monoclonal antibody specific for the Vβ4 peptide. Immunofluorescence experiments demonstrated that this antibody selectively reacts with T cells expressing the Vβ4 gene product, therefore demonstrating that the peptide mimics a Vβ4 epitope that is exposed on the native molecule. Interestingly, the culturing of PBMCs from normal donors in the presence of the antipeptide monoclonal antibody resulted in the selective expansion and growth of Vβ4-positive T cells.

Taken collectively, these results suggest that an important component of the immune response against gp120 is characterized by cross-reactive antibodies capable of interacting with particular Vβ segments. The consequence of these interactions, in association with the binding of gp120 to CD4, may be the selective expansion or deletion of those cells expressing the Vβ recognized by the cross-reactive antibodies. The real potential of this mechanism in promoting cell death is just beginning to be revealed, and to be fully appreciated it will be necessary to wait for the availability of a complete panel of Vβ recombinant proteins.

CONCLUSIONS

We have reviewed some of our opinions about the mechanisms responsible for the pathogenesis of AIDS. Some of the arguments presented are still highly speculative, but they are all based on our conviction that the disease is probably not caused by an unique mechanism but, on the contrary, by several pathological events acting together in synergy. We have considered the existence of a virus-induced superantigen, the possibility that gp120 may interact with both CD4 and some Vβ elements, and, finally, the existence of autoantibodies directed against TcR-variable regions. The common denominator of our speculations is the alteration of the TcR Vβ repertoire observed in AIDS patients that leads us to believe that this receptor molecule may play a previously unsuspected role in the development of the disease. If the TcR becomes a new protagonist on the AIDS scene, it is possible that a better understanding of the interplay between HIV and the TcR molecule may finally provide the missing link in the complete understanding of the pathogenesis of AIDS.

ACKNOWLEDGMENTS

This work was supported by Sorin Biomedica and the V Progetto AIDS of the Istituto Superiore di Sanità.

REFERENCES

1. Schnittman SM, Psallidopoulos MC, Lane HC, Thompson L, Baseler M, Massari F, Fox CH, Salzman NP, Fauci AS. The reservoir for HIV-1 in human peripheral blood is a T cell that maintains expression of CD4. Science 1989; 245:305–308.
2. Brinchmann JE, Albert J, Vartdal F. Few infected CD4$^+$ T cells but a high proportion of replication-competent provirus copies in an asymptomatic HIV-1 infection. J Virol 1991; 65:2019–2024.
3. Medley GF, Anderson RM, Cox DR, Billard L. Incubation period of AIDS in patients infected via blood transfusion. Nature 1987; 328:719–721.
4. Lui KJ, Darrow WW, Rutherford GW III. Model-based estimate of the mean incubation period for AIDS in homosexual men. Science 1988; 240:1333–1335.
5. Watanabe M, Ringler DJ, Fultz P, Mackey JJ, Boyson JE, Levine CG, Letvin NL. A chimpanzee-passaged human immunodeficiency virus isolate is cytopathic for chimpanzee cells but does not induce disease. J Virol 1991; 65:3344–3348.
6. Lusso P, Ensoli P, Markham PD, Ablashi DV, Salahuddin SZ, Tschachler E, Wong-Staal F, Gallo RC. Productive dual infection of human CD4 lymphocytes by HIV-1 and HHV-6. Nature 1989; 337:370–373.
7. Fauci AS. The human immunodeficiency virus: infectivity and mechanisms of pathogenesis. Science 1988; 239:617–622.
8. Van Noesel CJM, Gruters RA, Terpstra FG, Schellekens TPA, van Lier RAW, Miedema F. Functional and phenotypic evidence for a selective loss of memory T cells in asymptomatic human immunodeficiency virus-infected men. J Clin Invest 1990; 86:293–299.
9. Kion TA, Hoffmann GW. Anti-HIV and anti-anti-MHC antibodies in allo-immune and autoimmune mice. Science 1991; 253:1138–1140.
10. Stott EJ. Anti-cell antibody in macaques. Nature 1991; 353.
11. Langlois AJ, Weinhold KJ, Matthews TJ, Greenberg ML, Bolognesi DP. The ability of certain SIV vaccines to provoke reactions against normal cells. Nature 1992; 255:292–293.

12. Ameisen JC, Capron A. Cell dysfunction and depletion in AIDS: the programmed cell death hypothesis. Immunol Today 1991; 4:102–105.
13. Groux H, Torpier G, Monté D, Mouton Y, Capron A, Ameisen JC. Activation-induced death by apoptosis in CD4$^+$ T cells from human immunodeficiency virus-infected asymptomatic individuals. J Exp Med 1992; 175:331–340.
14. Acha-Orbea H, Shakhov AN, Scarpellino L, Kolb E, Muller V, Vessaz-Shaw A, Fuchs R, Blochlinger K, Rollini P, Billotte, J Sarafidou M, MacDonald HR, Diggelmann H. Clonal deletion of Vβ14-bearing T cells in mice transgenic for mammary tumour virus. Nature 1991; 350:207–211.
15. Choi Y, Kappler JW, Marrack P. A superantigen encoded in the open reading frame of the 3′ long terminal repeat of mouse mammary tumour virus. Nature 1991; 350:203–207.
16. Dyson PJ, Knight AM, Fairchild S, Simpson E, Tomonari K. Genes encoding ligands for deletion of Vβ11 T cells cosegregate with mammary tumour virus genomes. Nature 1991; 349:531–532.
17. Frankel WN, Rudy C, Coffin JM, Huber BT. Linkage of Mls genes to endogenous mammary tumour viruses of inbred mice. Nature 1991; 349:526–528.
18. Marrack P, Kushnir E, Kappler J. A maternally inherited superantigen encoded by a mammary tumour virus. Nature 1991; 349:524–526.
19. Woodland DL, Happ MP, Gollob KJ, Palmer E. An endogenous retrovirus mediating deletion of αβ T cells? Nature 1991; 349:529–530.
20. Fleischer B, Schrezenmeier H. T cell stimulation by Staphylococcal enterotoxins. Clonally variable response and requirement for major histocompatibility complex class II molecules on accessory or target T cells. J Exp Med 1988; 167:1697–1707.
21. Janeway CA Jr, Yagi J, Conrad PJ, Katz ME, Jones B, Vroegop S, Buxser S. T-cell responses to Mls and to bacterial proteins that mimic its behavior. Immunol Rev 1989; 107:61–88.
22. Choi Y, Herman A, DiGiusto D, Wade T, Marrack P, Kappler J. Residues of the variable region of the T-cell-receptor β-chain that interact with S. aureus toxin superantigens. Nature 1990; 346:471–473.
23. Pullen AM, Wade T, Marrack P, Kappler JW. Identification of the region of T cell receptor β chain that interacts with the self-superantigen Mls-1a. Cell 1990; 61:1365–1374.
24. Kappler JW, Staerz U, White J, Marrack P. Self-tolerance eliminates T cells specific for Mls-modified products of the major histocompatibility complex. Nature 1988; 332:35–40.
25. MacDonald HR, Pedrazzini T, Schneider R, Louis JA, Zinkernagel RM, Hengartner H. Intrathymic elimination of Mlsa-reactive (Vβ6 +) cells during neonatal tolerance induction to Mlsa-encoded antigens. J Exp Med 1988; 167:2005–2010.

26. White J, Herman A, Pullen AM, Kubo R, Kappler JW, Marrack P. The Vβ-specific superantigen staphylococcal enterotoxin B: stimulation of mature T cells and clonal deletion in neonatal mice. Cell 1989; 56:27-35.
27. Janeway CA Jr. Self-superantigens? Cell 1990; 63:659-661.
28. Marrack P, Kappler J. The staphylococcal enterotoxins and their relatives. Science 1990; 248:705-711.
29. Janeway C. Mls: makes a little sense. Nature 1991; 349:459-461.
30. Imberti L, Sottini A, Bettinardi A, Puoti M, Primi D. Selective depletion in HIV infection of T cells that bear specific T cell receptor Vβ sequences. Science 1991; 254:860-862.
31. Haase AT, Jenkins MK, Peng H, Urdahl K. nef-naf nexus? Curr Biol 1992; 2:130-132.
32. Grassi F, Meneveri R, Gullberg M, Lopalco L, Rossi GB, Lanza P, De Santis C, Brattsand G, Buttò S, Ginelli E, Beretta A, Siccardi AG. Human immuno-deficiency virus type 1 gp120 mimics a hidden monomorphic epitope borne by class I major histocompatibility complex heavy chains. J Exp Med 1991; 174:53-62.
33. Newell K, Haughn LJ, Maroun CR, Julius MH. Death of mature T cells by separate ligation of CD4 and T-cell receptor for antigen. Nature 1990; 347:286-289.
34. Wilks D, Walker LC, Habeshaw JA, Youle M, Gazzard B, Dalgleish AG. Anti-CD4 autoantibodies and screening for anti-idiotypic antibodies to anti-CD4 monoclonal antibodies in HIV-seropositive people. AIDS 1990; 4:113-118.
35. Sekigawa I, Groopmen JE, Allan JD, Ikeuki K, Biberfield G, Takatsui K, Byrn RA. Characterization of autoantibodies to the CD4 molecule in human immunodeficiency virus infection. Clin Immunol Immunopathol 1991; 58:145-153.
36. Weimer R, Daniel V, Zimmermann R, Schimpf K, Opelz G. Autoantibodies against CD4 cells are associated with CD4 helper defects in human immuno-deficiency virus-infected patients. Blood 1991; 77:133-140.
37. Golding H, Robey FA, Gates FT III, Linder W, Beining PR, Hoffman T, Golding B. Identification of homologous region in human immunodeficiency virus 1 gp41 and human MHC class II β 1 domain. J Exp Med 1988; 167:914-923.

13

Expression of Heat-Shock Proteins in HIV-1 Infection

Fabrizio Poccia, Roberta Placido, Giorgio Mancino, Francesca Mariani, Lucia Ercoli, Silvia Di Cesare, and Vittorio Colizzi
University of Rome "Tor Vergata"
Rome, Italy

INTRODUCTION

The human immunodeficiency virus (HIV) was identified as the etiological agent of acquired immunodeficiency syndrome (AIDS) some years ago; nevertheless the pathogenesis of the disease is still unclear. The main question remains how the presence of HIV genome in a minority of cells can lead to the progressive destruction of the immune system.

The finding that other T-cell-cytopathic viruses, e.g., HHV-6, do not cause immunodeficiency in infected hosts (1) together with the observation that HIV-infected chimpanzees support HIV growth but do not develop AIDS (2) had led to the speculation that factors other than virus-induced cytopathogenicity may be involved in the massive T-cell depletion observed in AIDS. The possibility that HIV proteins and other exogenous and endogenous cofactors may contribute to altering of the T-cell signaling, causing "unphysiological" activation of the immune system with subsequent T-cell depletion, has been recently discussed (3). In fact, several—but no mutually exclusive—hypotheses on mechanisms by which T-cell loss occurs in AIDS has been proposed, namely: cofactor and apoptosis (4), graft-versus-host and alloepitope (5), superantigen and T-cell-receptor (TcR) depletion (6,7), and autoimmunity and idiotypic network (8,9).

In this chapter, we present recent data on the expression of heat-shock proteins (HSPs) in the course of HIV infection, and discuss the role of HSPs in AIDS pathogenesis. The major finding in preliminary experiments was the surface expression of HSPs on HIV-infected cells in vitro (10). This observation was considered surprising as HSPs are cytoplasmatic and nuclear molecules, which only a few reports have shown to be also localized on the cell membrane (11,12). The evidence that HSPs are expressed on the membrane of HIV-infected cells prompted us to investigate in more detail their role as immunological targets, also raising the question of the involvement of HSPs as endogenous cofactors responsible for HIV-induced T-cell activation.

PHYSIOPATHOLOGY OF HSP

HSPs are a family of highly conserved molecules that play an important physiological role in folding and unfolding of proteins and are overexpressed under conditions of stress (13). They are encoded inside the major histocompatibility complex (MHC) genes (14), bind antigenic peptides (15,16), and show a secondary structure similar to the antigen-binding domain of MHC class I and II molecules (17,18). HSPs also represent superantigens and autoantigens involved in the induction of several autoimmune diseases (19), resulting from cross-reactivity between host HSPs and the HSPs of infecting organisms. These molecules are relevant antigens recognized by T cells carrying both the $\alpha\beta$ and the $\gamma\delta$ TcR, the latter shown to be increased in AIDS patients, suggesting their activation by HSPs (20,21).

HSP synthesis is strictly related to cell cycle and oncogene activation (22). In fact, myc-overexpressing cells show viral myc-proteins nuclearly colocalized with nuclear HSP70 (23). It has also been reported that the adenoviral E1a product induces HSP70 family synthesis by acting as a transcriptional activator, but it is not yet clear whether increased levels of HSP may facilitate tumoral and viral proliferation (24). HSP70 is able to bind to mutant p53, and the stability of this interaction was proposed as influencing transformation (25). Normal p53 acts as a "molecular policeman,'' monitoring the integrity of the genome. If DNA is damaged, p53 accumulates and switches off replication to allow extra time for its repair. If the repair fails, p53 may trigger cell suicide by apoptosis (26). Tumor cells in which p53 is inactivated by mutation, or by binding to host or viral proteins, cannot carry out this function. HSPs are also tumor-associated antigens (11), and we recently described the recognition and killing of tumor cells expressing surface HSP65 with specific immunotoxin containing saporin (27).

Moreover, the production of HSPs is increased by microbial and viral infection. In humans, antibodies and T cells directed against HSP65 can be isolated from persons infected with *M. leprae* or *M. tuberculosis* (28). The infection with HSV-2 induces HSP90 expression at cytoplasmic and membrane levels (12,29). Simian virus and polyoma virus (30) induce HSP synthesis as well as paramyxoviruses (31), vescicular stomatitis virus (32), and Newcastle virus (33). HSP expression during adenoviral infection seems to be mediated by transcriptional activation of HSPs at the genomic level (34). All these observations show that cell response to different pathological situations consists in an increase of HSP synthesis and that surface expression of these molecules is a characteristic signal for altered/damaged cells.

MEMBRANE EXPRESSION OF HSPs ON CELLS INFECTED WITH HIV-1

We recently reported that T cells chronically infected with HIV express abnormal levels of membrane HSP72 (10). The membrane expression of HSPs on the H9 cell infected with HIV has been documented using flow cytometric analysis, antibody-dependent cell-mediated cytotoxicity (ADCC), and an in vitro binding method using immunotoxin specific for HSP65 (27). A panel of monoclonal antibodies (MAbs) has been used for cell-surface staining in indirect immunofluorescence. MAb H60.15 is an IgG_{2b} that recognizes a 28-kDa protein from *M. tuberculosis* and cross-reacts with 12 other species of mycobacteria except *M. leprae* but does not react with proteins of other bacteria (35). MAb ML30 (IgG_1) recognizes amino acids 275–295 of the 65-kDa HSP from *M. leprae, M. tuberculosis,* and other species of mycobacteria and cross-reacts with human HSP65 (36,37). MAb H105 (IgG_1) recognizes an epitope in the region of amino acids from 20 to 54 in the sequence of the 65-kDa recombinant protein from *M. leprae* (35). HSP72 has been detected by using the monoclonal antibody RPN 1197 of IgG_1 class (Amersham) that specifically recognizes human HSP72 and the HSP72/73 Ab-1 (oncogene) that reacts with HSP72/73 of mammalian cells.

The second step of labeling was performed using a fluorescein-conjugated goat anti-mouse antibody, and cells were analyzed using a FACScan (Becton Dickinson). As can be seen in Figure 1, no or very few uninfected cells were positive for membrane fluorescence with anti-HSP72 MAb, while a net increase was observed after HIV infection. As positive control we used heat-treated H9 cells. The membrane expression of HSP28 has been investigated during the acute infection of H9 cells by flow cytometry using a MAb specific for HSP28. A significant surface expression of HSP28 could be observed after 2 days, becoming more relevant 7–10 days after infection (Figure 2). A similar kinetic curve of HSP65 membrane expression after HIV infection has been detected using an immunotoxin anti-HSP65 (Poccia et al., in preparation).

Evaluation of ADCC was performed using a 4-hour ^{51}chromium-release assay. Effector cells consisted of peripheral blood mononuclear cells (PBMCs) obtained from healthy donors, isolated by density-gradient centrifugation on Ficoll Hypaque. Uninfected, heat-shock-treated, and HIV-infected H9 cells showed similar spontaneous release. For ADCC

Figure 1 Cytofluorimetric analysis of HSP72 expression on the membrane of HIV-infected H9 cells. The HTLV-IIIB strain derived from H9/HTLV-III$_B$ cells was used to infect cells in vitro. Flasks containing 10^7 cells were incubated 4 hours with stock virus. HIV-1 replication was assessed by monitoring cultures for viral cytopathic effect (multinucleated giant cell formation) and p24 antigen production (HIV-1 EIA, Abbott Laboratories, North Chicago, IL). The percentage of productively infected cells was determined by indirect immunofluorescence for gp120 antigen using anti-gp120 monoclonal antibodies (M38, Biosoft, Paris).

For cytofluorimetric analysis, cells were resuspended in 100 ml of PBS with 1% FCS and incubated with the first antibody (anti-HSP) for 30 minutes at 4°C. Cells were then centrifuged, washed twice, and incubated for 30 minutes in the presence of the second antibody, consisting of FITC-conjugated goat anti-mouse IgG$_1$ (GAM-Zymed). Intensity of fluorescence was analyzed with a flow cytometer (FACScan, Becton Dickinson). Fluorescence of negative controls (samples stained only with the second fluoresceinated antibody) is shown in the left panels. The right panels show the positive staining with first and second antibodies (anti-HSP72 and fluoresceinated goat anti-mouse). (a) H9 cells; (b) H9 cells after heat shock; (c) HIV-infected H9 cells.

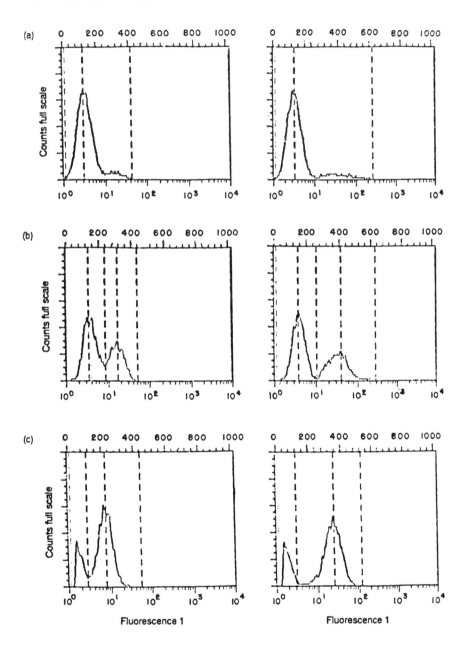

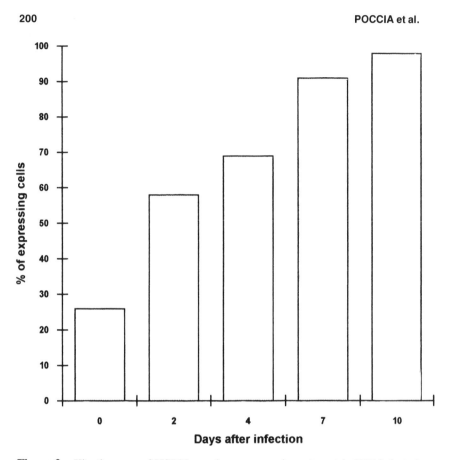

Figure 2   Kinetic curve of HSP28 membrane expression on acutely HIV-infected H9 cells. Samples 2, 4, 7, and 10 days after HIV infection were analyzed for membrane HSP28 expression. The fluorescence of controls (samples with only the second fluoresceinated antibody) was subtracted from the percentage of staining with the first and second antibodies (anti-HSP28 and fluoresceinated goat antimouse).

analysis, effector cells were incubated with different dilutions of the anti-72kDa HSP MAb. An E/T ratio of 10/1 has been proven to be optimal for detection of cellular cytotoxicity. All target cells—uninfected, HIV-infected, or heat-stressed—are similarly sensitive to NK activity. Figure 3 shows the ADCC activity exerted by PBMCs against all three types of target cell in the presence of different dilutions of anti-72kDa HSP MAb. This MAb mediates ADCC activity, which is significantly higher against

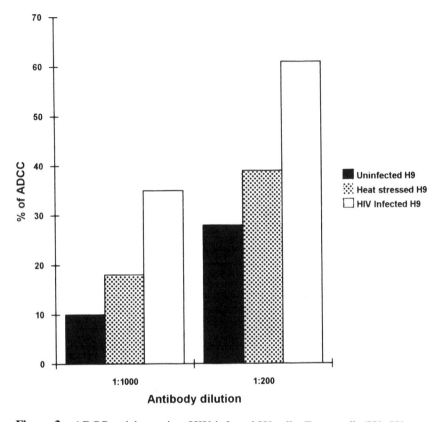

Figure 3 ADCC activity against HIV-infected H9 cells. Target cells (H9, H9—heat-shocked, H9-HIV-infected) were incubated for 1 hour at 37°C with 5% CO_2 in the presence of ^{51}Cr (NEN Research Products, 100 μCi). Effector cells consisted of PBLs obtained from healthy donors, isolated by density gradient centrifugation on Ficoll Hypaque. Labeled target cells were incubated in 96-well, round-bottom microtiter plates in the presence or absence of antibodies for 30 minutes at 37°C before effector cells (PBLs) were added. The release of ^{51}Cr after 4 hours due to cytotoxic cell lysis was measured with an LKB-γ counter. Specific cytotoxicity was expressed using the following formula:[(Experimental counts − spontaneous counts)/(total counts − spontaneous counts)] × 100. The spontaneous release of all target cells was always less than 10% of the total release. Uninfected and HIV-infected H9 cells showed similar spontaneous release. For ADCC analysis, target cells were preincubated with different dilutions of the anti-72kDa HSP MAb for 30 minutes. An E/T ratio of 10/1 has been proven to be optimal for detection of cellular cytotoxicity. The results are expressed as percentage of increase in NK activity (i.e., in the presence of anti-HSP antibody).

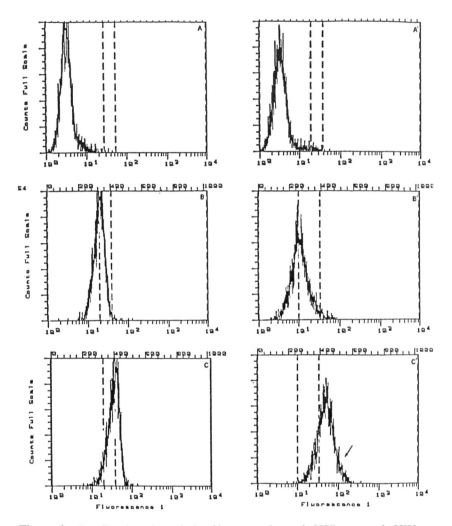

Figure 4 Cytofluorimetric analysis of intracytoplasmatic HSP on acutely HIV-infected PBMCs. Lymphocytes' isolation by Ficoll gradient were cultured at a concentration of 10^6 cells/ml in culture medium RPMI-1640, supplemented with L-glutamine, antibiotic, and 10% fetal calf serum. Cells were activated with PHA 4 μg/ml and after 2 days infected with HIV-1. Samples 2 or 3 days after infection were fixed in 70% ethanol and then analyzed for intracytoplasmic HSP expression. Left panels show the fluorescence of negative controls (stained only with the second antibody). Right panels show the positive staining with first and second antibodies (anti-HSP72 and fluoresceinated goat-anti mouse). (A) Uninfected PBMCs; (B) HIV-infected PBMCs (2 days after infection); (C) HIV-infected PBMCs (3 days after infection).

HIV-infected cells than against uninfected H9. It is interesting to note that similar specific killing of acutely HIV-infected H9 cells can be observed using a specific immunotoxin, anti-HSP65 (F. Poccia et al., in preparation). Our observations confirm that HSP membrane expression is characteristic for HIV-infected cells, whereas with uninfected cells no killing could be observed.

HSP PRODUCTION BY IN VITRO ACUTELY HIV-INFECTED PBMCs

Studies on PBMCs obtained from healthy donors, stimulated with PHA and infected with HIV-1 virus (HTLV-IIIB strain derived from H9/HTLV-IIIB cells), indicate that HIV infection in vitro induces an increase of intracytoplasmic levels of HSP after 72 hours, as shown by cytometric analysis of HSP72 (Figure 4) and Western blotting for HSP65 (Figure 5). In these experiments the previously described MAbs were directed against

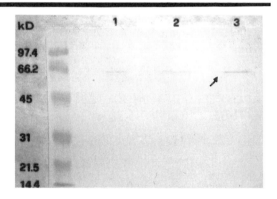

Figure 5   Western blotting of intracytoplasmic HSP on acutely HIV-infected PBMCs. PBMCs 3 days after HIV infection were lysed in lysis buffer (50 mM Tris pH 8, 62.5 mM EDTA, 2% Triton X-100). Protein concentration was determined using the BCA method. All samples were loaded on a sodium dodecyl sulfate-polyacrylamide gel electrophoresis (SDS-PAGE), and proteins were transferred to nitrocellulose paper. Anti-HSP65 MAbs were used first, and bands of immune complexes were revealed by adding goat anti-mouse IgG coupled to biotin (Zymed). Streptavidin was added and 4-chloronaphtol dissolved in ethanol was used as chromogenic substrate. To induce heat-shock response, cells were resuspended at a concentration of 5×10^5/ml and incubated for 15 minutes at 45°C. Cells were then centrifuged, resuspended at the same concentration in medium at 37°C, and incubated for 24 hours at 37°C in a 5% humidified CO_2 atmosphere before analysis. (1) Uninfected PBMCs; (2) uninfected and heat-treated PBMCs; (3) HIV-infected PBMCs (3 days after infection). It is possible to see that HSP-65 is never greatly expressed, but it is more evident on HIV-infected PBMCs (lane 3).

the major families of HSP. Less than 48 hours after infection, there is no significant increase of HSP synthesis, confirming that HSP expression needs virus replication. There is no evidence for HSP membrane localization in fresh or activated [PHA and interleukin-2 (IL-2)] PBMCs, confirming that HSP membrane expression represents a pathological factor for normal cells (Figure 6).

We then studied HSP surface expression on PBMCs and monocytes after acute HIV infection in vitro by flow cytometry. One week after infection, PBMCs showed a net increase of HSP expression on the cell surface (Figure 6). Similar observations have been made on monocytes 1 week after HIV infection, as shown in Figure 7. These findings demonstrate that HSP surface expression is a common feature of HIV-infected lymphocytes and monocytes. However, the number of HIV-expressing cells in all cases has been shown to be greater than the number of gp120 + cells, indicating that HIV infection in vitro also induces HSP membrane expression on uninfected cells. In fact, HSP surface expressing cells in the course of HIV infection are mainly CD3 + both in vivo and in vitro and carry either the CD4 + or the CD8 + phenotype (F. Poccia et al., submitted).

HSP PRODUCTION AND APOPTOSIS IN MONOCYTES INFECTED BY HIV AND *M. TUBERCULOSIS*

Heat-shock treatment of HIV-1-infected H9 cells and PBMCs increases viral replication (38). Moreover, it has been reported that U937 cells infected with HIV showed a 3–10-fold increase in reverse transcriptase activity 2–4 days after exposure to heat shock. Finally, it has been found that IL-6 was synergistic with heat treatment for viral replication in U937 cells (39). Thus, we conclude that cell lines can respond to stress induced by HIV infection with increased HSP synthesis, and high HSP levels will then increase sensitivity of cells to cytokine-mediated stimuli. These investigations suggest that HSPs induced by HIV infection could interact with HIV products and facilitate viral proliferation.

Infection with *M. tuberculosis* (MTB), representing a major HSP-inductive stimulus for macrophages (28), has been suggested to play an important role as an immunopathogenic factor associated with progression from HIV seropositivity to clinical disease (40). This could not be explained merely by an increased HIV replication by coinfected macrophages, since recent reports show that concurrent HIV and *M. tuberculosis* infection of macrophages in vitro does not increase HIV replication (41).

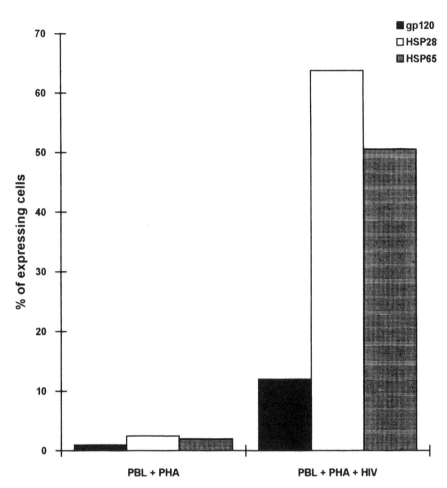

Figure 6   HSP membrane expression on in vitro HIV-infected PBLs. Cells were isolated on a Ficoll gradient and cultures at a concentration of 10^6 cells/ml in RPMI-1640, supplemented with L-glutamine, antibiotic, and 10% fetal calf serum. Cells were activated with PHA 4 μg/ml, infected with HIV-1 after 2 days, and kept in culture with IL-2 at 5 U/ml. Samples were analyzed by flow cytometry as previously described, using anti-HSP28 and anti-HSP65 MAb. The HIV-infected cells were stained for membrane gp120 (HIV-envelope protein) expression using a specific anti-gp120 MAb. The number of HSP membrane-expressing cells was shown to be higher than the percentage of HIV-infected cells. As a negative control, the membrane expression of HSP on PBLs was cultured in the presence of cytokines for 1 week.

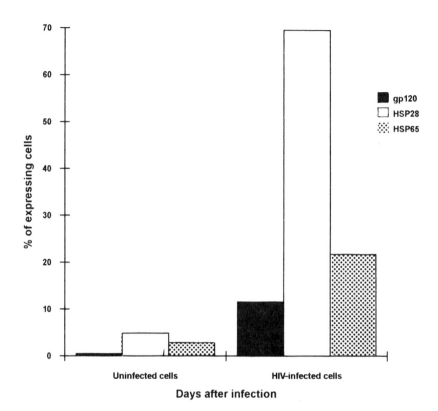

Figure 7 HSP membrane expression on in vitro HIV-infected monocytes. Monocytes were obtained from PBMCs of healthy donors after 24 hours of adherence to a polystyrene flask and kept in culture with IL-1. One week after HIV infection, cells were analyzed for HSP membrane expression by flow cytometry as described, using anti-HSP28 and anti-HSP65 MAb. The HIV-infected cells were stained for membrane gp120 expression using a specific anti-gp120 MAb. As previously observed with PBLs, the number of monocytes expressing surface HSP was higher than the number of gp120-expressing cells. As a negative control, the membrane expression of HSP on monocytes cultured in the presence of IL-1 for 1 week.

However, the concomitant presence of infected monocytes expressing HSP and HIV peptides could be relevant in AIDS immunopathogenesis, considering a possible role of HIV peptide bound to HSPs in the induction of T-cell loss.

The involvement of HSPs in the induction of programmed cell death (apoptosis) has been suggested following the observation that cycloheximide added during hyperthermic stress inhibits the appearance of apoptotic bodies, indicating that heat-shock-induced apoptosis is dependent on protein neosynthesis (42). We then developed an in vitro model of *M. tuberculosis* and HIV infection of peripheral blood monocytes and the monocytic U937 cell line. Infections were followed by PCR technology using the primers P34.1–P34.2, which amplify a band of 710 bp, belonging to the *M. tuberculosis* insertion sequence (F. Mariani et al., submitted), and primers JA9–JA12, which amplify a band of 453 bp on the hypervariable V3 region of the *env* gene of HIV-1 used by J. Albert (43). Figure 8A shows the amplification of genomic DNA *M. tuberculosis* after monocyte infection. It can be seen that *M. tuberculosis* replication in U937 cells became relevant 7 days after infection and subsequently increased again after a latency period of 7 days.

Figure 8B shows a coinfection with HIV and *M. tuberculosis* on U937 cells. To distinguish specific from unspecific amplification with outer primers, we performed a "nested" PCR, with the primers JA10–JA53— which amplify an "inner" band of HIV-1 DNA—being highly specific.

The DNA fragmentation pattern of cells infected with *M. tuberculosis* or HIV was then evaluated by detection of the scale of 200 bp characteristic for apoptosis. Figure 9A shows that U937 became apoptotic after 18 days of MTB infection, while HIV-1 induced apoptosis after 5 days. Figure 9B compares the DNA migration pattern of a tumor cell line dying from overcrowdedness and DNA from MTB-infected cells with apoptosis. These observations indicate that MTB is an important cofactor able to induce apoptosis and the the induction of HSPs on monocyte membranes may help amplify this phenomenon, as HSPs may bind to p53-forming complexes able to regulate cell suicide (26) and HSP synthesis is required for cell apoptosis (42). Moreover, cytotoxicity mediated by T cells and antibodies may contribute to the disappearance of autologous CD4+ and CD8+ T cells expressing membrane HSP in patients at the AIDS stage of disease by direct killing or induction of programmed cell death (F. Poccia et al., submitted).

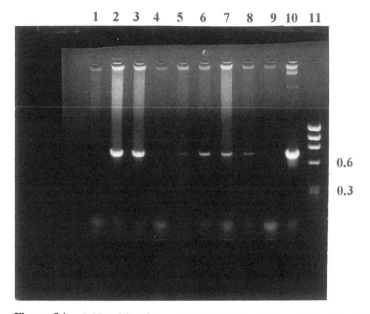

Figure 8A PCR with primers P34.1–P34.2, which amplify a band of 710 bp, belonging to the insertion sequence isolated in our laboratory. (F. Mariani, et al., submitted). Amplification was performed on genomic DNA extracted from U937 infected with *M. tuberculosis* and analyzed 5, 7, 10, 13, 18, 21, 24, and 27 days after infection (lanes 1 to 8). Lane 9: the same amplification on uninfected U937; lane 10: a positive control of amplification on the clone pFRk containing the insertion sequence; lane 11: molecular weight markers f × 174/Hae III. The primers' concentrations were 0.5 μM, dNTP 0.2 mM, and MgCl₂ 1.5 mM. 30 cycles of amplification were done (1 min at 94°C, 1 min at 65°C, and 3 min at 72°C). *M. tuberculosis* replication in U937 cells became relevant 7 days after infection, with a subsequent increase again after a latency period of 7 days.

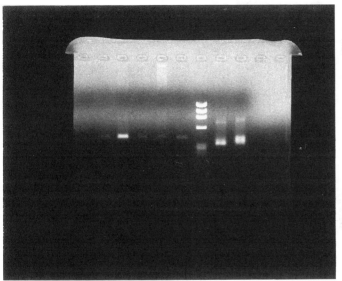

Figure 8B PCR of HIV-infected PBLs and "nested" PCR of HIV-MTB co-infected monocytes. PCR with primers JA9–JA12, which amplify a band of 453 bp on the hypervariable region V3 of the *env* gene of HIV-1 used by J. Albert (43). On this "outer" amplification it is possible to perform a "nested" PCR with the primers JA10–JA53, which amplify an "inner" band. The inner PCR is highly specific for HIV-1 DNA and allows us to distinguish specific from unspecific amplification with outer primers. Lane 1: a negative control (uninfected PBLs); lanes 2–5: outer amplification on HIV-1-infected PBLs; lane 6: similar amplification on chronically infected H9 cells; lanes 8 and 9: two nested PCRs on coinfected monocytes; lane 7: the same molecular weight markers as above.

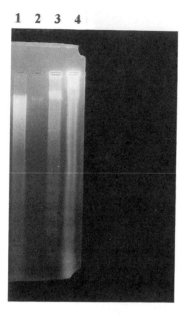

Figure 9A Analysis of DNA fragmentation pattern of cells infected with *M. tuberculosis* or HIV. Cells were lysed with Proteinase K (20 mg/ml), EDTA 0.2 M, and Triton 10%. The supernatant was extracted with phenol and chloroform before precipitation with ethanol. The samples were run in a 1.5% agarose gel electrophoresis and stained with ethidium bromide. Lane 1: U937 after 5 days of infection with HIV-1; lane 2: the same cells after 10 days; lane 3: U937 after 18 days of infection with *M. tuberculosis*; lane 4: H9 cells chronically infected with HIV.

HSP EXPRESSION BY PBMCs FROM AIDS PATIENTS

Recent findings show that viral and bacterial products can activate T cells interacting directly with the α or β chains of TcRs (44,45). These proteins, defined as superantigens, can induce massive T-cell activation with an eventual switch to anergy or apoptosis. Analysis of TCR rearrangements of peripheral blood lymphocytes (PBLs) from AIDS patients have shown selective TcR deletion (6,7). These findings suggest the possibility that superantigens such as viral proteins (envelope proteins, Nef) and/or infectious agents (mycoplasma, mycobacteria) could be involved in the pathogenesis of AIDS.

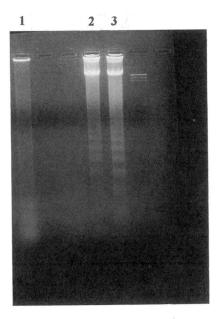

Figure 9B   A comparison between the DNA migration patterns of "suffering" and infected cells. Lane 1: DNA fragmentation of human pancreatic carcinoma cells growing slowly and showing great quantities of granolomatosus and necrotic cells; lanes 2 and 3: DNA degradation of U937 10 and 18 days after infection with *M. tuberculosis*, which generated ladders of 200 bp characteristic of apoptosis. These results confirm the relevance of MTB in inducing cell suicide by apoptosis.

We then analyzed the presence of surface HSPs on PBMCs from AIDS patients to support the possibility that endogenous proteins such as HSPs may act as superantigens (46). A high percentage of cells expressing membrane HSPs of 28, 65, and lower but significant levels of 72kDa are present in AIDS patients, while no HSP expression is observed on PBMCs from uninfected donors (Table 1). The HIV-infected cells expressing gp120 on the membrane in PBMCs from AIDS patients were about 16%, showing that the number of HSP membrane-expressing cells is always greater than the percentage of HIV-infected cells as we have previously described in vitro on PBLs and monocytes 1 week after HIV in-

Table 1 FACS Analysis of Membranes HSP28, HSP65, and HSP72 on PBMCs from AIDS Patients

Cells	% of expressing cells					Apoptotic nuclei (%)
	HSP28	HSP65	HSP72	gp120	CD3	
PBMCs (healthy donors)	10 ± 3	6 ± 4	1 ± 1	0.5 ± 0.2	76 ± 6	0.1 ± 0.1
PBMCs (AIDS patients)	50 ± 16	48 ± 19	25 ± 10	11 ± 3	66 ± 20	16 ± 9

The fluorescence of negative controls (samples stained only with the second fluoresceinated antibody) was subtracted from the percentage of staining with the first and second antibodies (fluoresceinated goat-anti mouse). MAbs directed against the major families of HSP and MAbs specific for gp120 HIV envelope protein and the CD3 T-cell marker have been used for staining.

The percentage of apoptotic nuclei was detected by propidium iodide staining as described in Ref. 49. The cell pellet was gently resuspended in 1.5 ml hypotonic fluorochrome solution (PI 50 mg/ml in 0.1% sodium citrate plus 0.1 Triton X-100, Sigma), and samples were incubated overnight at 4°C in the dark before flow-cytometric analysis. The fluorescence of individual nuclei was also measured using a FACScan flow cytometer (Becton Dickinson).

fection. Surface HSPs could also be induced by other stimuli such as increased cytokine levels (TNF-α) or opportunistic infections that normally occur at this stage of disease. Moreover, the intact immune system appears to require a delicate balance between pro-oxidant and antioxidant conditions; this balance is obviously disturbed in HIV infection (47) and may therefore contribute to stress conditions leading to HSP overexpression.

$\gamma\delta$ T CELLS IN HIV-1 INFECTION

Lymphocytes bearing TcR $\gamma\delta$ constitute 1–5% of human PBLs (21). These cells usually express the CD3 + CD4 – CD8 – or CD3 + CD4 – CD8 + surface phenotype. Unlike conventional TcR $\alpha\beta$ + cells, TcR $\gamma\delta$ cells are homogeneously cytolytic with non-MHC-restricted cytotoxic activity. Two subsets of human T $\gamma\delta$ lymphocytes are identifiable as accounting for >95% of all TcR $\gamma\delta$ + peripheral blood cells, the Vδ2 expressing cell fraction represents about 66%, and the Vδ1-expressing cells represent 33%. Although their precise function remains to be defined, some TcR $\gamma\delta$ + cells have been shown to recognize alloantigens, while others appear to recognize mycobacterial antigens and to proliferate specifically in response to mycobacterial extracts or HSPs (48). All T $\gamma\delta$ coexpressing the products of the variable region TcR gene segments $V\gamma9/V\delta2$ recognize antigens from some mycobacterial extracts and a GroEl homologous (HSP65) on the surface of Burkitt's lymphoma cells. The absolute number of peripheral blood TcR $\gamma\delta+$ cells, both $V\delta2+$ and $V\delta1+$, is increased in patients with HIV-1 infection compared with age-matched healthy controls, and these increases correlate with disease stages or CD8+ or CD4+ cell proportions (21).

PBMCs were obtained from five healthy donors, and each cell suspension was immediately analyzed for surface antigens or HIV-infected and cultured in the presence of IL-2. We analyzed the surface markers expressed after 2 weeks for each cell suspension. Table 2 shows the average plus the standard deviation obtained for each group of cells with the same treatment. It can be seen that, in the immediately analyzed PBLs, which express very low levels of membrane HSP, the number of T $\gamma\delta+$ cells is $4 \pm 3\%$, as is normally observed in healthy donors. No significant differences were observed after 2 weeks of culture in vitro in the presence of IL-2. In contrast, in HIV-infected lymphocytes, which express relevant levels of membrane HSP (22–34%), the number of T $\gamma\delta+$ cells is consis-

Table 2 Analysis of PBMCs from Five Healthy Donors

Cells	% of expressing cells							
	gp120	CD3	CD4	CD8	T$\gamma\delta$	Vγ9	Vδ2	Vγ4
PBMCs (from healthy donors)	0	78 ± 5	44 ± 8	27 ± 6	4 ± 3	3 ± 2	2 ± 2	2 ± 1
PBMCs (15 days culture in vitro)	0	75 ± 6	44 ± 6	29 ± 6	6 ± 5	5 ± 4	4 ± 2	1 ± 1
PBMCs + HIV (15 days culture in vitro)	25 ± 3	71 ± 9	35 ± 7	25 ± 5	19 ± 4	18 ± 3	17 ± 4	4 ± 2

The mononuclear cell fraction was isolated by Ficoll gradient and immediately analyzed or cultured at a concentration of 10^6 cells/ml in complete medium (RPMI-1640 medium, enriched with 10% inactivated fetal calf serum, 1% glutamine, and antibiotics) in presence of IL-2 20 U/ml. HIV-1 infection was performed and monitored as described.

A panel of MAbs was used for cell-surface staining in indirect immunofluorescence. B1 is an IgG$_1$ MAB that reacts with the T$\gamma\delta+$ cell subsets, while B3, 4G6, and 4A11 are all IgG$_1$ MAbs that specifically react with three molecular forms of $\gamma\delta+$ TcR (coded by Vγ9, Vδ2, or Vγ4 gene segments, respectively).

tently (more than fourfold) higher than in the uninfected controls. The expanded cell subset bears $V\gamma9$ and $V\delta2$ cells, suggesting that the HSP membrane expression induced by HIV may induce T $\gamma\delta+$ cell activation.

RELEVANCE OF HSP TO AIDS PATHOGENESIS

Current results show that HSP surface expression is a signal for serious cell damage (infection, transformation), raising the question about the role of HSPs in monitoring cell homeostasis and triggering cell suicide by apoptosis. In this context, the results presented here suggest that surface HSP may be a surrogate marker of HIV-1 infection, and the reduction of viral proliferation through selective killing of HIV-infected cells expressing membrane HSPs using specific immunotoxins may indicate a possible therapeutic approach for reducing the number of infected cells that spread HIV virus and give wrong signals to the immune system. In fact, HSPs might modulate the antigen presentation of viral antigens (15), inducing an α-helical conformation classically recognized by TcR.

Surface expression of HSPs is not a frequent event, and activated cells do not stain for membrane HSPs. On the contrary, cell damage related to oncogene activation or viral infection seems necessary to transfer HSPs from the intracellular compartment to the cell surface. HIV infection can induce HSP synthesis and translocation to the cell membrane showing a kinetic curve for HSP28 and 65. On in vitro infected PBMCs and on macrophages we found a net increase of HSP surface expression. This result is relevant mainly for the role of antigen-presenting cells in signaling T cells. Moreover, analyses of PBMCs from AIDS patients showed a high percentage of cells expressing membrane HSP that did not consist entirely of HIV-infected cells, probably as consequence of opportunistic infection and of immune balance alteration (autoreactivity, cytokine synthesis, immunocomplexes). These findings with PBMCs of AIDS patients also confirm that surface expression involves all the major families of HSP (28, 65, and 72kDa), as previously reported for chronically infected H9 cells. The ability of HSPs to bind to peptides could be crucial in the production of complexes (HSP/HIV peptides and/or HSP/opportunistic infectious agents) not present in the early stage of infection but highly expressed in the cytoplasma and on the membrane of PBMCs from AIDS patients. HSP may act as a cofactor inducing the immunopathological activation of T cells, as shown in Figure 10.

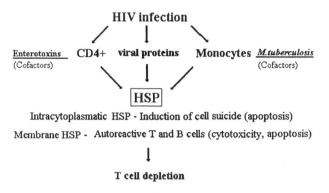

Figure 10 Schema of how HSP may act as a cofactor inducing the immunopathological activation of T cells.

Finally, HIV could induce the expression of an autoantigen and/or superantigen always present in the genome of host cells such as HSP (46). The possible involvement of HSP in triggering apoptosis (42), the role of HSP as superantigen in several autoimmune disease (19), and the recent observation of T Vβ deletion in AIDS (2) suggest that HSP expressed on lymphocyte or monocyte cell membranes in AIDS could play a central role as a cofactor leading to the degeneration of the immune system.

ACKNOWLEDGMENTS

We thank Professor G. Damiani of the Biochemistry Institute of the University of Genova and Professor J. Ivanyi of the Hammersmith Hospital of London for providing us with the anti-HSP monoclonal antibodies, Dr. G. De Libero of the Basel Kantonsspital for the panel of anti-γδ-T-cell monoclonal antibodies, and Ms. S. Bach for careful reading of the manuscript.

This work was supported by the AIDS Project of the Ministero della Sanità, the M.U.R.S.T., and the C.N.R. Progetto Finalizzato Fatma.

REFERENCES

1. Lusso P, Ensoli B, Markham PD, Ablashi DV, Salahuddin SZ, Tschachler E, Wong-Staal F, Gallo RC. Productive dual infection of human CD4 + T lymphocytes by HIV-1 and HHV-6. Nature 1989; 337:370–373.

2. Watanabe M, Ringler DJ, Fultz PN, Mac Key JJ, Boyson JE, Levine CG, Letvin NL. A chimpanzee passaged human immunodeficiency virus isolate is cytopathic for chimpanzee T cells but does not induce disease. J Virol 1991; 65:3344–3348.

3. Dalgleish AG, Colizzi V. Role of major histocompatibility complex recognition in the protection and immunopathogenesis of AIDS. AIDS 1992; 6:523–525.

4. Gougeon ML, Montagnier L. New concepts in the mechanisms of CD4 + lymphocyte depletion in AIDS, and the influence of opportunistic infections. Res Microbiol 1992; 143:362–368.

5. Habeshaw J, Hounsell E, Dalgleish A. Does the HIV envelope induce a chronic graft-versus host-like disease? Immunol Today 1992; 13:207–209.

6. Imberti L, Sottini A, Bettinardi A, Puoti M, Primi D. Selective depletion in HIV infection of T cells that bear specific T cell receptor Vβ sequences. Science 1991; 254:860–862.

7. Dalgleish AG, Wilson S, Gompels M, Ludlam C, Gazzard B, Coates AM, Habeshaw J. T-cell receptor variable gene products and early HIV infection. Lancet 1992; 339:824–828.

8. Kion TA, Hoffman GW. Anti-HIV and anti-anti-MHC antibodies in alloimmune and autoimmune mice. Science 1991; 253:1138–1140.

9. Lombardi W, Rossi P, Romiti L, Mattei M, Mariani F, Poccia F, Colizzi V. HIV gp120 epitope immunodominance in MRL/lpr mice. AIDS Hum Retrovir 1992; 6:671–672.

10. Di Cesare S, Poccia F, Mastino A, Colizzi V. Surface expressed heat shock proteins by stressed or HIV infected lymphoid cells represent the target for antibody dependent cellular cytotoxicity. Immunology 1992; 76:341–343.

11. Ullrich SJ, Robinson EA. A mouse tumor-specific transplantation antigen is a heat shock-related protein. Proc Natl Acad Sci USA 1986; 83:3121–3125.

12. La Thangue NB, Latchman SD. A cellular protein related to heat-shock protein 90 accumulates during herpes simplex virus infection and is overexpressed in transformed cells. Exp Cell Res 1988; 178:169–170.

13. Lindquist S, Craig EA. The heat shock proteins. Annu Rev Genet 1988; 22:631–677.

14. Sargent CA, Dunham I, Trowsdale J, Campbell RD. Human major histocompatibility complex contains genes for the major heat shock protein HSP70. Proc Natl Acad Sci USA 1989; 86:1968–1972.

15. De Nagel DC, Pierce SK. A case for chaperones in antigen processing Immunol Today 1992; 13:86–89.

16. Landry SJ, Gierasch LM. The chaperonin GroEL binds a polypeptyde in an α-helical conformation. Biochemistry 1991; 30:7360–7362.

17. Rippman F, Taylor WR, Rothbard JB, Green NM. A hypothetical model for the peptide binding domain of hsp70 based on the peptide binding domain of HLA. Embo J 1991; 10:1053–1059.

18. Landry SJ, Jordan R, McMacken R, Gierasch LM. Different conformation for the same polypeptide bound to chaperones DnaK and GroEL. Nature 1992; 355:455–457.

19. Kaufmann SHE. Heat shock proteins and the immune response. Immunol Today 1990; 11:129–136.

20. De Paoli P. A subset of $\gamma\delta$ lymphocytes is increased during HIV-1 infection. Clin Exp Immunol 1991; 83:187–191.

21. De Maria A, Ferrazin A, Ferrini S, Ciccone E, Terragna A, Moretta A. Selective increase of a subset of T cell receptor $\gamma\delta$ T lymphocytes in the peripheral blood of patients with human immunodeficiency virus type 1 infection. J Infect Dis 1992; 165:917–919.

22. Pechan PM. Heat shock proteins and cell proliferation. FEBS 1991; 280:1–4.

23. Koskinen PJ, Sistonen L, Evan G, Morimoto R, Alitalo K. Nuclear colocalization of cellular and viral *myc* proteins with HSP70 in *myc*-overexpressing cells. J Virol 1991; 65:842–851.

24. Ralston R. Complementation of transforming domains in E1a/*myc* chimeras. Nature 1991; 353:866–868.

25. Finlay CA, Hinds PW, Tain TH, Elyahu D, Oren M, Levine AJ. Activating mutations for transformation by p53 produce a gene product that forms a hsc-p53 complex with an alterated half-life. Mol Cell Biol 1988; 8:531–536.

26. Yonish-Rouach E, Resnitzky D, Lotem J, Sachs L, Kimchi A, Oren M. Wild type p53 induces apoptosis of myeloid leukaemic cells that is inhibited by interleukin-6. Nature 1991; 352:345–347.

27. Poccia F, Piselli P, Di Cesare S, Bach S, Colizzi V, Mattei M, Bolognesi A, Stirpe F. Recognition and killing of tumour cells expressing heat shock protein 65kD with immunotoxins containing saporin. Br J Cancer 1992; 65:427–432.

28. Shinnick TM, Vodkin MH, Williams JC. The *Mycobacterium tuberculosis* 65-kilodalton antigen is a heat shock protein which corresponds to common antigen and to the *Escherichia coli* GroEl protein. Infect Immun 1988; 56:446–451.

29. Notarianni EL, Preston CM. Activation of cellular stress protein genes by herpes symplex virus temperature sensitive mutants which overproduce immediate early polypeptides. Virology 1982; 123:113–122.

30. Khandjian EW, Turler H. Simian virus 40 and polyoma virus induce synthesis of heat shock proteins in permissive cells. Mol Cell Biol 1983; 3:1–8.

31. Peluso RW, Lamb RA, Choppin PW. Infection with paramyxo-viruses stimulates synthesis of cellular polypeptides that are also stimulated in cells transformed by Rous sarcoma virus or deprived of glucose. Proc Natl Acad Sci USA 1978; 75:6120–6124.

32. Garry RF, Ulug ET, Bose HR Jr. Induction of stress proteins in Sindbis virus- and vesicular stomatitis virus-infected cells. Virology 1983; 129:319–332.

33. Collins PL, Hightower LE. Newcastle disease virus stimulates the cellular accumulation of stress (heat shock) mRNAs and proteins. J Virol 1982; 44: 703–707.

34. Newins JR. Induction of the synthesis of a 70kD mammalian heat shock protein by the adenovirus EIA gene product. Cell 1982; 29:913–919.

35. Damiani G, Biano A, Beltrame A, Vismara D, Filippone Mezzopreti M, Colizzi V, Young BD, Bloom B. Generation and characterization of monoclonal antibodies to 28-, 35-, and 65-kD protein of *M. tuberculosis*. Infect Immun 1988; 56:1281–1287.

36. Ivanyi J, Sinha S, Aston R, Cussel D, Keen M, Sengupta U. Definition of species specific and cross-reactive antigenic determinants of *M. leprae* using monoclonal antibodies. Clin Exp Immunol 1983; 52:528–536.

37. Evans DJ, Norton P, Ivany J. Distribution in tissue section of the human groEL stress-protein homologue. APMIS 1990; 98:437–441.

38. Furlini G, Re MC, Musiani M, Zerbini ML, La Placa M. Enhancement of HIV-1 marker detection in cell cultures treated with mild heat shock. Microbiologica 1990; 13:21–26.

39. Stanley SK, Bressler PB, Poli G, Fauci AS. Heat shock induction of HIV production from chronically infected promonocytic and T cell lines. J Immunol 1990; 145:1120–1126.

40. Moch DJ, Roberts NJ Jr. Proposed immunopathogenic factors associated with progression from human immunodeficiency virus seropositivity to clinical disease. J Clin Microbiol 1987; 25:1817–1821.

41. Meylan PRA, Munis JR, Richmann DD, Kornbluth RS. Concurrent human immunodeficiency virus and mycobacterial infection of macrophages in vitro does not reveal any reciprocal effect. J Infect Dis 1992; 165:80–86.

42. Ghibelli L, Nosseri C, Oliverio S, Piacentini M, Autuori F. Cycloheximide can rescue heat-shocked L cells from death by blocking stress induced apoptosis. Exp Cell Res 1992; 201. In press.

43. Albert J, Fenyo EM. Simple, sensitive and specific detection of human immunodeficiency virus type 1 clinical specimens by polymerase chain reaction with nested primers. J Clin Microbiol 1990; 28:1560–1564.

44. Janeway CA Jr. Self superantigens? Cell 1990; 63:659–661.

45. Marrack P, Kappler J. The staphylococcal enterotoxins and their relatives. Science 1990; 248:705–711.

46. Littlefield JW. Possible supplemental mechanisms in the pathogenesis of AIDS. Clin Immunol Immunopathol 1992; 65:85–97.

47. Droge W, Eck HP, Mihm S. HIV-induced cysteins deficiency and T-cell dysfunction—a rationale for treatment with N-acetylcysteine. Immunol Today 1992; 13:211–214.

48. Heregewoin A, Soman G, Homan RC, Finberg RW. Human γδ T cells respond to mycobacterial heat shock proteins. Nature 1989; 340:309–312.

49. Nicoletti I, Migliorati G, Pagliacci MC, Grigniani F, Riccardi C. A rapid and simple method for measuring thymocyte apoptosis by propidium iodide staining and flow cytometry. J Immunol Meth 1991; 139:271–279.

14

γδ T Cells in the Pathogenesis of HIV-1 Infection

Rita Rossol, Georg Geissler, and Dieter Hoelzer

J. W. Goethe University
Frankfurt, Germany

Altered cellular function and depletion of $\alpha\beta$ receptor + T cells (e.g., CD4 + T cells) are the most important immunological events in HIV-related pathogenesis, but until now the role of T cells bearing the γδ-T-cell receptor (TcR) in HIV infection and other viral diseases has been unknown. This T-cell subset represents about 5% of T lymphocytes in the peripheral blood and bears an alternative form of TcR composed of γδ heterodimers. It is also found on a minor population of thymocytes, spleen cells, and lymph node cells. This population is recognized by TcR δ1, a pan-δ monoclonal antibody (MAb). Sixty to seventy percent of TcR δ1 + T cells react with TiγA and BB3, monoclonal antibodies directed against the Vγ9 and Vδ2 determinants, respectively. Separated, 20–30% of TcR δ1 + cells express Vδ1 (δTCS1 antibody). A possible role for γδ T cells in the pathogenesis of HIV-1 infection is worthy of discussion because it has been demonstrated that these cells may lyse autologous T cells.

INTRODUCTION

The majority of human T lymphocytes express a disulfide-linked receptor composed of a heterodimer of α and β chains (TcR $\alpha\beta$) on their cell surface in association with the CD3 molecular complex (1). A novel second form of T-cell subset expressing a CD3-associated $\gamma\delta$-T-cell receptor was recently identified by Brenner et al. (2) (Figure 1). In humans, but also in mice, these $\gamma\delta$ T cells represent a relatively minor population of the total T cells (2), whereas in chicken (3) and sheep (4) they are present in greater numbers. In the peripheral blood of humans, more than 95% of the T lymphocytes express the $\alpha\beta$ TcR and include the helper-inducer CD4 T-cell subset and the cytotoxic suppressor CD8 T-cell subset. However, $\gamma\delta$-TcR + T cells are usually CD4 −, and a small fraction express CD8 (5).

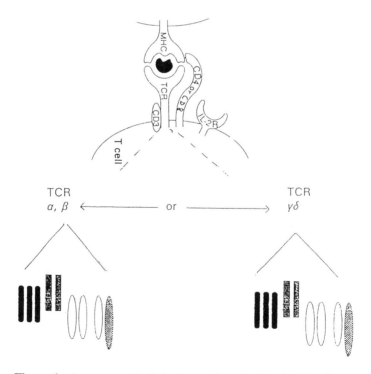

Figure 1   Structure and cellular interaction of $\alpha\beta$ and $\gamma\delta$ T-cell receptors. (From Ref. 2).

The majority of γδ T cells lack both CD4 and CD8 accessory molecules. γδ T cells in humans have been further subdivided by using MAbs BB3 (6) and δTCS-1 (7). In general, the BB3 + cells display γ and δ chains in disulfide-linked form, while the δTCS-1 + cells carry a nondisulfide-linked heterodimer. In addition, these cells can be distinguished morphologically (8) or by their C- and V-gene usage (9,10). The majority of peripheral blood γδ T cells are TigA (Vγ9) + and BB3 (Vδ2) + (7,10), whereas δTCS-1 (Vγ1) + cells are less frequently expressed (11).

Concerning their response to antigen, the repertoire of γδ TcR + cells seems to be more limited, and extrathymic positive selection has been demonstrated for many γδ-T-cell clones. Extrathymic positive selection is thought to be achieved by selective expansion of appropriate T-cell clones over extended periods of time. This type of selection implies a peripheral clonal expansion of γδ T cells, which could be faciliated by specific physiological properties exhibited by these cells (12). On the basis of their distribution in vivo and the properties described so far in vitro, several functions have been proposed for γδ T cells, e.g., primary specific cytotoxicity restricted to autologous or allogeneic tumor targets (13,14), epithelial surveillance against viral infection, and transformation.

Attempts to identify the ligands for γδ TcR have focused on major histocompatibility complex (MHC) class-I-like proteins, heat-shock proteins (HSP), and mycobacteria (10). It is believed that γδ T cells constitute a more primitive immunosurveillance system, able to recognize non-MHC-restricted antigens (15).

In contrast to mycobacteria-reactive human γδ T cells, no appropriate inducer is known that activates one of the two subsets of γδ T cells so far identified in the human system, termed δTCS-1 + T cells.

Data are accumulating on the role of γδ T cells in various inflammatory processes. For example, it has recently been demonstrated that γδ T cells that express the variable (V) gene segments V delta 1, V delta 2, and V gamma 2 (V gamma 9) accumulate in acute, demyelinating multiple sclerosis (MS) plaques and appeared to have undergone clonal expansion, probably through recognition of a specific CNS ligand. Furthermore, in these experiments it was shown that 60- and 90- kDa heat-shock proteins, which are believed to be target antigens for autoreactive γδ T cells, were found to be expressed in normal CNS tissue and overexpressed in acute MS plaques (16). Interestingly, during immune monitoring—e.g., after renal transplantation—treatment with azathioprine and cyclosporine caused marked diminution in αβ T cells but not in γδ T cells (17). γδ T

Table 1   Subpopulation of $\gamma\delta$ T Cells in the Human System

Subpopulation	Anatomical site	TcR usage	Characteristics	Refs.
Vγ1 Vδ1	Thymus	γ: VIC2	Predominant in thymus	35,36
		No S-S bridge	Rare in blood	35,36
		δ: V1 (MAb δTCS)	Proportion in blood decreases with age	36
			Most cells remain CD45RV	9
Vγ9 Vδ2	Blood	γ: V9C1	Rare in thymus	35,36
		S-S bridge (MAb Tiγa)	Predominant in blood	9,35, 36
		δ: V3 (MAb V3BB3)	Proportion in blood increases with age	36
			Most cells become CD45RO	9,11

cells have also been demonstrated to be involved in the lysis of autologous T cells during allogeneic bone-marrow transplantation, also suggesting some autoimmune activity (18). Table 1 summarizes recently published data on the activation of $\gamma\delta$ T cells.

$\gamma\delta$ T CELLS IN THE PERIPHERAL BLOOD OF HIV-1-INFECTED PATIENTS

Analysis on T-cell subsets in PBMCs of 123 patients infected with HIV-1 at different stages of the disease using MAbs binding to $\gamma\delta$ + T cells—as determined by FACS analysis with the TcR δ1 antibody, which precipitates the TcR δ subunit on all CD3 + cells—showed that there was no quantitative variation in any stage of the disease (Figure 2). However, as early as in stage WR 2 of HIV infection, there was a significant increase of up to 70% ($p < 0.001$) in $\gamma\delta$ + T cells reacting with the δTCS-1 antibody, which builds to a TCS-1 + subpopulation (Figure 3).

In healthy donors, the corresponding epitope Vδ1 was expressed on only a small subset (up to 30%) of peripheral $\gamma\delta$ + T cells. A tendency to

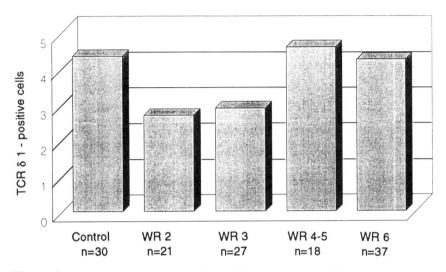

Figure 2   Analysis of TcR δ+ T cells in different stages of HIV-1 infection.

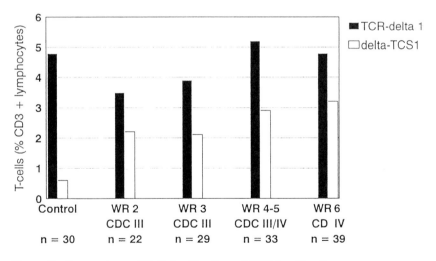

Figure 3   Comparison of TcR δ+ T cells and TCS-1+ T cells.

further elevation without statistical significance could be observed in patients with a more progressive CD4 + T-cell depletion and the clinical appearance of full-blown AIDS. Repeated testing of individual patients over time (8–12 months) revealed a stable behavior of the δTCS-1 + γδ T-cell population. In addition, there was no change of γδ TcR expression following AZT therapy. To determine whether phenotypical changes within the γδ + T cell population are a common feature of viral infections, we compared patients with chronic viral diseases—e.g., chronic viral hepatitis types B and C (posttransfusional hepatitis NonA–NonB) and chronic HSV-2 infection—demonstrating that only in patients with HIV-1 infection is there a strong and significant enhancement of δTCS-1-reacting γδ + T cells. These results indicate that HIV-1 itself and/or HIV-1-mediated mechanisms lead to a stimulation of a defined T-cell subset.

It is known that suppression of activation signals such as interleukin-2 receptors (IL-2R) and functional correlated markers (CD4) in T cells of patients progresses with the stage of HIV-1-related disease. Expression of HLA-DR, IL-2R, CD8, and CD4 on the surface of γδ + T cells (TcR δ1 +) and thereby a marked increase in the expression of HLA-DR ($p <$ 0.001) and a reduction of IL-2R ($p < 0.05$) could be defined (Figure 4). γδ + T cells have been characterized as being predominantly a double negative (CD4 and CD8) T-cell subset in healthy donors. In HIV-1 infec-

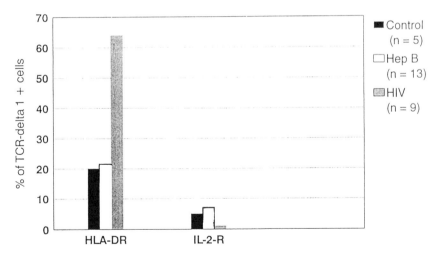

Figure 4 Activation marker on γδ T cells in different viral infections (hepatitis B, HIV-1).

tion, there was no reaction with the CD4 antibody. However, compared to the control, a higher proportion of the cells (50% in mean) expressed the CD8 antigen ($p < 0.05$). These results were obtained in patients at all stages of the disease tested.

Altered cellular function and depletion of $\alpha\beta$ receptor + T cells (e.g., CD4 + T cells) are important immunological events in HIV-related pathogenesis, but the role of peripheral T cells bearing the alternative γδ-T-cell receptor in HIV infection and other chronic viral diseases remains unknown. However, recent evidence has been presented that γδ + T cells and CD16 + thymocytes are not infectable with HIV-1, mediate non-MHC-restricted cytotoxicity, and might therefore contribute to further immunosuppression (15).

T-cell receptors using different constant-region gene segments may have altered functions in T-cell differentiation or may be responsive to different antigenic stimuli. Whereas increased expression of TcR δ1 has been reported following stimulation with either mycobacterial antigens or heat-shock proteins (10), no appropriate inducer for the δTCS-1 + subpopulation can be identified yet. Attempts to use viral proteins as a stimulatory agent did not result in the proliferation of the δTCS-1 + subpopulation (16). Recent results revealed a conservation of the mycobacteria responsible for the γδ + T-cell population characterized by the Ti-γA antibody. Since we have been able to show that enhanced δTCS-1 expression is associated only with HIV-1 infection and no other chronic infection (e.g., chronic hepatitis or HSV-2 infection), one might argue that δTCS-1 expression may be somewhat HIV-1-related. In addition, HIV-related viral opportunistic infection (e.g., Epstein-Barr virus and cytomegalovirus) is not correlated with an increasing population of γδ + T cells. However, besides direct interactions between virus and cells, HIV-1 infection does also produce autoimmune phenomena that might contribute to the pathogenesis of the disease. It is therefore possible that such mechanisms may be responsible for enhanced δTCS-1 expression. Moreover, it has been shown by others (17) that enhanced γδ-T-cell expression is correlated with autoreactive activity following autologous bone-marrow transplantation and therefore may suggest such mechanisms. Furthermore, it should be stressed that in our experimental situation most of the γδ + T cells were HLA-DR + and IL-2R − (Figure 3), indicating cellular activation, and, with the progression of the disease, we could observe higher proportions of CD8 + cells among the δTCS-1 fraction, suggesting some cytolytic activity. Only a limited series of activation signals is needed for the proliferation and IL-2 production of $\gamma\delta +$ T cells in vitro, and therefore it might be speculated that δTCS-1 + cells may be involved in the lysis of CD4 + $\alpha\beta$ T cells.

$\gamma\delta$ T CELLS IN THE BONE MARROW OF HIV-1-INFECTED PATIENTS

HIV-1-infected patients in progressive stages of the disease suffer from anemia, leukopenia, and neutropenia, all of which have been described as symptoms of a generalized bone-marrow deficiency (19). It has been speculated by many investigators that direct infection of bone-marrow progenitor cells may account for the observed malignancies. However, little is known about the exact mechanism mediating the observed hematological disorders. For example, altered cytokine production in patients' sera may contribute to changes in the cytokine network responsible for growth and maturation of lymphoid cells. Besides enhanced levels of interferon-γ, the enhanced production of TNF-α and TGF-β may regulate bone-marrow function. Moreover, it has been shown by Carlo Stella et al. (19) that an imbalance in the CD4/CD8 ratio of T lymphocytes and some enhanced suppressor function of CD8 lymphocytes may be responsible for hematological failure. Because $\gamma\delta$ T cells in HIV-1-infected patients are mostly CD8 +, we have asked whether this cell population might suppress bone-marrow cell function. In bone marrow aspirated from patients at progressive stages of the disease, significantly enhanced expression of δTCS-1 cells was observed (Figure 5). Bone-marrow aspirates of the posterior illiac crest were taken from patients at progressive stages of the disease mostly at risk for lymphoma. Low-density bone-marrow cells were isolated from these specimens by removing adherend cells and further panning. Hemopoietic colony formation was measured using CFU-GEMM, BFU-E, and CFU-GM. Selective elimination of δTCS-1 cells increased the proliferation of hemopoietic progenitor cells significantly (Table 2).

Retitration of δTCS-1 cells diminished proliferation. When other T cells such as CD4 cells and pan-$\alpha\beta$ T lymphocytes were depleted, no increase in hematopoietic colony formation was seen, neither in HIV-positive nor in HIV-negative individuals. There may be different explanations of the mechanism by which δTCS-1 + $\gamma\delta$ T cells mediate inhibition of colony formation in HIV-1-infected but not in healthy individuals. For example, as a sign of possible functional activation, up to 50% of the δTCS-1 + $\gamma\delta$

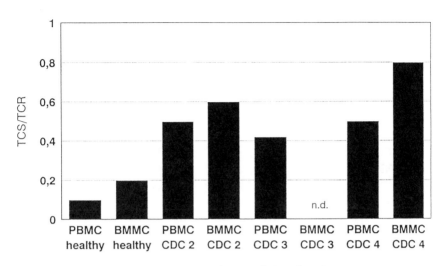

Figure 5   γδ T cells in bone marrow of HIV-1-infected patients.

T cells are CD8 + only in HIV-1 infection, whereas in healthy subjects these lymphocytes are CD8 − . CD8 + δTCS-1 + γδ T cells are believed to be more cytotoxic than their CD8 − counterparts (18), and therefore the presence of this subpopulation may account for the observed difference. Moreover, δTCS-1 + γδ T cells were shown to produce more TNF-α compared to αβ + T cells (16), and therefore high amounts of TNF-α in the bone marrow may inhibit hematopoietic progenitor cells. In a set of experiments in which we added neutralizing antibodies to the progenitor cell cultures in the presence of δTCS-1 + γδ T cells, an increase of CFU-GM colony growth in HIV-1-infected patients was observed. These data suggest that, besides a direct cellular suppressive effect, secretion of soluble inhibitors are involved in the hemopoietic failure in HIV-1 infection (Table 3).

TNF-α IN HIV-1 INFECTION:
ITS REGULATORY FUNCTION ON γδ T CELLS

Cytokines are thought to play a major role in the development and progression of HIV-1 infection. High levels of TNF-α have been detected in the sera of infected patients, and macrophages isolated from the periph-

Table 2 Role and Activation of γδ T Cells in Human Diseases

Disease	Inducing agent	Receptor repertoire/ subtype	Function or pathophysiological role	Ref.
Malaria	*Plasmodium falciparum*	V gamma 9 V delta α	TNF-α production	25
HIV-I infection	Unknown	δTCS-1		26
Mycobacterial infection		δTCS-1 (V delta 2)		27
Rheumatoid arthritis	Mycobacterial antiglus	V delta 1 CD45 Ro HLA-DR		28 29
LGL expansion (T-gamma lymphocytosis), neutropenia, thrombocytopenia	Not known (polyclonal expansion)	V gamma 9 V delta 2 J gamma 1.2 J delta 1		30
Viscercel leishmaniasis		CDy+ CD8– CD28, CD38, CD71, HLA-DR	Secrete BCGF, BCDF	31 32
Multiple sclerosis	Heat-shock proteins (HSP 60, HSP 90)	V delta 1 V delta 2 V gamma 2 V gamma 9	33	21
Schistosomiasis and carcinoma of the urinary bladder		CD25, CD38 CD71, HLA-DR	BDGF, BLDF Il-2-deficient	34

Table 3 Hematopoietic Colony Growth in % ±1 SEM of Controls Without T-Lymphocyte Depletion After Depletion of δTCS-1 +, CD-4 +, or $\alpha\beta$ + T Cells or After Depletion and Immediate Readdition of δTCS-1 + Cells in Methylcellulose Assay

Experiment	Colony	Growth in % from control	
		HIV-positive	HIV-negative
Control without	CFU-GEMM	100.0 ± 0.0	100.0 ± 0.0
depletion	BFU-E	100.0 ± 0.0	100.0 ± 0.0
	CFU-GM	100.0 ± 0.0	100.0 ± 0.0
δTCS-1 cell	CFU-GEMM	237.2 ± 40.1	99.0 ± 6.3
depletion	BFU-E	139.8 ± 4.8	100.4 ± 1.2
	CFU-GM	154.3 ± 9.2	100.4 ± 0.5
δTCS-1 cell deple-	CFU-GEMM	66.7 ± 60.0	102.6 ± 9.6
tion with re-	BFU-E	101.2 ± 4.3	102.8 ± 2.6
addition	CFU-GM	101.3 ± 2.2	99.6 ± 1.1
CD4 cell depletion	CFU-GEMM	100.0 ± 33.3	102.6 ± 4.8
	BFU-E	101.2 ± 6.2	100.2 ± 1.9
	CFU-GM	101.0 ± 1.7	100.0 ± 1.4
T-$\alpha\beta$-cell depletion	CFU-GEMM	66.7 ± 60.0	97.4 ± 6.6
	BFU-E	98.6 ± 8.3	101.2 ± 2.6
	CFU-GM	100.6 ± 0.5	100.0 ± 1.6

CFU-GEMM = colony-forming unit–granulocyte-erythrocyte-monocyte-megakaryocyte; BFU-E = burst-forming unit–erythrocyte; CFU-GM = colony-forming unit–granulocyte-monocyte.

eral blood of infected patients have been shown to produce significantly more TNF-α as compared to uninfected controls (20).

For example, monocyte-derived cytokines such as TNF-α have been shown to stimulate HIV-1 transcription via activation of the transcription factor NF-$\varkappa$B. Moreover, we have been able to show that TNF-α secretion by peripheral blood mononuclear cells (PBMCs) of HIV-1-positive patients is enhanced at late stages of the disease and is regulated on both the transcriptional and the translational levels (24). PBMCs that were stimulated with TNF-α (10 ng/ml) and mitogen were examined by FACS analysis. It turned out that the number of δTCS-1 + $\gamma\delta$ T cells increased, whereas the number of CD4 + cells and the number of TiγA + $\gamma\delta$ T cells (which represent the other of the two known subsets of $\gamma\delta$ T cells so far described in the human system) decreased. In the presence of TNF-α alone, the number of δTCS-1 + $\gamma\delta$ T cells remained unchanged, whereas the number of

TiγA + $\gamma\delta$ T cells and CD4 cells decreased. There was no change in the number of TiγA + T cells and CD4 cells when antibodies for TNF-a were added.

From these data, it may be hypothesized that local TNF-α production as a result of acute HIV-1 infection leads to enhanced proliferation of δTCS-1 + $\gamma\delta$ T cells at different anatomical sites. Since $\gamma\delta$ T cells have been shown to be able to lyse autologous $\alpha\beta$ T cells (e.g., during allogeneic bone-marrow transplantation), it may be hypothesized that an additional mechanism responsible for the elimination of CD4 cells and hematological disorders during HIV-1 progression may be active.

CORD BLOOD: A MODEL TO STUDY THE ROLE OF CYTOKINES IN THE GROWTH OF δTCS-1 + $\gamma\delta$ T CELLS

Compared to the amount of $\gamma\delta$ T cells in peripheral blood from adults, the frequency of $\gamma\delta$ T cells in cord blood cells (CBMCs) is higher, as well as the percentage of precursor cells. Therefore, cord blood may serve as a useful model with which to study growth conditions of $\gamma\delta$ T cells.

The proportion of δTCS-1 + cells in cultures of CBMCs can be enhanced by costimulation of CBMCs with a mitogenic-acting compound in association with TNF-α. Blocking experiments using antibodies recognizing TNF-α epitopes could completely abrogate the enhancement of the δTCS-1 + T-cell subpopulation. Since the δTCS-1 subpopulation is enhanced during HIV-1 infection, and since TNF-α plays a major role in HIV-1 virus replication associated with enhanced expression of this cytokine during infection with this virus, it is conceivable that TNF-α in combination with a mitogen can activate the δTCS-1 + cells. Moreover, enhanced δTCS-1 + cells have also been identified in the peripheral blood of cancer patients undergoing surgery who need several blood transfusions. Since the proportion of δTCS-1 + cells is enhanced during incubation with TNF-α, it may be hypothesized that these cells are more resistant to the toxic effects mediated by TNF-α as compared to the other subtype of $\gamma\delta$ T cells. For the proliferation of δTCS-1 + cells, the addition of a mitogen in combination with TNF-α is necessary, since the addition of antibodies to TNF-α in the presence of mitogen did not result in proliferation of δTCS-1 + cells. However, there was no increase in the percentage of HLA-DR + cells following TNF-α stimulation, indicating that TNF-α may act as a growth factor and the observed proliferation is not related to antigenic stimulation. Therefore, two mechanisms may be responsible for the enhanced presence of δTCS-1 + cells during HIV-1 infection: first, the TNF-α-dependent proliferation of δTCS-1 + cells and, second, the resistance of this subtype to the TNF-α-triggered cell death. High titers of TNF-α present in the sera of patients at late stages of the disease and opportunistic infections such as bacterial infections that may have mitogenic and TNF-α-inducing activity may therefore enhance proliferation of δTCS-1 + cells, not only in the peripheral blood but also at other anatomical sites such as the bone marrow or spleen.

REFERENCES

1. Allison JP, Lanier LL. Structure function and serology of the T-cell antigen receptor complex. Annu Rev Immunol 1987; 5:503–540.
2. Brenner et al. Identification of a putative second T cell receptor. Nature 1986; 322:145.
3. Sowder JT, et al. A large subpopulation of avian T cells express a homologue of the mammalian γ/δ receptor. J Immunol 1988; 167:315.
4. Mackay CR. γ/δ T cells express a unique surface molecule appearing late during thymic development. Eur J Immunol 1989; 19:1477.
5. Lanier LL, et al. The gamma T cell antigen receptor. J Clin Immunol 1987; 7:429.
6. Mingari M, et al. Eur J Immunol 1988; 18:1831.
7. Wu Y, et al. J Immunol 1988; 141:1476.
8. Grossi CE. Human T cells expressing the γ/δ T cell receptor (TCR-1): Cγ1- and Cγ2-encoded forms of the receptor correlate with distinctive morphology cytoskeletal organization, and growth characteristics. Proc Natl Acad Sci USA 1989; 86:1619.
9. Moretta L. A human T lymphocyte expressing γ/δ T cell antigen receptor. Clin Immunol Immunopathol 1989; 550:117.
10. Triebel F. Subpopulations of human peripheral T gamma delta lymphocytes. Immunol Today 1989; 10:186.
11. Foure F, et al. J Immunol 1988; 141:3357.
12. Rajasekar R, Augustin A. Selective proliferation of $\gamma\delta$-T lymphocytes exposed to high doses of Ionomycin. J Immunol 1992; 149:812–824.
13. Itoh K, Platsoucas CD, Balch CM. J Exp Med 1988; 168:1419.
14. Ioannides CG, Platsoucas CD, Rasheed S, Edwards C, Freedman RS. Cancer Res 1991; 51:4257.
15. Manzo G. Immunological correlations between ontogenesis and oncogenesis: theoretical implications and suggestions for tumor immunotherapy. Med Hypotheses 1992; 37:(3):166–170.

16. Rossol R, Hoelzer D, et al. Unpublished data.
17. Benussan A, et al. Immunodeficiency after bone marrow transplantation can be associated with autoreactive T-cell receptor gamma delta-bearing lymphocytes. Immunol Rev 1990; 116:5–13.
18. Morio T, et al. Phenotypia profile and functions of T cell receptor-gamma-delta-bearing cells from patients with primary immunodeficiency syndrome. J Immunol 1990; 144:1270–1275.
19. Carlo Stella C, Ganser A, Hoelzer D. Defective in vitro growth of the hemopoietic progenitor cells in acquired immunodeficiency syndrome. J Clin Invest 1987; 80:286–293.
20. Kabelitz D, et al. A large fraction of human peripheral blood g/d T cells is activated by Mycobycterium tuberculosis but not by its 65-kD heat shock protein. J Exp Med 1990; 171:667–679.
21. Wucherpfennig KW, Newcombe J, Li H, Keddy C, Cuzner ML, Hafler DA. γ/δ T-cell receptor repertoire in acute multiple sclerosis lesions. Proc Natl Acad Sci 1992; 89(10):4588–4592.
22. Nowaczyk M, et al. Immunomonitoring after renal transplantation. II. Posttransplant disturbances in the CD3 complex expression may be caused by immunosuppression. Arch Immunol Ther Exp Warsaw 1991; 39(3):297–299.
23. Benussan A. et al. Immunodeficiency after bone marrow transplantation can be associated with autoreactive T-cell receptor gamma delta-bearing lymphocytes. Immunol Rev 1990; 116:5–13.
24. Voth R, Rossol S, et al. Differential gene expression of IFN-α and tumor necrosis factor-α in peripheral blood mononuclear cells from patients with AIDS related complex and AIDS. J Immunol 1990; 144:970.
25. Goodier, et al. Int Immunol 1992; 4(1):33–41.
26. De Paoli P, et al. Clin Exp Immunol 1991; 83(2):187–191.
27. De Maria A, et al. J Infect Dis 1992; 165(5):917–919.
28. Bucht A, et al. Eur J Immunol 1992; 22(2):567–574.
29. USG, et al. Arthr Rheum 1992; 35(3):270–281.
30. Van Oostvem, et al. Leukemia 1992; 6(5):410–418.
31. Raziuddin S, et al. Eur J Immunol 1992; 22(5):1143–1148.
32. Vyemura K, et al. J Immunol 1992; 148(4):1205–1211.
33. Selmay K, et al. Neurology 1992; 42(4):795–800.
34. Raziuddin S, et al. Eur J Immunol 1992; 22(2):309–314.
35. Lanier LL, et al. Eur J Immunol 1988; 18:1985.
36. Casorati G, et al. J Exp Med 1989; 170:1521.

15

Autoreactivity and HIV Infection

Ryszard A. Hermaszewski and Angus G. Dalgliesh

St. George's Hospital Medical School
University of London
London, England

Elizabeth F. Hounsell

Clinical Research Centre
Harrow, England

INTRODUCTION

Immunodeficiency and the decline of CD4 levels in HIV infection may involve mechanisms other than direct cytopathic cell killing. One argument used in favor of this is that HIV infects only small numbers of the overall circulating CD4 + lymphocyte population. Recently it has been shown that, although the number of peripheral lymphocytes infected is low, the number of infected cells in the lymph nodes is extremely high even in asymptomatic people (1,2) with a reservoir of infection in the follicular dendritic cells (3). After the initial infective episode (which follows an acute pattern one would expect of a cytopathic virus), HIV can be detected in only one in 10^5 peripheral blood cells of asymptomatic persons and one in 10^3 patients with AIDS (4). Considering the reproductive capacity of hemopoietic stem cells, it is unlikely that this low frequency of infection can induce immunodeficiency or a persistent decline in CD4 cells without invoking additional mechanisms. Furthermore, there are other ubiquitous viruses, such as human herpes virus 6, cytomegalovirus, and measles, that are as cytopathic for CD4 cells in vitro but do not cause profound CD4 cell loss and immunodeficiency in vivo. Moreover, the specific dysfunction of memory CD4 cells seen within a few weeks of becoming HIV-infected is not consistent with a gradual decline of immunocompetence caused by steadily decreasing numbers of CD4 cells killed in a random fashion by a cytopathic virus. The long time from infection to the development of AIDS is in contradistinction to the marked cytotoxicity of HIV for CD4 cells in vitro. The most striking feature of HIV-related disease is the fact that children of HIV-positive mothers do not inevitably develop AIDS even though viral genome is detectable in circulating lymphocytes (5), which argues for variable host factors. Chimpanzees whose lymphocytes and monocytes are readily infectable in vitro do not become ill (6). This strongly suggests the need for specific host factors in order to initiate disease. The fact that not all infected humans progress to disease, and that this applies to children, implies additional mechanisms other than pure viral pathogenesis.

AUTOREACTIVITY

One potential mechanism for immunodeficiency and loss of CD4 cells includes an HIV-induced immunological perturbation that causes autoreactivity against CD4 cells or their precursors. Support for this hypothesis may be found in the clinical picture of AIDS, animal models of HIV infection, other retroviral-mediated diseases, and in vitro studies of reactivity against HIV and its components. Features consistent with autoimmunity in HIV infection are shown in Table 1.

Although autoantibodies are common in a number of virus infections, autoreactivity or serious organ damage is rare. Moreover, the prevalence of any one autoimmune feature—for example, idiopathic thrombocytopenic purpura (ITP)—in a population of HIV-infected patients is rarely over 10%. However, all these features looked at together suggest a significant incidence of HIV-induced autoreactivity. HIV-infected humans develop cytotoxic lymphocytes that can lyse CD4 + cells. These are not present in chimpanzees infected with HIV, and these animals do not develop AIDS (7). It is therefore possible that susceptibility to disease is somehow linked with the presence of these cytotoxic lymphocytes.

Table 1 Features of Autoimmunity in HIV Infection

Autoimmune condition	Ref.
Skin disease Seborrheic dermatitis, psoriasis, pemphigoid	24,25
Joint disease Reiter's syndrome, psoriatic arthritis	26,27
Hematological disease ITP, neutropenia, aplastic anemia	28–32
Neurological disease Acute and chronic inflammatory demyelinating polyneuropathy, sensory ganglioneuritis, polyradiculopathy, distal symmetrical polyneuropathy, mononeuritis multiplex	33,34
Vascular and connective tissue Chronic active hepatitis, vasculitis, myopathies, ocular myositis, Sjögren's syndrome, SLE-like syndrome	27,35,36
Immunological findings Immune complexes, polyclonal B-cell activation with hypergammaglobulinemia, autoantibodies (e.g., to CD4, platelets, antinuclear, rheumatoid factors), anticollagen antibodies	21,37,38

OTHER LENTIVIRUSES

The fact that HIV may be able to induce autoreactivity should not be surprising. All the other lentiviruses induce autoreactive pathology (8):

Equine infectious anemia virus causes an autoimmune reaction directed at erythrocyte cell surface antigens.

Visna virus of sheep is thought to precipitate an immune response to neural antigens.

Caprine arthritis encephalitis virus causes synovitis and multisystem disease.

Another human retrovirus (HTLV-I) is clearly connected with tropical spastic paraparesis (TSP), which does not appear to be due to direct viral-induced myelin damage.

The in vivo cell tropism of HTLV-I is predominantly CD4, CD45RO+ cells (9), and in TSP this is accompanied by extremely high-titer serological and cell-mediated responses compared to asymptomatic infected or adult T-cell-leukemia/lymphoma patients (10). This suggests that the immune response itself may be responsible for the pathology in TSP, and indeed there is marked lymphocytic infiltration in the pathological lesion in the absence of evidence (using MABS and PCR) of direct viral infection of neurological tissue. Furthermore, HTLV-I-induced neuropathology had been correlated with a particular amino acid sequence of HLA DRB1 (11), and HTLV-I *tax* gene product–directed CD8+ lymphocytes show a similar restriction to those patients with neurological disease (12). Further credence to the hypothesis that TSP is caused not by direct viral cytopathic effect but by immune-mediated damage is provided by the finding that even in endemic areas HTLV-I-negative cases may be found, indicating other possible cross-reacting trigger factors. Therefore, it is not unlikely that HIV may induce at least part of its pathology by autoreactive mechanisms.

MECHANISMS OF HIV-INDUCED AUTOREACTIVITY

Mechanisms by which HIV may induce autoreactivity include the following:

1. Chronic antigenic stimulation, leading to B-cell hyperactivity with concomitant autoantibody production.
2. The presence of MHC sequence homologies in gp120 and gp41 provides molecular mimicry at peptide level with crucial host proteins (13) (Table 2).
3. Functional mimicry of MHC, leading to chronic allogeneic stimulation. Evidence for both humoral and cytotoxic recognition of conserved domains between HIV and MHC has recently been proposed (14). If this functional mimicry was recognized as allogeneic MHC, this would lead to proliferation, autocytotoxicity, and autosuppression, resulting in anergy in a manner similar to that induced by allogeneic challenge in F1 hybrid mice (13).

EXPERIMENTS SUGGESTING A ROLE FOR HIV
IN PERTURBATING TcR RECOGNITION

The fact that HIV, and in particular gp120, can interfere with antigen recognition and lead to anergy in vitro has been demonstrated in a series

Table 2 Conserved Sequences of HIV gp160 with HLA Class I or Class II Homology

AA no.	Sequence	Ref.
247	R V QCTHGIKPIVSTQLLNGSLAE	45
432	Y A P P I	20
444	LI SNITGILLTRDGG	46, DR β1
468	D R GGGNMKDNW	20; HLA-A2
479	V ELYKYKVI	20; Beretta, unpublished observation
488	V R Q IEPLGIAPTKAKRRVVEREKRA	14; Beretta, unpublished observation
837	EGTDRVI	47

of experiments by Manca et al. (15–19). Briefly, they showed that T cells exposed to antigen in the presence of HIV or gp120 are functionally deleted when rechallenged in an activation assay with the same antigen but in the absence of HIV/gp120. This is accompanied by selective loss of reactive T cells, although the mechanism is unclear. No cytopathic effect or viral replication was detected, suggesting that clonal anergy due to suppression and/ or apoptosis may be of greater significance.

Inhibition of antigen-specific responses by gp120 is MHC-restricted, reversible (unlike whole HIV, which leads to irreversible functional deletion of antigen-specific responses), and not transferred to bystander cells. gp120 does not interfere with antigen pulsing of presenting cells but is inhibitory during the proliferation assay in this system. This suggests that the inhibitory activity is mediated by CD4.

Soluble gp120 inhibits specific human T-cell lines that respond to gp120-pulsed autologous antigen-presenting cells. This inhibitory activity of gp120 may be abolished by preventing CD4-gp120 interaction by either denaturation of gp120 or use of soluble CD4 or polyclonal antibodies. Furthermore, these effects may be mimicked by other CD4-binding agents such as anti-Leu3a MAbs. Again, the effect is reversed by soluble CD4 and denaturation of both molecules, indicating that the inhibition is mediated via CD4 binding. This reversible inhibition of CD4 cell function may facilitate the induction of tolerance in the presence of antigen. gp120 itself induces a T-cell response that is restricted to a selected immunodominant epitope in individuals. This site varies from person to person. Silent epitopes may be detected by using peptide fragments (16).

Following these experiments, we postulated that gp120 may interfere with antigen presentation either by acting like an anti-CD4 antibody or by inhibiting and/or stimulating inappropriate signals through the CD3/T-cell receptor (TcR) complex (15). Analysis of gp120 sequences revealed, in conserved regions, several areas of homology with MHC. These could interact with CD4 and the TcR complex in two ways. First, gp120-derived peptides with homology to MHC bound to self-MHC could stimulate an allogeneic response. Second, particularly in view of several areas of homology, we proposed that the tertiary structure of gp120 may mimic MHC and this too might function by means of stimulation as an alloepitope.

PROPOSED STRUCTURE OF THE CARBOXY TERMINUS OF gp120

The crystallographic structure of gp120 is unresolved. To elucidate whether the tertiary structure of gp120 could approximate areas of MHC, we modeled the carboxy terminal region using computational protein chemistry. Without placing prior restrictions on the computed structure with respect to known class I MHC structure, we found that this region of gp120 folded to produce a β-strand region adjacent to a major and minor α-helix-type sequence that bears a strong resemblance to the known structure of HLA-A2 (20). Cell-surface gp120 exists as a dimer, and it is possible that the combined structure resembles allo-MHC sufficiently to directly stimulate an alloreactive response (21).

CONSEQUENCES OF ALLOSTIMULATION

This type of allogeneic response would be expected to produce hypergammaglobulinemia secondary to nonspecific activation of B cells under the influence of responding T cells as well as the induction of autosuppressive and autocytotoxic T cells (21).

One of the consequences of an allostimulation hypothesis of HIV-induced pathogenesis is that individuals would be expected to have varying responses to gp120 and whole HIV. Indeed, hyperresponsiveness to gp120 is seen in some people only (16). The limited studies to date indicate that progression to AIDS may be strongly influenced by MHC haplotype (22) (see Table 3 for review). Furthermore, there is preliminary evi-

Table 3 Effect of MHC Haplotype on Progression to AIDS

Haplotype	Effect	Ref.
HLA A1 B8 DR3	Progression	22
HLA DR5	Progression	39
HLA DRB1*0702, DQA1*0201	Absence of disease	40
B35 CW5	Progression	41
B35	Progression	42
B51	Susceptibility to infection	43
B52, B44	Resistance to infection	43
Absence of C4 null alleles	Reduced progression	44

dence for disturbance of the T-cell repertoire in early asymptomatic HIV-infected patients before the onset of clinically significant immunosuppression (23).

Clearly, lymphocyte response to presentation of HIV surface glycoproteins on the surface of presenting cells will be influenced by the surrounding milieu. Inappropriate activation may result in anergy or the elimination of T cells by autocytotoxic lymphocytes or secondary to autoantibody production. Additionally, activation of lymphocytes in itself will promote viral replication and cytotoxicity.

CONCLUSION

HIV-induced disease has features seen in autoimmune mediated diseases and many similarities to experimental chronic allogeneic disease.

Despite the lack of large numbers of circulating HIV-infected lymphocytes, there is evidence of a reservoir of infection in the thymus and lymph nodes, critical areas for the induction and suppression of immune responses where the exposure of lymphocytes to an allostimulus would be at a premium. Sequence and structural homologies between HIV surface glycoproteins and MHC may cause allostimulation of host lymphocytes. The resulting autocytotoxicity and autosuppression may account for many of the features of early HIV infection before the establishment of AIDS, at which point control over virus replication is diminished.

It is important to appreciate that HIV does not necessarily have to mimic the intact MHC molecule in a way proposed by the Hounsell et al. model to induce the described changes in AIDS. The model also predicts areas of gp120 that may be processed in a way similar to MHC in the cell and presented as peptide antigen mimics of foreign MHC sequences (of which HIV contains several) presented by self-MHC. This would also lead to the chronic inappropriate antigen stimulation that results in the activation of all the components of the immune response. It is possible that chronic superantigen stimulation (for which murine AIDS—caused by a defective murine leukemia virus—is a good model) and antibodies against the TcR could also lead to a similar clinical picture; these possibilities are discussed in other chapters in this volume. However, AIDS pathogenesis is likely to be multifactorial, and more than one of these mechanisms may be more crucial at different stages of disease. For instance, in the murine AIDS model CD4 + cells are never depleted to 200 and extrapolation to the HIV model must take into account that HIV is a cytopathic virus capable of acting as its own opportunistic infection following in the wake of its own indirect destruction of the immune system.

Our proposals are not inconsistent with the ideas expressed by Hoffman (see Chapter 17).

REFERENCES

1. Pantaleo G, Graziosi G, Butini L, et al. Lymphoid organs function as major reservoirs for HIV. Proc Natl Acad Sci USA 1992; 88:9838.
2. Fox CH, Tenner-Racz K, Racz P, et al. Lymphoid germinal centers are reservoirs of human immunodeficiency virus type 1 RNA. J Infect Dis 1991; 164(6): 1051.
3. Spiegel H, Herbst H, Niedobitek G, Foss HD, Stein H. Follicular dendritic cells are a major reservoir for human immunodeficiency virus type 1 in lymphoid tissues facilitating infection of CD4 + T-helper cells. Am J Pathol 1992; 140(1):15.
4. Harper ME, Marsell LM, Gallo RC, Wong-Staal F. Detection of lymphocytes expressing HIV in lymph nodes and peripheral blood for infected individuals by in situ hybridization. Proc Natl Acad Sci USA 1986; 83:772.
5. Escaich S, Wallon M, Baginski I, et al. Comparison of HIV detection by virus isolation in lymphocyte cultures and molecular amplification of HIV DNA and RNA by PCR in offspring of seropositive mothers. J AIDS 1991; 4(2): 130.
6. Watanabe M, Ringler DJ, Fultz PN, et al. A chimpanzee-passaged human immunodeficiency virus isolate is cytopathic for chimpanzee cells but does not induce disease. J Virol 1991; 65(6):3344.
7. Zarling JM, Ledbetter JA, Sias J, et al. HIV-infected humans, but not chimpanzees, have circulating cytotoxic T lymphocytes that lyse uninfected CD4 + cells. J Immunol 1990; 144(8):2992.

8. Schattner A, Rager ZB. Virus-induced autoimmunity [see comments]. Rev Infect Dis 1990; 12(2):204.

9. Richardson JH, Edwards AJ, Cruickshank JK, Rudge P, Dalgleish AG. In vivo cellular tropism of human T-cell leukemia virus type 1. J Virol 1990; 64(11):5682.

10. Dalgleish AG, Matutes E, Richardson J, et al. HTLV-1 infection in tropical spastic paraparesis: lymphocyte culture and enhanced serological response. AIDS Hum Retrovir 1988; 4(6):475.

11. Usuku K, Nishizawa M, Matsuki K, et al. Association of a particular amino acid sequence of the HLA-DR beta 1 chain with HTLV-I-associated myelopathy. Eur J Immunol 1990; 20(7):1603.

12. Jacobson S, Shida H, McFarlin DE, Fauci AS, Koenig S. Circulating CD8+ cytotoxic T lymphocytes specific for HTLV-I pX in patients with HTLV-I associated neurological disease. Nature 1990; 348(6298):245.

13. Habeshaw J, Hounsell E, Dalgleish A. Does the HIV envelope induce a chronic graft-versus-host-like disease? Immunol Today 1992; 13(6):207.

14. Grassi F, Meneveri R, Gullberg M, et al. Human immunodeficiency virus type 1 gp120 mimics a hidden monomorphic epitope borne by class I major histocompatibility complex heavy chains. J Exp Med 1991; 174(1):53.

15. Manca F, Habeshaw JA, Dalgleish AG. HIV envelope glycoprotein, antigen specific T-cell responses, and soluble CD4. Lancet 1990; 335(8693):811.

16. Manca F, Habeshaw J, Dalgleish A. The naive repertoire of human T helper cells specific for gp120, the envelope glycoprotein of HIV. J Immunol 1991; 146(6):1964.

17. Manca F. Selective functional depletion of HIV gp120 peptides complexed with MHC from antigen-presenting cells engaged with specific T lymphocytes. J Immunol 1992; 149(3):796.

18. Manca F, Newell A, Valle M, Habeshaw J, Dalgleish AG. HIV-induced deletion of antigen-specific T cell function is MHC restricted. Clin Exp Immunol 1992; 87(1):15.

19. Manca F, Walker L, Newell A, Celada F, Habeshaw JA, Dalgleish AG. Inhibitory activity of HIV envelope gp120 dominates over its antigenicity for human T cells. Clin Exp Immunol 1992; 88(1):17.

20. Hounsell EF, Renouf DV, Liney D, Dalgleish AG, Habeshaw J. A proposed molecular model for the carboxy terminus of HIV-1 gp120 showing structural features consistent with the presence of a T-cell alloepitope. Molec Aspects Med 1991; 12(4):283.

21. Via CS, Morse H3, Shearer GM. Altered immunoregulation and autoimmune aspects of HIV infection: relevant murine models. Immunol Today 1990; 11 (7):250.

22. Simmonds P, Beatson D, Cuthbert RJ, et al. Determinants of HIV disease progression: six-year longitudinal study in the Edinburgh haemophilia/HIV cohort [see comments]. Lancet 1991; 338(8776):1159.

23. Dalgleish AG, Wilson S, Gompels M, et al. T-cell receptor variable gene products and early HIV-1 infection [erratum appears in Lancet 1992; 339(8798): 942] [see comments]. Lancet 1992; 339(8797):824.

24. Staughton R. Skin manifestations in AIDS patients. Br J Clin Prac (symp suppl) 1990; 71(109):109.

25. Kinloch-de Loes S, Didierjean L, Rickhoff-Cantoni L, Imhof K, Perrin L, Saurat JH. Bullous pemphigoid autoantibodies, HIV-1 infection and pruritic papular eruption. AIDS 1991; 5(4):451.

26. Kaye BR. Rheumatologic manifestations of infection with human immunodeficiency virus (HIV). Ann Intern Med 1989; 111(2):158.

27. Buskila D, Gladman D. Musculoskeletal manifestations of infection with human immunodeficiency virus. Rev Infect Dis 1990; 12(2):223.

28. Stricker RB. Hemostatic abnormalities in HIV disease. Hematol/Oncol Clin N Am 1991; 5(2):249.

29. Baranski BG, Young NS. Autoimmune aspects of aplastic anemia. In Vivo 1988; 2(1):91.

30. Telen MJ, Roberts KB, Bartlett JA. HIV-associated autoimmune hemolytic anemia: report of a case and review of the literature. J AIDS 1990; 3(10): 933.

31. Karpatkin S, Nardi M. Autoimmune anti-HIV-1gp 120 antibody with anti-idiotype-like activity in sera and immune complexes of HIV-1-related immunologic thrombocytopenia. J Clin Invest 1992; 89(2):356.

32. Ribera E, Ocana I, Almirante B, Gomez J, Monreal P, Martinez-Vazquez JM. Autoimmune neutropenia and thrombocytopenia associated with development of antibodies to human immunodeficiency virus. J Infection 1989; 18(2): 167.

33. Kennedy PGE. Neurological aspects of lentiviral infection in animals. In: Rudge P, ed. Neurological Aspects of Human Retroviruses. London: Bailliere Tindall, 1992:41.

34. Parry GJ. Peripheral neuropathies associated with human immunodeficiency virus. Ann Neurol 1988; 23(suppl):S49.

35. Cabello A. Myopathy associated to human immunodeficiency virus (HIV) infection. Archivos de Neurobiologia 1989; 52(suppl 1):104.

36. de Clerck LS, Couttenye MM, de Broe ME, Stevens WJ. Acquired immunodeficiency syndrome mimicking Sjögren's syndrome and systemic lupus erythematosus. Arth Rheum 1988; 31(2):272.

37. Martinez A, Marco M, de I Hera A, et al. Immunological consequences of HIV infection. Lancet 1987; ii:454.

38. Kyriakis K, Tosca A, Katsantonis J, Hatzivasiliou M, Eliopoulos G, Stratigos J. Detection of autoimmunity parameters in the acquired immunodeficiency syndrome (AIDS). Int J Dermatol 1992; 31(2):113.

39. Cruse JM, Brackin MN, Lewis RE, Meeks W, Nolan R, Brackin B. HLA disease association and protection in HIV infection among African Americans and Caucasians. Pathobiology 1991; 59(5):324.

40. Louie LG, Newman B, King M. Influence of host genotype on progression to AIDS among HIV-infected men. J AIDS 1991; 4(8):814.
41. Jeannet M, Sztajzel R, Carpentier N, Hirschel B, Tiercy JM. HLA antigens are risk factors for development of AIDS. J AIDS 1989; 2(1):28.
42. Itescu S, Mathur WU, Skovron ML, et al. HLA-B35 is associated with accelerated progression to AIDS. J AIDS 1992; 5(1):37.
43. Fabio G, Scorza R, Lazzarin A, et al. HLA-associated susceptibility to HIV-1 infection. Clin Exp Immunol 1992; 87(1):20.
44. Hentges F, Hoffman A, Oliveira De Auraujo F, Hemmer R. Prolonged clinically asymptomatic evolution after HIV-1 infection is marked by the absence of complement C4 null alleles at the MHC. Clin Exp Immunol 1992; 88(2): 237.
45. Young JAT. HIV and HLA similarity (letter). Nature 1988; 333(6170):215.
46. Brinkworth RI. The envelope glycoprotein of HIV-1 may have incorporated the CD4 binding site from HLA-DQ beta 1. Life Sci 1989; 45(20).
47. Golding H, Robey FA, Gates F3, et al. Identification of homologous regions in human immunodeficiency virus I gp41 and human MHC class II beta 1 domain. I. Monoclonal antibodies against the gp41-derived peptide and patients' sera react with native HLA class II antigens, suggesting a role for autoimmunity in the pathogenesis of acquired immune deficiency syndrome. J Exp Med 1988; 167(3):914.

16

The Immune System Network and the Pathogenesis of AIDS

J. A. Habeshaw

London Hospital Whitechapel
London, England

INTRODUCTION

The virus HIV-1 is a sufficient first cause of the acquired immunodeficiency syndrome (AIDS). The purpose of this chapter is to explore the immune mechanism by which this retrovirus induces progressive immunodeficiency.

The integrity of the immune system is enforced by the evolutionary selection of the variable components in the presence of an invariant framework. Loss of the invariant framework [provided by the major histocompatibility complex (MHC) class I and II molecules] deprives the immune system of the necessary connectivity between the variable elements necessary to maintain specificity of response and the immunological memory of previous responses. We hypothesize that HIV-1 mimics the structurally invariant components (namely, MHC classes I and II) in humans, and thereby causes an alteration in the "self-referential" basis for signal generation within the immune system.

Recent data from studies involving whole HIV and SIV vaccines have led to an apparent paradox that protective immune responses against the virus (as exemplified by immune responses to key viral components) may have no direct relevance to resistance to the immunodeficiency disease caused by the virus.

In these studies, antibodies to the cells in which the virus was produced apparently reduce the susceptibility to the disease and make it more difficult for the virus to infect immune or vaccinated individuals. In other words, an effective immune response solely against retroviral components is not protective against disease caused by the same virus. The mechanisms of immunodeficiency induction are therefore not equivalent to a failure of the individual concerned to make an effective immune response against viral components.

Susceptibility to the development of AIDS, subsequent to infection with HIV-1, has little to do with the strength, type, or class of antiviral immune response. We may, however, reason that susceptibility to AIDS is a function of the constitution of the invariant (self-referential) component of immune system which can be imitated (mimicked) by the virus. Recognition of this paradox will allow development of effective therapy and protection against AIDS by specifically altering the susceptibility of individuals using techniques that are unrelated to the conventional means of inducing antiviral immunity.

DISTINGUISHING BETWEEN VIRUS-INDUCED CYTOPATHIC EFFECTS AND AIDS INDUCTION

The HIV-1 retrovirus is capable of infecting and reproducing in a variety of nonhuman primate cells. The chimpanzee is very closely related, genetically, to the human, yet human pathogenic strains of HIV-1 do not cause AIDS, or AIDS-like diseases, in chimpanzees.

Initially it was believed that subtle differences in the ability of HIV-1 to infect or kill chimpanzee T cells or other cell types accounted for this difference between the species in susceptibility to AIDS. It is now known that despite the relative resistance of chimpanzee T cells and bone-marrow macrophages to infection with HIV-IIIB, RF, or MN laboratory isolates, adapted strains of HIV-1 are cytopathic for chimpanzee T cells, and replicate as efficiently within the cells of this species, as in humans. However, such strains do not induce AIDS in the chimpanzee (1).

A further difference between the species is that HIV-1-infected humans, but not chimpanzees, develop cytotoxic CD8 + lymphocytes which kill uninfected human and chimpanzee CD4 + T lymphocytes (2). The development of HIV-specific cytotoxic T cells in humans is, in contrast to other viral infections, not dependent on prior exposure to HIV, and the frequencies of such T cells in the human T-cell repertoire are high (from 0.5 to 8% of the total lymphoid population in lung, blood, and lymph node) (3). Unprimed human T cells are capable of reacting to gp120 by the generation of T-cell lines restricted to single defined epitopes within the molecule. (4)

These data show that T-cell responses to HIV differ between humans and chimpanzees, and only the former species develops AIDS. Importantly, this difference is not due to any known characteristic of the virus, but must be due to constitutional differences between the species. Thus, the human T-cell repertoire contains T cells (both CD4 + and CD8 + subsets) that spontaneously interact with gp120/41, and in some individuals these T cells are present in high frequency. The chimpanzee T-cell repertoire lacks such cells. There is therefore a case for arguing that the spontaneous presence of T cells recognizing HIV-1 envelope glycoprotein gp120/41 in the human T-cell repertoire determines susceptibility to AIDS, irrespective of the intrinsic cytopathic attributes of HIV-1.

THE NATURE OF THE INTRINSIC STIMULUS TO HUMAN T CELLS BY HIV-1

The gp120 glycoprotein of HIV-1 binds to the CD4 molecule on the CD4 + T-cell subset (5) and on the other immune cells such as macrophages and antigen-presenting cells. CD4 is the T-cell surface receptor for MHC class II molecules (7), and there is evidence of functional equivalence of the CD4 region involved in MHC class II binding and gp120 binding (6). gp120 binding to CD4 prevents adherence between artificial target cells bearing MHC class II molecules and T-cell CD4 (8).

The fact that such inhibition is gp120-concentration-dependent and competitive further illustrates the conformational similarity between the MHC class II and gp120 molecules and their respective binding sites on CD4. Antibodies in HIV-1-seropositive individuals directed against the gp41 transmembrane component of the cell-surface-expressed gp120/41 heterodimer have been shown to cross-react with MHC class II antigens (9). An HLA-DR derived peptide (DRβ141-155) has the ability to inhibit HIV-1 syncytial induction. This sequence is homologous to the AA254–268-conserved, DR-mimicking sequence of gp120 (10). The same envelope sequence enhances PPD-specific and autoreactive activation of T cells in seronegative individuals (11). It has also been shown that a monomorphic MHC class I epitope expressed on activated T cells is mimicked conformationally by gp120 (12).

Thus, gp120/gp41 binds to CD4 using a binding site conformationally similar to MHC class II, and cross-reacts with antibodies directed toward monomorphic determinants of both MHC classes I and II. As previously recognized, the existence of CD4 binding and mimicry of MHC components by gp120 might conceivably constitute an "allogeneic" stimulus to the human T-cell receptor (TcR) (13). Such an interpretation would fit many of the known features of HIV-1-induced disease. In particular, the existence of spontaneously gp120-specific cytotoxic T cells from HIV-seronegative individuals and the spontaneous T-cell recognition of gp120 epitopes in HIV-seronegative individuals establish that a pre-existing pool of HIV-reactive T cells is present in the majority of the unprimed human population. Such cells occur in frequencies greater than can be accounted for by "accidental" priming with cross-reactive T-cell epitopes of extrinsic origin. By contrast, alloreactive systems are characterized by a high frequency of spontaneously reactive T cells of helper-T-cell (CD4 +) and cytotoxic (CD8 +) type.

Most cytotoxic T cells derived from alloreactive mixed-lymphocyte culture are CD8 + and recognize class I alloantigens. However, precursor frequencies of CD4 + alloreactive T cells recognizing MHC class II alloantigens or minor locus (MLS) antigens can be 6- to 20-fold higher than class I alloreactive CD8 + T cells (14). The expected frequencies of T cells reactive to allogeneic stimuli in unprimed individuals (0.3% for CD8 + / class I; 1.8 to 6% for CD4 + /class II or MLS combinations) are remarkably similar to the observed frequencies of spontaneously reactive CD4 + and CD8 + T cells to HIV + targets in HIV-1-seronegative individuals.

On this basis, several research groups now argue that AIDS subsequent to HIV-1 infection is analogous to chronic allogeneic reactivity as exemplified by experimental graft-versus-host disease (15). Further functional evidence supporting this viewpoint is available.

In HIV infection, allospecific self-MHC-restricted T-cell activation is defective, while allo-restricted T-cell activation is preserved (16). In mice immunized with allogeneic cells, antibodies are generated that cross-react with both gp120 and p24 antigens of HIV (17). Spontaneous anti-gp120 antibodies from MRL/Lpr mice react with the same gp120 epitopes that represent the main neutralizing domains in humans. This effect is apparently not linked to the presence of murine retrovirus mimicry of gp120 (18), and no such anti-gp120 activity is found in the closely related AKR mouse strain. Monoclonal anti-idiotypic antibodies to human anti-gp41 cross-react with pooled and single HIV-seropositive sera containing anti-gp120 and anti-p24 antibodies (19). The HIV gp120/gp41 antigens appear to mimic serologically determined alloepitopes in mice as well as in humans. The idiotype of antibodies to the gp120/gp41 epitopes is restricted and conserved between outbred HIV-seropositive humans.

These data together lead to the conclusion that:

1. T-cell activation by gp160/gp41 is qualitatively and quantitatively like activation by alloantigens.
2. The "alloantigenic" gp120/gp41 component is conserved in HIV-1 virus strains.
3. Murine antibodies generated to the HLA-mimicking determinants upon gp120/gp41 are cross-reactive with human HLA class I.
4. Alloimmune and autoimmune mice spontaneously express antibodies cross-reactive with gp120.
5. The idiotype of anti-gp120 antibodies is conserved (restricted) in HIV-seropositives humans.

The question of why nonrandom events in mice, such as allogeneic challenge or genetically induced autoimmune disease, should give rise to immune responses that imitate the human response to HIV-1 retrovirus is of basic biological significance. What kind of pathogenic process relates these apparently distinct entities? The hypothesis that HIV-1 induces graft vs. host disease (GVHD) in humans is one possible explanation, implying that mechanisms for allorecognition and alloreactivity are in some way "conserved" evolutionarily. How this might be is examined later. Initially the characteristics of HIV-1 envelope as an MHC mimic and the functional consequences of MHC mimicry are considered.

COMPUTER MODELING OF CONSERVED REGIONS OF gp120 AND STRUCTURAL HOMOLOGIES WITH MHC ANTIGENS

The gp120 sequence is very variable between laboratory strains (cloned isolates) of HIV-1. Apart from conservation of cysteine residues important in maintaining molecular conformation (and hence function), there are only six regions of gp120 highly conserved between the 16 or so available sequenced strains. These are:

```
         R   V
247  Q C T H G I K P I V S T Q L L N G S L A E

432  Y A P P I

         L I
444  S N I T G I L T R D G G

         D   R
468  G G G N M K D N W

             V
479  E L Y K Y K V I

             V       R           Q
488  I E P L G I A P T K A K R R V V E R E K R A
```

The sequence AA 247–269 is known to share sequence homology with human HLA class II (20). The sequence AA 426–432 (including valine 425 and tryptophan at 432—βRU strain) is critical for CD4 binding and infectivity (21). Previously Brinkworth (22) had noted the similarity of the gp120 sequence to HLA DQβI. The region AA 442–508 of the ELI gp120 shows some striking homology with both the HLA-A2 sequence (101–164) and HLA DRβI (15–80).

The sequence S N I T G L L T R D G I N has homology with the DRβI sequence N G T - - L - R C - I Y N. The sequence W T A D M of HLA-A2 has homology with the gp120 sequence P G G D M, the former being the site of the minor α helix of HLA-A2. When modeled using conventional algorithms for determining protein structure from sequence, the carboxy terminal portion of gp120 shows the same general structural features as both MHC class I and class II (23):

1. A terminal α helix.
2. An underlying β-pleated sheet made up of three antiparallel strands.
3. A conserved tryptophan residue at position 477 in gp120 occupies the same spatial orientation to a "minor α-helical" region (468 G G D M) that the conserved tryptophan at AA 147 (HLA-A2) does to the minor α helix of class I (AA 135 T A A D M).
4. A conserved glycosylation site at gp120 N 442 corresponds to a similar glycosylation site at HLA-A2 N86. The sequences of the α-helical structures of the C terminus of gp120 (496–508) compared with those of HLA-A2 (152–165) and class II DRβI (68–81) show

that the nonpolymorphic residues of HLA-A2 and HLA DRβI that interact with the TcR are either mimicked by the gp120 α helix or expressed as an arginine residue as below (22):

HLA-A2	V A E Q L R A Y L E G T C V
DRβI	L L E Q R R A A V D T Y C A
gp120	T R A K R R V V E R E K R

The existence in reality of a gp120 structure conforming to this model would account for:

1. The CD4 binding characteristics of gp120.
2. The cross-reactivity of anti–class I and II antibodies against conserved HLA-like determinants within gp120.
3. The reactivity of T cells with gp120. This is due to the CD4 binding characteristics together with the TcR's being engaged by the residues in the gp120 α helix homologous to those in the equivalent location in class I and II antigens (24).

The gp120/gp41 glycoprotein therefore mimics HLA to the human TcR with a high degree of probability.

THE MOLECULAR IMMUNOLOGY OF ALLORECOGNITION

All (or the vast majority) of T cells in an adult individual interact with "self"-MHC. This interaction forms the basis of the immune system's ability to discriminate at a molecular level between peptide fragments presented to the T-cell V-region receptor. Self-proteins are cleaved into peptides, bind to the appropriate MHC molecule (class I or II), and engage the TcR following interaction of the CD4 or CD8 ligand with the MHC class I or II molecule on the peptide-presenting cell (25).

Since the MHC is invariant and the self-peptide is also invariant, the same MHC will bind the same invariant peptide in the same way. This encounter (self-MHC + self-peptide) constitutes an "expected signal" to the T cell, and no proliferative response ensues. Conceptually, peripheral T cells fail to respond to the "self-MHC–self-peptide" combination either because T cells responding by proliferation to this combination are no longer present in the adult or because such interactions are suppressed by feedback circuits.

However, the "self" interaction is necessary, in some way, to maintain homeostasis of the T-cell repertoire. It is as if the continued existence of self-restricted T cells depends on their receiving a continuous signal from encounters with self-MHC–self-peptide-presenting cells. In vitro, highly purified CD4+ or CD8+ lymphocytes deprived of syngeneic MHC class I or II positive antigen-presenting cells die unless activated through TcR-independent pathways.

The most common form of immune reactivity occurs when a peptide presented by self-MHC has an amino acid sequence that differs from those previously encountered by the TcR repertoire. In this case, the interacting T cell proliferates, since an altered (i.e., not self) amino acid sequence of an MHC-presented peptide constitutes a "signal" to the T cell.

Normally only a very small proportion of T cells can interact with a non-self peptide sequence (probably fewer than one in 10^4) presented on self-MHC (26). If the same non-self sequence is repeatedly presented to the T-cell repertoire, the proportion of peptide-specific T cells rapidly increases.

Although different allelomorphic forms of MHC bind peptides differently (27), provided that the self-MHC and peptides of self origin are invariant (since in the individual all self-proteins other than the V regions of the TcR or the Ig molecule are invariant), only proteins with a peptide sequence differing from the library of self-peptides "learned" by the TcR repertoire will produce proliferation of a specific subset of T cells.

In physiological terms, most of the signal input to the self-recognizing T-cell subsets occurs through peptides derived from variable-region gene expression. High mutation rates in these proteins constitute a continuous signal to the self-peptide-maintained T-cell pool. The flanking sequences of the peptide in the whole protein are of importance in determining how peptides are cleaved, and the allelomorphic forms of the MHC determine which of the many peptide sequences will be bound. The specificity of T-cell proliferation to "foreign" proteins, as measured in the laboratory, is therefore a function of:

1. The invariance of self-MHC.
2. The repertoire of TcRs maintained in the peripheral lymphoid tissues by the self-MHC–self-peptide presentation.
3. The variation in amino acid sequence of the "foreign" peptides derived from the protein in question in comparison with the repertoire of peptides presented as invariants derived from self-proteins. Sequences of "foreign" protein-derived peptides that are identical with invariant self-protein-derived peptides do not constitute a signal and produce no T-cell proliferation (28).

T-cell specificity for an antigen, as measured by T-cell proliferation, is therefore a measure of which antigenic peptide sequences differ from self sequences when presented by self-MHC. Because all individuals (except identical twins) have "different" MHC molecules, few peptide sequences are equivalently antigenic in all humans. Those that are constitute promiscuous or universal antigenic epitopes to the T cell (28).

The polymorphic nature of the MHC permits diversity of T-cell response to foreign epitopes, as can be seen from the individual variability of responses to gp120 in unprimed (naive) individuals (4).

Three classes of response by T cells appear not to be dependent upon peptide presentation; that is, responses occur without antigen processing to peptides and are therefore not restricted by self-MHC. These three classes of response are:

1. Responses due to "superantigens," otherwise known as VbSE (variable-region β-chain selective elements) (29,30)
2. Responses due to non-self-MHC; the allogeneic response (31)
3. Responses to antibody molecules that interact directly with the TcR without prior processing (anti-T-cell idiotype responses)

The effects of such non-MHC-restricted responses depend on T-cell activation or suppression without specificity being dictated by a self-MHC–peptide complex. In all three cases, direct interaction of the whole protein with the TcR occurs. The effects produced are out of proportion to the stimulus presented, since the frequency of reactive T cells is higher than for self-MHC–peptide combinations.

When the sequences of MHC molecules supporting the proliferation of alloreactive T-cell clones are examined, two types of variation representing the specific "alloepitope" are seen: substitution in the α helix of the class I or II molecule that projects "upward" to the face of the TcR and substitution in the α helix that projects "inward" to the peptide-binding groove, or that occurs in the β-pleated sheet that forms the base of the peptide-binding groove (27,31). Current knowledge therefore indicates that alloreactivity occurs when:

1. Peptides derived from the allogeneic MHC are presented by self-MHC; this is self-MHC-restricted allospecific reactivity equivalent to a T-cell response to any foreign peptide sequence.
2. The allogeneic or foreign MHC presents a different class of self-peptide to the TcR. There is variation in the capacity of different

MHC molecules to present a specific peptide; thus, a different selection of self-peptides will be presented by a foreign MHC, and responses will be allorestricted (i.e., dependent on the class of allogeneic MHC presenting the self-peptide) and peptide-specific.

3. Where differences between self-MHC and foreign MHC involve those portions of the α helix projecting toward the face of the TcR, the alloresponse will occur irrespective of which peptide is present in the antigen-binding groove.

These are "allospecific" responses that lack defined HLA restriction, but responses are restricted by the available TcRs and independent of the peptide presented.

Allospecific reactions of the third type are similar to the class of T-cell response produced by the superantigens (or VβSE). They differ in two respects:

1. The superantigen requires MHC for its presentation (as a whole molecule) to the TcR (32).
2. The superantigen interacts with regions of the TcR that are not involved in direct interaction with the MHC peptide complex (32–34).

The interaction between the superantigen and the TcR is specific for a single element (usually the β-chain V region) of the TcR. In class III allospecific reactions, the TcR and foreign MHC interact theoretically without bias toward a single element of the TcR (31). However, where the allogeneic MHC is present from birth or is allowed to select "allorestricted" T cells in vitro, the resulting TcR repertoire is functionally different and differs in the frequencies of usage of the Vβ components of the TcR, in comparison to repertoires evolved in the absence of the allogeneic MHC (reviewed in Refs. 35 and 36).

CONSERVATION OF TcRs MEDIATING MHC-RESTRICTED ANTIGEN RESPONSES

It is known that for individuals who share an MHC class I phenotype, the same TcR Vα and Vβ sequences are used to recognize a single antigenic peptide (31,37).

Most of the variability observed in the TcR Jα and Jβ segments in peptide-specific, MHC-restricted responses indicates that TcR selection in such responses is achieved by the peptide MHC complex itself and not solely by the MHC class presenting the peptide (38). If responses are due primarily to the presentation of many different self-peptides by the allogeneic MHC (as in the second class of alloreactivity), then TcR Vα or Vβ selection by the allo-MHC would not be an expected feature of alloreactivity (28). Thus, if gp120/41 were an exact mimic of MHC class I or II, presenting self-peptide to the TcR following its interaction with CD4, one would not expect to find bias in TcR Vα-Vβ gene expression in seropositive individuals (31).

When highly purified CD4+ T cells are cocultured with gp120/41-expressing CHO KI cells, no proliferative response is seen. In contrast, CD4+ T cells will proliferate when exposed to allogeneic antigen-presenting cells (39). Thus, gp120/41 does not induce alloreactivity of the second class (allorestricted self-peptide-specific). Reactions to envelope glycoprotein do occur in about 50% of naive individuals, provided the CD4-blocking effect of gp120 on HLA class II–restricted responses is removed (4). Therefore, the proliferative effect of gp120/41 on human T cells involves more than a direct encounter between this molecule and the CD4+ T cell.

Data from molecular modeling and serological studies strongly suggest MHC mimicry by gp120/41. Moreover, the capacity of gp120 to bind CD4 directly implies that self-MHC class II is not necessary to present intact gp120 to the TcR complex, as is found with superantigens. The major pathogenic effect of HIV-1 mimicry of MHC is therefore to induce non-MHC-restricted responses in the target T-cell population. The fact that most individuals respond in the same way to the gp120/41 complex strongly suggests that the mimicry is of some conserved, nonpolymorphic domain of MHC class I or II. Such domains have been implicated in GVHD protection (35,36,68) and in autosupressive and autoreactive immune states (50–53,58).

THE PREDICTED EFFECTS OF MHC MIMICRY BY HIV-1 gp160

Is There Selective Bias for Particular TcR Vα or Vβ Elements?

With conventional alloreactivity, one would expect the TcR repertoire of animals exposed to allogeneic MHC to be functionally different from the TcR of unexposed animals, but one would not expect to find strongly biased usage of a single class of TcR V region. This is because the majority of the TcR V-region elements are used in generation of the TcR repertoire for each individual, and because conventional alloantigens are so closely related structurally that the same TcR repertoire can interact more or less completely with the self-peptide allogeneic MHC combinations encountered (40). Because of close structural similarity between MHC antigens (38) and because of the invariance in most endogenous proteins within a single strain, any "selective" effect of the allogeneic MHC will act upon a substantial fraction of the entire TcR repertoire (perhaps 10–20% of T cells), effectively precluding selection by proliferation of a single TcR V-region class.

In the case of the defined superantigens (VβSE), negative selection of some Vβ elements can occur in fetal thymus culture, but this is observed only when the appropriate MHC class II– expressing antigen-presenting cell is present (30,33,34,37,41). When VβSE is presented by medullary epithelial cells, there is no reduction in the Vβ component that interacts with the superantigen. Another mechanism, dependent on transmission of superantigen or maternal antibody to the fetus, also results in deletion of the VβSE-interactive portion of the TcR repertoire. Such deletion can be transmitted via lactation and suckling in a passive manner.

In the case of the proposed mimicry of MHC by gp120/41, it is evident that the proportions of T cells in any individual interacting with gp120/41 will be smaller than in conventional allogeneic reactions (that is, self-restricted allospecific reactivity and allorestricted peptide-specific reactivity). Thus, the T-cell populations responding by proliferation to the MHC mimic may exhibit TcR V-gene restriction to the extent that they form, initially, only a small proportion of the TcR repertoire.

Whether or not any such gp120/41 interactive T cells exist initially in the individual may be a function of either the individual MHC genotype or the MHC haplotype. Individuals lacking such T cells from their repertoire will not progress to AIDS when infected with HIV-1. In others, susceptibility to AIDS will depend on the proportion of TcRs in the repertoire reacting to gp120/41 in a "non"-MHC-restricted manner. Here we postulate that the only restrictive element is the reactive TcR. Thus, in patients who are HIV-1 positive but progress to AIDS slowly (i.e., have the smallest proportion of reactive T cells in the repertoire), one is more likely to find TcR V-region restriction than in patients with rapid progression to AIDS.

In a recent study, positive selection of Vβ5 was shown in a selected population of HIV-1-seropositive patients with normal CD4 counts (42). It is unlikely that Vβ5 is the only selected element as, in contrast to superantigen deletion, allospecific reactions probably involve both Vα- and

Vβ-specific motifs. Thus, Vβ selection is predicted to be apparent only in those HIV-1-seropositive individuals who are least susceptible to AIDS.

Is T-Cell Depletion in AIDS Restricted to Certain TcR Vα or Vβ Elements?

The mechanisms of T-cell depletion in the presence of an allogeneic MHC are not well understood. In the thymus, depletion of "self-reactive" T cells depends on whether the immature T cell encounters a peptide presented on thymic epithelial cells (in which case positive selection occurs) or whether presentation of peptide is by specialized medullary dendritic cells (in which case negative selection or depletion occurs). Depletion occurs by apoptosis of the thymocyte (34).

These considerations are relevant to HIV-1 infection since the virus occurs within dendritic cells in lymph nodes and spleen, and encounters between virus and T cells in these sites have been advanced as a cause of CD4 + T-cell depletion. Moreover, preapoptotic T cells have been demonstrated in up to 80% of HIV-seropositive patients; apoptosis is triggered either in the presence of a superantigen or by nonspecific polyclonal T-cell activators such as PHA.

Evidence for selective depletion of TcR Vα or Vβ elements by gp120/41 is currently available (43), but since the envelope glycoprotein does not demonstrably have "superantigen" characteristics, it appears unlikely that specific depletion is easily detected. The issue is further clouded by the overall loss of T cells due to mechanisms other than direct interaction with gp120/41.

Haplotype Versus MHC Genotype in Determining AIDS Susceptibility

Mimicry of HLA class I or II antigens by gp120/41 implies that susceptibility to AIDS must relate to the HLA genotype or the HLA haplotype of the seropositive individual. There is substantial evidence of such linkage (44–47) but no quite definite association with a single genotype or haplotype. If gp120/41 mimicked a known HLA alloantigen, then distinct linkage should have been established by now. What if the mimicry of HLA was of a conserved domain, common to many genotypes but absent in a few MHC alleles? Here one would predict that only those individuals whose genotype contained those alleles lacking the "conserved domain" would be resistant to AIDS development following HIV infection. The fact that the great majority of humans are AIDS-susceptible to some degree, and the fact that no evidence of direct linkage to HLA genotype has yet been established, strongly suggest that the HLA component mimicked by gp120/41 is common to the majority of MHC class I or II alleles; i.e., that it is a "self-MHC" restriction element.

If this is so, it leads to the question of whether such mimicry of what amounts to a cryptic "self-MHC domain" could give rise to GVH-like disease, bearing in mind that autologous (self)-reactive T cells supposedly are eliminated during fetal and neonatal life or are otherwise "suppressed" in the adult (48,49). A definitive answer to this question is not currently available, but there is evidence for the existence of both autoreactive CD4 + and autocytotoxic CD8 + T cells in the normal T-cell repertoire, and the occurrence of such cells has been documented in both autoimmune disease and some bacterial or viral infections (11,50–53).

The fact that such autoreactive T cells can be demonstrated in disease implies a selective process in T-cell ontogeny that results in their survival as antigen-specific T-cell clones, while inducing tolerance of their reactivity to self-MHC.

MATERNAL RESPONSES TO PATERNAL ALLOANTIGENS

Specific reactivity of T cells to allogeneic MHC is an acquired characteristic. The immune system of the newborn mammal contains T cells that react directly with both self- and foreign MHC. Such priming of the fetal immune system by the mother depends on the maternal antibody response made to paternal MHC alloantigens expressed on placenta. Conversely, when paternal MHC alloantigens are presented on lymphocytes or spleen cells are directly injected into the mother (54,55), alloreactive priming does not occur, although pregnancy in such alloimmune mothers appears to progress normally. Small doses of allogeneic immunocompetent cells have very similar protective effects in neonatal animals subsequently re-exposed to GVHD induction by the same cells.

The absence of "alloreactive" priming seen in such immunization prevents the occurrence of GVHD in neonates challenged with paternal strain cells (35,36). This occurs for GVHD induced in semiallogeneic, allogeneic (55), and minor locus (54) incompatible mouse strain combinations. In in vitro MLR, the T cells from F_1 mice born to preimmunized mothers adopt the reactive profile of T cells from the paternal strain; i.e., they are unreactive to cells from the donor strain. In contrast, when co-cultured with lymphocytes from the syngeneic strain, the lymphocytes of F_1 mice born to preimmunized mothers stimulate but do not themselves react to lymphocytes of syngeneic origin (55). These data indicate that alloreactivity is a property associated with the network of interactive TcR V-region gene products and is only indirectly a reaction dictated by the MHC. The agent responsible for selection of the "alloreactive" TcR repertoire is maternal antibody.

In terms of immune network responses to alloantigens, the MHC haplotype (MHC paternal + MHC maternal) incompatibility is of more significance than the genotype of the F_1 (MHC F_1) because:

1. Maternal antipaternal MHC responses occur universally during pregnancy.
2. Maternal antibody forms the major source of diverse peptide presentation within the developing fetal thymus and in the neonate.
3. The neonatal TcR repertoire needs to be reactive with the inherited haploid set of paternal MHC for the lymphocytes of F_1 genotype to generate self-restricted antigen specific responses using those components of the paternal MHC haplotype that differ from maternal MHC haplotype as restriction elements.
4. The absence of paternal immunocompetent cells in normal pregnancy and hence the presence of self-restricted F_1 TcRs interactive with paternal alloantigen ensure that alloreactivity is conserved in the F_1 generation.

In contrast, if the mother is immunized with paternal lymphocytes that are alloreactive to maternal MHC, then condition 4 no longer applies and the F_1 is not susceptible to GVHD induced by semiallogeneic challenge from paternal lymphocytes, despite remaining tolerant of them as self in condition 3. Similar effects are induced by injection of small numbers of parental-strain T cells into susceptible neonatal rats (68).

These experimental data are relevant to HIV infection. The transmission of HIV from a seropositive mother to her offspring occurs with varying frequency (6–30%). Since some MHC class II alleles are not found in infected children, one component of effective transmission of HIV-1 appears to be the MHC genotype of the offspring. There is also evidence in the adult that both infectability with HIV-1 and susceptibility to AIDS are MHC-linked. If AIDS is caused by molecular mimicry of MHC molecules by gp120/41, then MHC linkage is explained and a prediction of how susceptibility to AIDS occurs can be made.

If the cause of AIDS is TcR interaction with a gp120/41 molecule that mimics a conserved nonpolymorphic (cryptic) determinant of MHC, then susceptibility will be greatest in the population that has a high proportion of "allo"- or "auto"-reactive TcRs, capable of interacting with gp120/41. The frequency of such TcRs may be predictable from the HLA haplotype if the maternal genotype and that of the individual concerned are known. The "alloreactive" TcR frequency will be determined by the response of the mother to paternal alloantigens. The inheritance of susceptibility to AIDS is therefore predicted to be a maternal dominant characteristic.

In view of the very large number of potential haplotype combinations giving rise to alloreactive TcRs in outbred human F_1 generations, cross-reactivity of T cells with an MHC mimic such as HIV-1 gp120/41 will occur in high frequency. Moreover, MHC linkage is explained since only some of these alloreactive T cells will recognize gp120/41 as "their" particular alloepitope. Therefore, although reactivity toward gp120/41 may be frequent in the human population, the severity of the resulting susceptibility to AIDS will vary directly with maternal antipaternal allotype response and indirectly with the genotype of the affected individual.

SUPPRESSION, CYTOTOXICITY, AND THE ALLOGENEIC EFFECT

One striking feature of allogeneic reactivity (GVHD) is the existence of allocytoxic and autocytotoxic T-cell activities detectable in circulating lymphocyte populations. Under normal conditions, the "autocytotoxic" populations are subject to control by an "autosuppressor" population (56).

Autocytotoxic T-cell populations are generated in the intact animal following allogeneic challenge (57); they are normally suppressed by an autosuppressor population, which does not suppress the cytotoxic response to allogeneic cells. Autoreactive cytotoxic T-cell clones, specific for MHC class II and capable of polyclonal B-cell activation, have been described following allogeneic challenge or response to influenza virus (51). The B-cell helper function of these clones is HLA-DR-restricted, and the target for cytotoxicity is MHC class II DR (50). Since MHC class II is expressed on activated T cells, these autocytotoxic T-cell clones might be expected to functionally suppress any activated T cells expressing MHC class II (59). They do not apparently suppress T cells expressing syngeneic MHC class II, even when such cells are activated, but do kill EBV-transformed syngeneic B-cell targets. In general terms, suppressor circuits exist, whereby activated T cells expressing MHC class II are suppressed or killed when such activation occurs through contact with syngeneic non-T cells expressing self-antigens (60). The suppression occurs only when the MHC class II expressed by the activated cell and by the suppressor cell are the same. Such autoreactive T cells are not activated by allogeneic MHC (50, 51,56) but occur spontaneously in a number of viral and bacterial infections (Figure 1) (53,58). A further component of GVHD is the allogeneic effect, which refers to the capacity of an allogeneic MHC to convert an unresponsive animal to a responsive one in association with a defined antigenic determinant.

In haptene carrier responses in guinea pigs, unprimed allogeneic cells, when transferred, can restore carrier function in animals primed with BGG and subsequently challenged with BGG-DNP. In the syngeneic situation, unprimed syngeneic cells do not transfer carrier function. For the allogeneic effect to exist, the inducing cells (the allogeneic cells) must elicit a response on the part of the host. If the host is unreactive to the allogeneic cells, no immunological priming for haptene carrier responses occurs. In this respect, the TcR of the responding host must be capable of interacting with the MHC of the allogeneic cell for the allogeneic effect to occur. The allogeneic effect is unidirectional—which illustrates that the phenomenon cannot be due to cytokine release. It also shows that the surface receptor of the allogeneic cell (Ig V region in B cells, TcR in T cells)

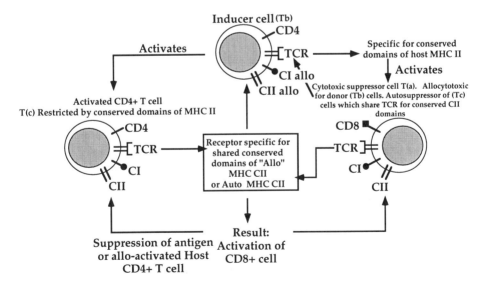

Figure 1 Donor GCH inducer cell: CD4+ host allospecific.

is not required to elicit the allogeneic effect. The allogeneic effect alone does not produce progressive immune deficiency, and is therefore not the cause of GVH-like immunodeficiency induced by HIV-1. As already discussed, the structure of gp120/41 is MHC-like with a high degree of probability. It is not necessary for cells expressing or presenting gp120/41 to the host T cell to express an additional receptor (such as Ig or TcR) for the allogeneic effect to occur. The host TcR must interact with the intact (unprocessed) allogeneic MHC to induce GVHD (61) or to induce the allogeneic effect and is also predicted to interact directly with unprocessed HIV gp120/41. Finally, resistance to virus, in the SIV model, can be elicited by the allogeneic cells used as a vehicle for virus production (62). As with the allogeneic effect, priming an animal with allogeneic cells before attempting to elicit an allogeneic effect by subsequent transfer of allogeneic cells abolishes the allogeneic effect. The allogeneic effect is seen as an important component of autoantibody formation, allowing antibody responses to develop in nonresponder (tolerant) recipients of allogeneic MHC.

In practice, the mimicry of MHC by gp120/41 explains several hitherto obscure features of HIV infection. HIV-1-seropositive patients are found to lack self-restricted antigen-specific CD4 + T cells that respond to gp120 (63), although such cells are present in at least half of uninfected individuals (4).

Since the majority of HIV-infected individuals do exhibit some form of serological response (which requires CD4-mediated T-cell help) to gp120 (64), it is pertinent to ask where such help comes from in the absence of the self-restricted gp120-specific CD4 + T-cell priming. The hypothesis of mimicry by gp120/41 of an MHC antigen, producing the allogeneic effect, accounts for the presence of antibody to gp120 in the absence of self-restricted antigen-specific T-cell help (65,66). The allogeneic effect also accounts for the hypergammaglobulinemia seen in both alloreactivity and HIV infection.

In terms of the mechanism of the immunodeficiency induced by HIV, the key observation relevant to 1) HIV infection, 2) the allogeneic effect, and 3) the related GVHD is that all depend on the existence of a host TcR population that interacts with (or can be activated by) the "allogeneic" stimulus directly, without processing of the alloantigen.

GRAFT VERSUS HOST DISEASE

GVHD differs from the allogeneic effect in that it is a progressive immunodeficiency, requiring an immunologically competent T cell for its induction.

In the experimental situation, such inducer T cells (donor T cells) are of allogeneic or semiallogeneic origin and have TcRs that interact with host MHC. The host MHC components must activate the donor T cell. The progressive immunodeficiency of GVHD requires the persistence of the donor T cell, which means GVHD is easily induced only in the neonatal period or requires prior immunosuppression for its induction. In the special case of semiallogeneic GVHD, elimination of the donor inducer T cells is defective, since part of the MHC haplotype is shared between donor and host. Given that an allogeneic immunocompetent T cell exists, such that its TcR can interact with and be activated by host MHC and that the allogeneic T cell cannot be eliminated from the host, progressive immunodeficiency ensues.

Host T cells have been shown to recognize determinants on the allogeneic GVHD inducer T-cell population. These determinants are related to the specificity of the GVHD inducer cell for host MHC–peptide complexes. It appears that the specificities recognized are in the form of a conserved idiotype on all TcRs interacting with a particular MHC class II product. In the case where GVHD protection is induced by prior immunization with low doses of inducer T cells or by other means, cytotoxic T cells occur that lyse all T cells with specificity for the donor TcR recognizing host (i.e., allogeneic) MHC. The determining factor is not the donor MHC background but the specificity of the TcR for a particular allelomorphic form of MHC. The host cytotoxic T cells, induced by donor antihost T cells, have specificity for conserved domains of TcR idiotypes recognizing host MHC class II. Since, in immune responses, the MHC class II–restricted self–T cell expresses the same TcR idiotype (one that recognizes self–MHC class II), the induction of anti-TcR cytotoxic T cells by immunizing with allogeneic T cells produces profound immunosuppression. Indeed, it has been demonstrated that T cells (Ta) specific for a shared or conserved determinant on MHC class II–specific T cells (Tb) and on the same class of MHC class II–restricted T cells (Tc) will suppress both the GVHD induced by Tb and antigen-specific T-cell responses by Tc (reviewed in Ref. 68) (Figure 1).

If gp120/41 of HIV-1 envelope is expressed on the surface of an infected host CD4 + T cell and if the mimicry of MHC class I or II is sufficient to ensure interaction with host TcR, then the situation is analogous to that with GVHD. The "inducer" cell (Tb)—the HIV-1-infected host T cell—has a TcR specific for MHC class II interaction. The HLA mimic (gp120/41) will induce host T suppressor cells (Ta) specific for conserved TcR domains of MHC class II–specific T cells (Tb) and also those expressed on antigen-specific MHC class II–restricted T cells (Tc). Thus, the effect of HLA mimicry by gp120/41 is to induce suppressor cytotoxic T cells that eliminate antigen-specific HLA class II–restricted T-cell responses. gp120/41 has an additional activity. Normally, inactive CD4+ T cells do not interact since they do not express MHC class II. Activation signals are therefore transmitted only by MHC class II–expressing antigen-presenting cells. However, when activated by the antigen-presenting cells, the CD4+ T cell expressing MHC class II can interact with any other CD4+ T cell, active or inactive. Since gp120/41 binds to CD4, it ensures T cell–to–T cell interaction as though the gp120/41-expressing T cells were activated. Therefore, the gp120/41-expressing CD4+ T cells in an infected individual shows all the criteria required for the induction of GVHD defined experimentally:

1. Expression of a TcR interactive with "host" MHC
2. Expression of an activation signal
3. Expression of an "allogeneic" MHC, in this case a mimic of HLA

By this sequence, such cells will induce autocytotoxic and autosuppressor T-cell populations which, in this case, will have anti-TcR specificity for TcR domains shared by all MHC class II–restricted host T cells. Such T-suppressor cells have previously been described in a variety of clinical conditions in addition to GVHD.

Autoreactive MHC class II–specific CD4+ T cells can activate MHC-restricted T-suppressor cells, provided the suppressor cell has the same MHC restriction as that of the autoreactive T cell (56). Such suppressor cells act to suppress antigen-specific MHC class II–restricted T-cell responses irrespective of the nominal antigen specificity of these clones (52). In mycobacterial infections, such responses are known to be restricted by MHC class II DQ (58) (Figure 2).

CONCLUSIONS, PREDICTIONS, AND NEW CONCEPTS ARISING FROM THE HYPOTHESIS THAT HIV MIMICS MHC ANTIGENS

The HIV virus would be a nonpathogenic, sporadically transmitted RNA fragment were it not for two characteristics. First, its envelope glycoprotein, which functionally (and probably structurally) resembles human MHC antigen, binds to CD4 and interacts with a subclass of human TcRs. Second, the virus itself propagates best within activated T cells and so ensures its survival and transmission by bearing an envelope that activates the T cells it infects.

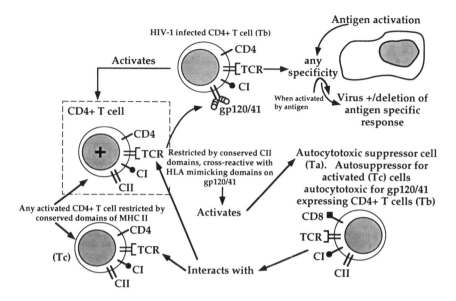

Figure 2 HIV-induced immunosuppression and CD4 + T-cell depletion.

If these two characteristics of the virus could be easily and effectively countered, the organism would no longer constitute a threat to the human population individually or collectively. Much of the pathogenesis of AIDS derives from the way the immune system reacts to what may loosely be termed allogeneic challenge. By analogy with a computer network, the immune network as a whole is quite tolerant of faults in the individual processing units linked in the network. However, apparently trivial faults, such as may occur in a program running on a network, can cause the whole network to crash. Immune network "programming" is continuously updated by the day-to-day accumulation of environmental antigenic stimuli. The observed complexity of immune responses, as defined by the immunoregulatory circuits of T-cell help and suppression and idiotype regulation, ensures that the program is kept "clean" by appropriate adjustments to the interacting cell populations, which we categorize as "immune responses." Environmental stimuli are therefore directed through the network in different pathways which are themselves defined by the progressive facilitation of responses to common stimuli, until these stimuli no longer evoke a response. The system is then described as "immune" or "tolerant," depending largely on the extrinsic or intrinsic origin of the stimulus.

This daily reprogramming of specific immune responses depends on the existence of the phenomenon known as "T -cell restriction." T-cell restriction operates because the TcRs show specificity of response only in the context of self-MHC. However, the MHC domains mediating restriction in the individual may be common to many individuals. The immune network program is therefore uniquely vulnerable to allogeneic challenge.

Neonatally induced GVHD is a fatal immunodeficiency with many features in common with AIDS. The failure to discriminate between self-MHC and foreign (allogeneic) MHC occurs at the individual—idiotypic—T-cell level.

Theoretically, it is possible that there is a relationship between the presence of alloreactive T cells in the neonate (and adult) and the maternal response to paternal alloantigens that occurs during normal pregnancy. The vehicle of transmission appears to be maternal immunoglobulin derived from the maternal antipaternal MHC response. Since the vehicle is an antibody, then interaction with the developing fetal TcR repertoire will be by direct anti-idiotypic interaction either between the TcR and the antibody or between TcR self-MHC and variable peptides derived from the Ig V region.

In either case, the "allogeneic" image transmitted will be distinct from that transmitted by physical encounters between a syngeneic MHC molecule and the same TcR. The cryptic, or hidden, nature of the allo-antigenic domain and its apparent conservation in both "self"-MHC and the allogeneic MHC may be explained by the physical transmission of alloreactivity as an immunoglobulin variable-region domain. Part of the gp120 glycoprotein has a structure homologous to the Ig variable-region domain (23,67). T cells bearing receptors for such shared MHC domains will not be eliminated during thymic selection, and hence they are detectable as "autocytotoxic," "autosuppressive," or "alloreactive" T-cell populations in the adult.

If gp120/41 acts as an MHC mimic in humans, one can predict from the above that previous pregnancy may protect a mother by reducing susceptibility to HIV infection and AIDS induction as a consequence of the maternal antipaternal MHC allotype response. The hypothesis also predicts that agents that interfere with gp120/41 interaction with the TcR, or agents that block T-cell activation by such interaction, will prevent the development of AIDS in HIV-seropositive individuals.

Susceptibility to AIDS development following HIV infection is predicted to correlate with the proportion of T cells in an individual that are activated by HIV gp120/41. It is likely that such T cells have a common TcR Vα Vβ constitution or exhibit common TcR motifs for gp120/41 interaction. Depletion of these cells will permanently prevent the development of AIDS in HIV-seropositive individuals.

In transmission of AIDS during pregnancy and in determining susceptibility of children of HIV-seropositive mothers to HIV infection and AIDS, it can be predicted that resistance in the child will be a product of the paternal MHC haplotype (maternal, antipaternal MHC haplotype response) rather than a direct correlate of the HLA genotype of the child.

These predictions can be tested. Furthermore, the concept that AIDS, alloreactivity, and autoaggressive reactivity may have similar origins from maternal dominant transmission of archaic antipaternal MHC immune responses opens a door to novel systematic approaches to the immunotherapy of such conditions.

ACKNOWLEDGMENT

J. A. H. is supported by Hiver Ltd.

REFERENCES

1. Watanabe M, Ringler DJ, Fultz PN, MacKey JJ, Boyson JE, Levine CG, Letvin NL. A chimpanzee-passaged human immunodeficiency virus isolate is cytopathic for chimpanzee T cells but does not induce disease. J Virol 1991; 65:3344–3348.
2. Zarling JM, Ledbetter JA, Sias J, Fultz PN, Eichberg J, Gjerset G, Moran PA. HIV-infected humans, but not chimpanzees, have circulating T lymphocytes that lyse uninfected CD4+ cells. J Immunol 1990; 144:2992–2998.
3. Hoffenbach A, Langlade-Demoyen P, Dadaglio G, Vilmer E, Michel F, Mayaud C, Autran B, Plata F. Unusually high frequencies of HIV-specific cytotoxic T lymphocytes in humans. J Immunol 1989; 142:452–462.
4. Manca F, Habeshaw JA, Dalgleish AG. The naive repertoire of T cell responses to gp120. J Immunol 1991; 146:1964–1971.
5. Dalgleish AG, Beverley PC, Clapham PR, Crawford DH, Greaves MF, Weiss RA. The CD4 (T4) antigen is an essential component of the receptor for the AIDS retrovirus. Nature 1984; 312:763.
6. Piatier-Tonneau D, Gastinel LN, Moussy G, et al. Mutation in the D strand of the human CD4 VI domain effect CD4 interactions with the human immunodeficiency virus envelope glycoprotein gp120 and HLA class II antigens similarly. Proc Natl Acad Sci USA 1991; 88:6858–6862.

7. Ledbetter JA, June CH, Rabinovitch PS, Grossman A, Tsu TT, Imboden JB. Signal transduction through CD4 receptors: stimulatory vs. inhibitory activity is regulated by CD4 proximity to the CD3/T cell receptor. Eur J Immunol 1988; 18:525–532.

8. Rosenstein Y, Burakoff S, Herrmann SH. HIV gp120 can block CD4 class II MHC mediated adhesion. J Immunol 1990; 144:526–531.

9. Golding H, Robey FH, Gates FT, Linder W, Beining PR, Hoffman T, Golding B. Identification of homologous regions in human immunodeficiency virus I gp41 and human MHC class II B1 domain. J Exp Med 1988; 167:914–923.

10. Lewis DE, Ulrich RG, Atassi H, Atassi MZ. HLA-DR peptide inhibits HIV-induced syncytia. Immunol Lett 1990; 24:127–132.

11. Israel-Biet D, Venet A, Beldjord D, Andrieu JM, Even P. Autoreactive cytotoxicity in HIV-infected individuals. Clin Exp Immunol 1990; 81:18–24.

12. Grassi F, Menerveri R, Gullberg M, Lopalco L, Rossi GB, Lanza P, De Santis C, Brattsand G, Butto S, Ginelli E, Beretta A, Siccardi AG. Human immunodeficiency virus type I gp120 mimics a hidden monomorphic epitope borne by class I major histocompatibility complex heavy chains. J Exp Med 1991; 174:53–62.

13. Habeshaw JA, Dalgleish AG. The relevance of HIV ENV/CD4 interactions to the pathogenesis of acquired immune deficiency syndrome. J AIDS 1989; 2:457–468.

14. Lutz CT, Glasebrook AL, Fitch FW. Enumeration of alloreactive helper T lymphocytes which co-operate with cytolytic T lymphocytes. Eur J Immunol 1981; 11:726–734.

15. Ziegler JL, Stites DP. Hypothesis: AIDS is an autoimmune disease directed at the immune system and triggered by a lymphotropic retrovirus. Clin Immunol Immunopathol 1986; 41:305–313.

16. Shearer GM, Bernstein DC, Tung KSK, Via CS, Redfield R, Salahuddin SZ, Gallo RC. A model for the selective loss of major histocompatibility complex self-restricted T cell immune responses during the development of acquired immune deficiency syndrome (AIDS). J Immunol 1986; 137:2514–2521.

17. Kion TA, Hoffman GW. Anti-HIV and anti-anti-MHC antibodies in alloimmune and autoimmune mice. Science 1991; 253:1138–1140.

18. Lombardi V, Rossi P, Mattei M, Mariani F, Colizzi V. HIV gp120 epitope immunodominance in MRL/lpr mice. 1992. Submitted.

19. Muller S, Wang HT, Kaveri SU, Kohler H. Generation and specificity of monoclonal anti-idiotypic antibodies against human HIV specific antibodies. I. Cross reacting idiotypes are expressed in subpopulations of HIV-infected individuals. J Immunol 1991; 147:933–941.

20. Young JAT. HIV and HLA similarity. Nature 1988; 333:215.

21. Cordonnier A, Montagnier L, Emerman M. Single amino-acid changes in HIV envelope affect viral tropism and receptor binding. Nature 1989; 340:571–574.

22. Brinkworth RI. The envelope glycoprotein of HIV-1 may have incorporated the CD4 binding site from HLA DQNI. Life Sci 1989; 45(20):iii–ix.

23. Hounsell EF, Renouf DV, Liney D, Dalgleish AG, Habeshaw JA. A proposed molecular model for the carboxy terminus of HIV-1 gp120 showing structural features consistent with the presence of a T-cell alloepitope. Mol Aspects Med 1991; 12:283–296.

24. Rosen-Bronson S, Yu WY, Karr RW. Polymorphic HLA-DR7 β.1 chain residues that are involved in T cell allorecognition. J Immunol 1991; 146:4264–4270.

25. Rudensky AY, Preston-Hurlburt P, Hong SC, Barlow A, Janeway CA. Sequence analysis of peptides bound to MHC class II molecules. Nature 1991; 353:622–627.

26. Nanda NK, Apple K, Sercarz E. Limitations in plasticity of the T-cell receptor repertoire. Proc Natl Acad Sci 1991; 88:9503–9507.

27. Panina-Bordignon P, Corradin G, Roosnek E, Sette A, Lanzavecchia A. Recognition by class II alloreactive T cells of processed determinants from human serum proteins. Science 1991; 252:1548–1550.

28. Moss PAH, Moots RJ, Rosenberg WMC, Rowland-Jones SJ, Bodmer HC, McMichael AJ, Bell JI. Extensive conservation of α and β chains of the human T cell antigen receptor recognising the HLA-A2 and influenza α matrix peptide. Proc Nat Acad Sci USA 1991; 88:8987–8990.

29. Coffin JM. Superantigens and endogenous retroviruses: A confluence of puzzles. Science 1992; 255:411–413.

30. Tomai MA, Aelion JA, Dockter ME, Majumdar G, Spinella DG, Kotb M. T cell receptor V gene usage by human T cell stimulated with the superantigen streptococcal M protein. J Exp Med 1991; 174:285–288.

31. Bill J, Ronchese F, Germain RN, Palmer E. The contribution of mutant amino acids to alloantigenicity. J Exp Med 1989; 170:739–746.

32. Herman A, Labrecque N, Thibodeau J, Marrack P, Kappler JW, Sekaly RP. Identification of the staphylococcal enterotoxin A superantigen binding site in the β domain of the human histocompatibility antigen HLA-DR. Proc Natl Acad Sci USA 1991; 88:9954–9958.

33. Jenkinson EJ, Kingston R, Owen JJT. Newly generated thymocytes are not refractory to deletion when the α/β component of the T cell receptor is engaged by the superantigen staphylococcal enterotoxin β. Eur J Immunol 1990; 20:2517–2520.

34. Kawabe Y, Ochi A. Programmed cell death and extrathymic reduction of Vβ8 + CD4 + T cells in mice tolerant to *Staphylococcus aureus* enterotoxin B. Nature 1991; 349:245–248.

35. De Giorgi L, Habeshaw JA. Prevention of graft versus host disease by maternal antibodies. Bull Inst Pasteur 1990; 88:265–288.

36. Wilks D. The CD4 receptor: Post-binding events, conformational change and the second site. Mol Aspects Med 1991; 12:255–265.

37. Kotzin BL, Karuturi S, Chou YK, Lafferty J, Forrester JM, Better M, Nedwin GE, Offner H, Vandenbark AA. Preferential T-cell receptor β-chain variable gene use in myelin basic protein reactive T-cell clones from patients with multiple sclerosis. Proc Nat Acad Sci 1991; 88:9161–9165.
38. Davis MM. T cell receptor gene diversity and selection. Annu Rev Biochem 1990; 59:475–496.
39. Merkenschlager M, Ikeda H, Wilkinson D, Beverley PCL, Trowsdale J, Fisher A, Altmann DM. Allorecognition of HLA-DR and -DQ transfectants by human CD45RA and CD45RO CD4 T cells: repertoire analysis and activation requirements. Eur J Immunol 1991; 21:79–88.
40. Fan W, Kasahara M, Gutknecht J, Klein J, Mayer WE, Jonker M, Klein J. Shared class II MHC polymorphisms between humans and chimpanzees. Hum Immunol 1989; 26:107–121.
41. O'Neill HC. Preferential expression of a common T cell receptor structure by T cells induced to proliferate in vitro with a murine retrovirus. Cellular Immunol 1991; 136:54–61.
42. Dalgleish AG, Wilson S, Ludlum C, Gazzard B, Pinching A, Coates AM, Habeshaw JA. Positive selection of Vβ5 in patients with early HIV infection. Lancet. 1991. In press.
43. Imberti L, Sottini A, Bettinardi A, Puoti M, Primi D. Selective depletion in HIV infection of T cells that bear specific T cell receptor Vβ sequences. Science 1991; 254:860–862.
44. Cameron PV, Mallal SA, French MAH, Dawkins RL. Major histocompatibility complex genes influence the outcome of HIV infection. Ancestral haplotypes with C4 null alleles explain diverse HLA associations. Hum Immunol 1990; 29:282–295.
45. Kilpatrick DC, Hague RA, Yap PL, Mok JYQ. HLA antigen frequencies in children born to HIV-infected mothers. Dis Markers 1991; 9:21–26.
46. Fabio G, Scorza Smeraldi R, Gringeri A, Marchini M, Bonara P, Mannucci PM. Susceptibility to HIV infection and AIDS in Italian haemophiliacs is HLA associated. Br J Haematol 1990; 75:531–536.
47. Kaslow RA, Duquesnoy R, Vanraden M, Kingsley L, Marrari M, Friedman H, Su S, Saah AJ, Detels R, Phair J, Rinaldo C. A1, CW7, B8, DR3 HLA antigen combination associated with rapid decline of T-helper lymphocytes in HIV-1 infection. Lancet 1990; 335:927–930.
48. Crispe IN, Owens T. Veto in vivo. Immunol Today 1985; 6:40–41.
49. Rammensee HG, Bevan MJ, Fink PJ. Antigen specific suppression of T-cell responses—the veto concept. Immunol Today 1985; 6:41–43.
50. Tilkin AF. Vinci G, Michon J, Levy JP. Autoreactive HLA-DR-specific autoreactive T cell clones: Possible regulatory function for B lymphocytes and haematopoetic precursors. Immunol Rev 1990; 116:171–181.
51. Tilkin AF, Michon J, Juy D, Kayibanda M, Hein Y, Sterkers G, Betuel H, Levy JP. Autoreactive T cell clones of MHC class II specificities are pro-

duced during responses against foreign antigens in man. J Immunol 1987; 1338:674-679.

52. Rosenkrantz K, Dupont B, Flomenberg N. Generation and regulation of autocytotoxicity in mixed lymphocyte cultures: Evidence for active suppression of autocytotoxic cells. Proc Natl Acad Sci 1985; 82:4508-4512.

53. Del Gallo F, Lombardi G, Piccolella E, Montani MSG, Del Porto P, Pugliese O, Antonelli G, Colizzi V. Increased autoreactive T cell frequency in tuberculous patients. Int Arch Allergy Appl Immunol 1990; 91:36-42.

54. Matossian-Rogers A, De Giorgi L. Unresponsiveness to MLS^a induced in newborn MLS^b mice by maternal preimmunisation. Immunology 1991; 72: 219-225.

55. De Giorgi L, Matossian-Rogers A, Habeshaw JA. Cellular mechanisms of Graft Versus Host Disease in a mouse model. Scand J Immunol 1991; 33: 567-574.

56. Sano K, Fujisawa I, Abe R, Asano Y, Tada T. MHC-restricted minimal regulatory circuit initiated by a class II-autoreactive T cell clone. J Exp Med 1987; 165:1284-1295.

57. Gleichmann E, Pals ST, Rolink AG, Radaszkiewicz T, Gleichmann H. Graft-versus-host reactions: clues to the etiopathology of a spectrum of immunological diseases. Immunol Today 1984; 5:324-332.

58. Salgame P, Convit J, Bloom BR. Immunological suppression by human CD8 + T cells is receptor dependent and HLA DQ restricted. Proc Natl Acad Sci 1991; 88:2598-2602.

59. Sakamoto H, Michaelson J, Jones WK, Bhan AK, Abhyankar S, Silverstein M, Golan DE, Burakoff SJ, Ferrara JLM. Lymphocytes with a CD4 + CD8 − CD3 − phenotype are effectors of experimental cutaneous graft-versus-host disease. Proc Natl Acad Sci 1991; 88:10890-10894.

60. Lehmann PV, Drexler K, Tary-Lehmann M, Falcioni F, Hurtenbach U, Nagy ZA. Graft-versus-host resistance induced by class II major histocompatibility complex-specific T cell clones. J Exp Med 1991; 173:333-341.

61. Claesson MH, Rudolphi A, Tscherning T, Reimann J. CD3 + T cells in severe combined immunodeficiency (Scid) mice IV. Graft-versus-host resistance of H-2^d scid mice to intravenous injection of allogeneic H-2^b (C57 BL6) spleen cells. Eur J Immunol 1991; 21:2057-2062.

62. Langlois AJ, Weinhold KJ, Matthews TJ, Greenberg ML, Bolognesi D. The ability of certain SIV vaccines to provoke reactions against normal cells. Science 1992; 255:292-293.

63. Krowka JF, Stites DP, Jain S, Steimer KS, Nascimento CG, Gynes A, Barr PJ, Hollander H, Moss AR, Homsy JM, Levy JA, Abrams DI. Lymphocyte proliferative responses to human immunodeficiency virus antigens in vitro. J Clin Invest 1989; 83:1198-1203.

64. Lasky LA, Groopman JE, Fennie CW, Benz PM, Capon DJ, Dowbenko DJ, Nakamura GR, Nunes WM, Renz ME, Berman PW. Neutralisation of

the AIDS retrovirus by antibodies to a recombinant envelope glycoprotein. Science 1986; 233:209–212.

65. Clerici M, Via CS, Lucey DR, Shearer GM. Functional dichotomy of CD4 + T helper lymphocytes in asymptomatic human immunodeficiency virus infection. Eur J Immunol 1991; 21:665–670.

66. Clerici M, Landay AL, Kessler HA, Zajac RA, Boswell RN, Muluk SC, Shearer GM. Multiple patterns of alloantigen presenting/stimulating cell dysfunction in patients with AIDS. J Immunol 1991; 146:2207–2213.

67. Veljkovic V, Metlas R. HIV and idiotypic T-cell regulation: another view. Immunol Today 1992; 13:38.

68. Rammensee HG. GVHD protection and I.J. Immunol Today 1988; 9:70–72.

17

Allogeneic Lymphocytes as Cofactors in AIDS Pathogenesis and the Concept of Coselection

Geoffrey W. Hoffmann and Tracy A. Kion
University of British Columbia
Vancouver, British Columbia, Canada

BASIC SCIENCE

Introduction

Much data now supports the idea that AIDS is primarily an immunological disease. Model builders are thus confronted by two kinds of complexity: the complexity of HIV and AIDS is compounded by the complexity of the immune system, with the result that finding credible models of AIDS pathogenesis is not a trivial task. The problem is further compounded by the fact that there is currently no consensus on many basic theoretical questions in immunology. So, as part of the process of formulating models of AIDS pathogenesis, we cannot avoid addressing basic immunology questions. Martinez et al. wrote in 1988, "AIDS is a prime example of a major clinical problem, the solution of which depends on basic research. AIDS might well be one of the first cases in which views on the idiotypic network will have practical importance (1). We review here some idiotypic network ideas that we believe are important for a better understanding of AIDS pathogenesis. We then speculate about the problems of HIV diversity and latency in the context of an idiotypic network model of AIDS pathogenesis.

What are the important basic science issues? We are faced with a circular problem: which facts and phenomena are important depends on the theoretical framework we choose, and which theory we choose depends on what facts and phenomena we wish to explain. In these circumstances, it makes sense to focus on the phenomena that are most paradoxical in the context of the reigning orthodoxy. Our AIDS pathogenesis model was formulated in the wake of trying to resolve an intriguing paradox of basic cellular immunology, namely, the I-J paradox in the mouse. It is a model that involves allogeneic lymphocytes as a cofactor (2,3).

In addition to HIV and allogeneic lymphocytes (2–4), mycoplasma (5–10) have been implicated in AIDS pathogenesis. In all three cases (HIV, lymphocytes, mycoplasma) molecular mimicry leading to autoimmunity has been postulated to be the underlying mechanism. In this chapter we will focus on the theoretical basis for a cofactor role for the allogeneic lymphocytes.

Interactions in Idiotypic Network Models of Regulation: Stimulation, Inhibition, and Killing

Three types of specific interactions are important in models of network regulation: stimulation, inhibition, and killing. The network model that we have developed includes explicit postulates concerning the mechanisms that underlie these interactions. For example, specific stimulation is assumed to involve the cross-linking of specific receptors, and inhibition is assumed to involve the blocking of specific receptors by antigen-specific T-cell factors. Inhibition by specific T-cell factors can have a positive effect on the size of a clone if killing is inhibited—or a negative effect, if stimulation is inhibited. Antigen-specific factors are molecules that have a molecular weight of about 50,000 to 70,000 and are assumed to have a single V region. To our knowledge the first report of such molecules was by Nelson (11), and many immunologists have since contributed to their characterization (12,13).

Several mechanisms can give rise to specific killing; our model requires the existence of at least one mechanism with a rate that is linear in the concentration of effector cells and a second mechanism that is quadratic (or of higher order) in the concentration of effector cells or molecules. For example, IgM plus complement or cytotoxic T cells can be expected to kill at rates that are linear in their respective concentrations, while IgG plus complement or antibody-dependent cellular cytotoxicity (ADCC) can be expected to have a killing rate that is quadratic or higher in the concentration of the antibodies. These mechanisms lead to qualitatively distinct terms in mathematical models of the system (14).

The above postulates can be shown to give rise to multiple stable states of the system, and to the possibility of an antigen causing switching between the stable states. For each antigen the system has to have the possibility of being in a virgin state, an immune state, or a suppressed (or otherwise unresponsive) stable state. In our model, a term that can be interpreted as simulating IgM-mediated killing is important in the virgin state, while a term that can be interpreted as simulating IgG-mediated killing is important in the immune state (14).

MHC Restriction of T Cells: An Inherent Trait of All T Cells or a Consequence of Selection of Antigen Fragments?

The cross-linking-of-receptors postulate leads to the idea that idiotypic interactions between lymphocytes are symmetrical. If, for example, a multivalent form of the V regions of a lymphocyte A can cross-link the V regions acting as receptors of lymphocyte B, then the converse will also be true; that is, a multivalent form of the V regions made by a lymphocyte B can cross-link the V regions acting as receptors of lymphocyte A. The phenomenon of MHC restriction raises the question of whether this argument applies also to the stimulation of T cells. Our model is based on symmetrical interactions between T cells as well; there are reasons to believe that the phenomenon of MHC restriction of T cells may have been overinterpreted, and the dogma that T cells recognize only antigen fragments in MHC clefts may be an unjustified generalization, as we have discussed elsewhere (15). It is true that experiments with primed T cells give the impression that primed T cells recognize only antigen fragments in MHC clefts, but is this due to an intrinsic limitation of the virgin T-cell repertoire? It may instead be partly due to a survival-of-the-fittest process for antigen fragments; those fragments that are protected from proteolytic degradation by binding to an MHC cleft will stimulate T cells (whose V regions have been positively selected to recognize MHC or MHC-like shapes in the thymus) for a much longer time than other antigen fragments that are not so protected. The idea that T cells are not intrinsically limited to recognizing only antigen fragments in clefts is shown by, first, the fact that responses to allogeneic MHC are not restricted in this way, second, the phenomenon of superantigens, which stimulate T cells in an MHC-unrestricted fashion, and third, monoclonal antibodies against T-cell receptors that are able to stimulate T cells (17).

I-J

In 1976 a considerable amount of excitement was generated by the discovery of what appeared to be a new genetic subregion of the murine MHC (18,19). Called the I-J region, it was defined most rigorously on the basis of a serological difference between two recombinant mouse strains: B10.A(5R) and B10.A(3R), called 5R and 3R for convenience. Reciprocal immunizations of these strains leads to the production of anti-I-J antibodies that have interesting properties. The antisera (and subsequently monoclonal antibodies derived from these or similar immunizations) were able to kill suppressor T cells, and specific T-cell factors were found to express I-J determinants. 5R anti-3R serum reacted with suppressor T cells and specific T-cell factors from H-2^b mice, so 3R was assumed to have the I-J^b genotype and phenotype, while 3R anti-5R serum reacted with suppressor T cells and specific T-cell factors of H-2^k mice, so 5R was assumed to have the I-J^k genotype and phenotype. Anti-I-J reagents were featured prominently at that time in many papers published in the leading immunology journals.

The excitement turned to puzzlement, however, when it was shown that there was no I-J gene at the expected location within the MHC class II region that could encode for I-J, in spite of clear and consistent mapping of I-J (in many different strains, not just 3R and 5R) to that part of the MHC (20). The absence of an I-J gene in the MHC became known as the I-J paradox. An important step toward the resolution of the paradox was made when it was shown that a particular I-J phenotype is somatically acquired by T cells in the presence of the corresponding MHC haplotype (21–23). For example, H-2^b T cells maturing in an H-2^k thymus acquire the I-J^k phenotype. This suggested that I-J could actually be determinants on certain T-cell receptors (part of the T-cell idiotype), and that particular T-cell clones with particular I-J idiotypes are positively selected in the presence of a given MHC class II haplotype.

There are, then, two possibilities that come to mind in the context of idiotypic network models: I-J determinants are idiotopes that are complementary either to the MHC-II determinants or to helper-T-cell V regions, which are in turn anti-MHC-II. The latter case fits best with the rest of the symmetrical network model that we developed (2). The most probable picture appears to be that I-J determinants are idiotypic determinants on suppressor T cells that resemble MHC-II in that they recognize and are recognized by MHC-II-restricted helper T cells. In other words, I-J is an "image" of MHC only in the sense that helper-T-cell receptors have some complementarity to both MHC and the I-J determinants; the part of the T-cell receptor that recognizes MHC and the part that recognizes the I-J determinants are not necessarily identical. The mapping of I-J determinants to the MHC would then have been due to MHC providing an environment that permits particular I-J suppressor-T-cell idiotypes to be selected. The I-J determinants on suppressor-T-cell V regions would actually be genetically encoded together with the rest of the T-cell V regions, but the selection within a particular MHC-II environment would result in the appearance of these idiotypic determinants mapping to MHC-II. The inheritance of the different I-J phenotypes in 3R and 5R mice may be due to a maternal effect on the spectrum of selected T-cell idiotypes (2).

Coselection of Idiotypes

A single monoclonal anti-I-J antibody (24) is capable of functionally eliminating suppressor T cells or absorbing specific suppressor-T-cell factors. The only way that this seems possible is for the suppressor T cells to have in common a single antigenic determinant. Such a shared determinant could be the consequence of a coselection process that restricts the repertoires of both the suppressor T cells and the helper T cells they interact with. In this model, only those suppressor T cells that express an emergent I-J determinant or determinants are selected, and furthermore only those helper T cells are selected that have V regions with some degree of complementarity to the suppressor-T-cell I-J determinants.

These considerations led to the idea that the T-cell repertoire can be likened to a tent in which the center pole (T cells expressing MHC image, that is, MHC-mimicking, I-J-bearing determinants) holds up the canvas (anti-MHC T cells) and vice versa. This idea of MHC-related network self-stabilization leads in turn to the idea that each immune system has a "major axis" in shape space. [Shape space is a mapping of shapes in a highly dimensioned space such that similar shapes are close to one another and very different shapes are far apart (25).] The major axis is the sequence of shapes MHC/anti-MHC/MHC image/anti-MHC image, as shown in

Figure 1. In this figure, MHC and MHC image are similar in the sense that both have complementarity to anti-MHC, yet they are different in the sense that anti-MHC image has complementarity to MHC image but not to MHC. Anti-MHC and MHC-image T cells are believed to play a central role in the stability of the immune system. An extension of this idea is that strong perturbations of the immune system that excite it along or close to this major axis could destabilize the system.

Two kinds of stimuli can potentially excite the system along the major axis and thus contribute to either the destabilization or (depending on the magnitude of the perturbation) the stabilization of the system (3,4). The first class consists of substances that are themselves MHC-mimicking. They may include HIV components (reviewed in Ref. 3) and mycoplasma components (Chapter 7). The immune response to these could in principle cross-react with either MHC itself or MHC-image determinants on suppressor T cells. The second class consists of substances with complementarity to the first class. These include the V regions of anti-MHC allogeneic lymphocytes that recognize host MHC, and induce the production of MHC-image antibodies (26). To understand the possible role of allogeneic lymphocytes in AIDS pathogenesis, we need to understand the idiotypic relationships between the various antibodies that are present in alloimmune sera. In the next section we present a model of these relationships.

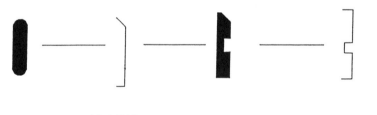

MHC   anti-MHC   MHC-image   anti-MHC-image

Figure 1   A model of the shapes along the MHC/anti-MHC/MHC-image/anti-MHC-image "major axis" of shapes in the immune system. MHC and MHC image on suppressor-T-cell idiotypes are produced by two completely different sets of genes—MHC and T-cell V genes, respectively—and they are similar from the perspective of anti-MHC idiotypes, but may nevertheless be different from the perspective of anti-MHC-image antibodies that do not bind MHC.

Second Symmetry

If two strains of mice—let us call them A and B—are cross-immunized with lymphocytes (A is immunized with B lymphocytes, and B with A lymphocytes), they each make three kinds of MHC-related antibodies, as shown in Table 1 for the A and anti-B serum. Most familiar are the conventional anti-foreign MHC antibodies, namely, A anti-(B MHC) and B anti-(A MHC). The second class are the MHC mimicking ("MHC-image" or "anti-anti-self") antibodies that are made against the receptors of the injected lymphocytes that recognize the host. The anti-foreign antibodies in an A anti-B serum have V regions that are complementary to the anti-anti-self antibodies of a B anti-A serum and vice versa (Figure 2). The anti-anti-self antibodies are MHC-image antibodies, and they can be detected in an inhibition of cytotoxicity assay (26). The anti-anti-self antibodies in one antiserum interact with anti-(foreign MHC) antibodies in the converse antiserum. The third kind of antibodies are anti-I-J antibodies (18,19). For now we will focus on just the anti-(foreign MHC) and anti-anti-self antibodies.

Extensive absorption of an alloimmune serum with fixed lymphocytes from the immunizing strain, such that all the cytotoxic anti-foreign antibody activity is removed, fails to remove the MHC-image antibodies. This has been shown with both inhibition of cytotoxicity (26) and the ELISA assay (T. A. Kion, unpublished). The V regions that could absorb the MHC-image antibodies in the naive absorbing lymphocytes may therefore be present at only a very low concentration. This may be partly because of the dynamic nature of immunization using viable lymphocytes. Dur-

Table 1 MHC-Related Antibodies in an A Anti-B Alloimmune Serum

1. Conventional anti-class I MHC and anti-class II MHC antibodies
   A anti-(B MHC)
   = Anti-*foreign*

2. MHC-image antibodies
   A anti-(B anti-A)
   = Anti-anti-*self*

3. Anti-I-J^B
   Postulated to be anti-(MHC image of B)
   = Anti-(*foreign* MHC image)

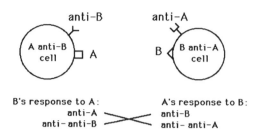

Figure 2   The immunogenic structures on the surface of lymphocytes of strain A that are injected into a mouse of strain B include the A-strain MHC antigens and anti-B receptors of the A-strain lymphocytes that recognize and are stimulated by the B-strain MHC antigens. If A- and B-strain mice are cross-immunized, the anti-foreign antibodies made in A are complementary to the anti-anti-self antibodies made in B, and the anti-foreign antibodies made in B are complementary to the anti-anti-self antibodies made in A.

ing the immune response, two population distributions change in an interdependent way, first, the population distribution in the inocculum lymphocytes whose V regions constitute the antigen, and second, the population distribution of the host clones that recognize the foreign idiotypes. Hence, V regions that are initially present at a very low level may eventually become dominant antigens, and absorption of antibody using naive immunogen may consequently be inefficient.

It is probable that T-cell receptors with anti-MHC specificity are the main idiotypic antigens for the production of MHC-image antibodies, rather than the analogous B-cell receptors, because T cells within the injected cells make a more vigorous response to the allogeneic host MHC than B cells do. The fact that the MHC-image antibodies nevertheless interact with the anti-(foreign MHC) *antibody* V regions in the converse antiserum would follow from the MHC-image antibodies having V regions that are a good imitation of self-MHC.

We find that there is a lot of cross-reactivity of MHC-image antibodies in their interactions with various anti-MHC antibodies (26). The specificity of MHC-image antibodies can most clearly be defined in terms of what they do not react with. In particular, the A anti-(B anti-A) antibodies (that is, anti-anti-self) do not interact with the A anti-B antibodies (anti-foreign) in the same serum, but they do react with many other antiforeign alloantibodies besides their nominal complement, namely, B anti-

A. This is a case of "hole specificity." The absence of any A anti-(A anti-B) antibodies in the anti-idiotypic set can be most simply ascribed to the cytotoxic effect of the A anti-B (i.e., anti-foreign) antibodies eliminating the subset of clones that are complementary to themselves.

The third kind of antibody that has been detected in alloimmune sera is anti-I-J (18,19). Anti-I-J antibodies are the basis of the definition of I-J. If these antibodies are made against the V regions of allogeneic MHC-image suppressor-T-cell idiotypes, they are anti-(foreign-MHC-image) antibodies. This idea leads to Figure 3, which is a model for the relationships between six classes of antibodies present in the pair of complementary alloimmune sera, A anti-B and B anti-A. This model is a generalization of "second symmetry," the idea that the total set of antibodies in an A anti-B serum is complementary to the total set of antibodies in the converse serum, B anti-A (26). The model predicts that anti-I-J antibodies should bind to MHC-image determinants on anti-anti-self antibody V regions, and we have some preliminary data showing that this is so.

MHC-image and anti-(MHC-image) immunity are central to our AIDS model of pathogenesis (below). Reports that anti-I-J antibodies react with a subset of CD8-bearing human lymphocytes (27) are consistent

A anti-B serum

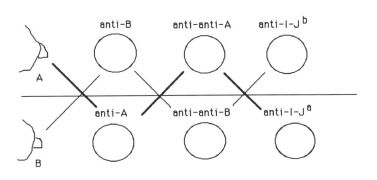

B anti-A serum

Figure 3 A model of the antibodies in two complementary alloimmune sera, A anti-B and B anti-A. Each component in one serum is complementary to one or more components in the other serum.

with the idea that there is cross-reactivity between MHC-image determinants on suppressor-T-cell V regions in mice and humans. Hence anti-
I-J antibodies may prove to be a useful tool for analyzing alloimmunity
and HIV-induced pathogenesis in humans.

AIDS

An Idiotypic Network Pathogenesis Model

Ideas about autoimmunity (28–32) and the idiotypic network (33–35),
together with the similarities between AIDS and graft-versus-host disease
(4) and the presence of MHC-image antibodies in alloantisera (26), have
led to an explicit model of AIDS pathogenesis that involves allogeneic
lymphocytes as a cofactor (2,3). HIV components appear to have MHC-
image properties, so an anti-MHC-image component of the immune response to HIV may synergize with the MHC-image component of the immune response to allogeneic lymphocytes, since each of these responses
is specific for the other. The MHC-image (class II) response is also directed
against helper-T-cell idiotypes, and the anti-MHC-image response is directed against suppressor T-cell idiotypes that normally stabilize the helper
T cells. The combination of these two responses may thus destabilize the
normally self-stabilizing system. Several lines of evidence from our laboratory support or are consistent with this idea.

Anticollagen Antibodies in Homosexuals

In a cross-sectional study of sera from homosexuals we detected anti-
collagen antibodies in all 17 of the homosexual AIDS patients' sera that
we tested (36). We also saw these antibodies in 32% of HIV-negative homosexuals ($n = 44$) and in 66% of HIV-positive homosexuals ($n = 24$), in
contrast with 0% of normal heterosexual controls ($n = 8$). A tentative
connection between these results and our model is based on the fact that
anti-collagen is also found in graft-versus-host disease, a form of alloimmunity that has similarities with AIDS (4). Anticollagen may thus be a
marker for alloimmunity, and hence a convenient marker for the presence
of this putative AIDS cofactor.

MHC-Image and Anti-HIV Antibodies in Alloimmune Mice

We found that alloimmune mice, but not normal, unimmunized mice,
contain both MHC-image antibodies (26) and anti-HIV antibodies (37),

namely, anti-gp120 and anti-p24. These mice have not been exposed to HIV or HIV components. It has been widely speculated that gp120 may be an MHC-mimicking substance, so anti-gp120 could be anti-MHC or anti-MHC-image antibodies that cross-react with gp120. We interpret the presence of anti-p24 in the sera in the light of evidence that several different HIV components—gp120, gp41, and Nef—have similarities with MHC (reviewed in Ref. 3), and we speculate that p24 may be another member in this class. Perhaps there is evolutionary pressure on HIV components to have MHC-image features. The more closely that HIV proteins resemble MHC or the internal image of MHC, the more difficult it is for the immune system to respond to HIV with a humoral immune response. The fact that it can take many weeks for a person to seroconvert following HIV infection would appear to fit with that idea. The coselection model described in the final section of this chapter provides a possible mechanism for HIV proteins to be selected to mimic MHC and/or endogenous MHC-image.

Anti-gp120 and anti-p24 antibodies appear to be anti-MHC-image rather than anti-MHC in that they are not readily absorbed out of the sera by the cells used to immunize the mice (T. A. Kion, unpublished), in contrast to anti-MHC antibodies. This is a feature that these putative anti-MHC-image antibodies have in common with MHC-image antibodies, which are also not readily absorbed out of the serum by the immunizing cells (26). As discussed above for MHC-image antibodies, this may be due to the antigenic T-cell idiotypes on the immunogen being present at a very low concentration in naive lymphocyte populations.

MHC-Image and Anti-MHC-Image Antibodies
in Autoimmune Mice

We found that the same two kinds of immunity that were postulated to be important in AIDS—MHC-image and anti-HIV (putative anti-MHC-image)—are present in the MRL-lpr/lpr mouse, an autoimmune strain that is a model for systemic lupus erythematosus (SLE) (37). Like the alloimmune mice, these mice have not been exposed to HIV or HIV components. We detect mainly anti-gp120 of HIV in MRl-lpr/lpr mice, in contrast with both anti-gp120 and anti-p24 in alloimmune mice. The presence of both the MHC-image and presumptive anti-MHC-image antibodies in these mice means that the model we formulated for AIDS may be relevant also for lupus pathogenesis. In this case there is no obvious external stimulus that triggers the disease. The disease may be due simply to the fact that the initial conditions (in particular, the initial conditions of the N-dimensional clonal population vector, where N is the number of clones) are such that a critical threshold in the clonal population space is exceeded. The system may have an initial trajectory in the N-dimensional idiotypic space that leads to elevated levels of MHC-image and anti-MHC-image antibodies. Such an explanation involving a fairly deterministic trajectory could account for the fairly narrow range in the life expectancy (with a mean of about 6 months) that typically characterizes MRL-lpr/lpr mice. It also suggests that a small perturbation in the initial conditions may suffice to deflect the trajectory away from the undesired region of the N-dimensional clonal population space.

Low Doses of HIV Components Injected into MRL Mice as a Model for an AIDS Vaccine Approach

We have been using the MRL-lpr/lpr mouse as a model for testing a novel AIDS vaccine concept that is designed to inhibit rather than provoke immunity to HIV proteins. If the anti-MHC-image antibodies are important in MRL-lpr/lpr pathogenesis, the suppression of the production of these antibodies should suppress pathogenesis. We have therefore been injecting subimmunogenic amounts of gp120 or p24 to see whether this suppresses the pathogenesis. The initial experiments gave promising results, especially using p24. This work is ongoing.

AIDS Without HIV?

If AIDS is typically caused by synergy between immunity to HIV and immunity to allogeneic lymphocytes, one might wonder whether there are circumstances (within the context of our MHC-image-anti-MHC-image picture) in which AIDS might be caused by HIV alone or by allogeneic lymphocytes alone. If the definition of AIDS includes the presence of HIV, there can of course be no AIDS without HIV, so the question is then short-circuited by the definition. There are, however, a considerable number of reports of AIDS-like conditions in HIV-negative individuals (38–50); these include Kaposi's sarcoma in young homosexual/bisexual men and depressed CD4 counts in transfusion recipients. A definition of AIDS that includes the presence of HIV may artificially distinguish between pathologies that would more appropriately be considered part of the same syndrome.

Thinking about the problem in the context of the MI-anti-MI model might lead one to guess that the probability of AIDS being transmitted by immune lymphocytes alone would be enhanced when there is a close match between the MHC of the infecting and the infected persons. Immune lymphocytes may then have a better chance of activating the system exactly along the MI-anti-MI axis. On the other hand, in the context of models in which nonspecific immune activation or the amount (rather than the nature) of allogeneic stimulation is critical, pathogenesis might be expected to occur more readily when there is a strong HMC mismatch between donor and recipient.

On Viral Diversity and Latency:
Coselection of Idiotypes and HIV?

During the final session at the Lake Annecy meeting, Patricia Fultz pointed out a paradoxical aspect of the rapid mutation rate of HIV. She noted that the usual idea that the virus mutates to evade the immune response would apply equally well to any virus or bacterium, so why don't they all mutate rapidly? In contrast to extremely accurate replication, a rapid mutation rate would appear to be something that could be easily acquired. All you need is a polymerase with a low fidelity of replication.

The question, then, is whether there may be some other advantage of the rapid mutation rate for HIV. An alternative to the "escape from recognition" model is one in which immune recognition of a particular viral strain actually favors the selection of that strain. Rapid mutation could be in the direction toward being recognized by as many T cells as possible, rather than not being recognized at all by antibodies. This would be the case if the T-cell receptor is involved in the cell-infection process, such that only T cells with specificity for HIV take it up and help it to propagate. If at the same time the virus were to stimulate these same T cells to proliferate, we would have a coselection scenario involving both T cells and virus. There could be positive selection for strains of virus that are recognized by as many T cells as possible, and for T cells that recognize as many of the viruses present as possible.

This coselection scenario is the same kind of dynamic process that we described in the model for the development of the helper-T-cell/suppressor-T-cell topology (canvas/center pole model). A prediction that would follow from this idea is that the fraction of T cells that are specific for the virus would increase with time (within an infected individual), and the fraction of the virus that is "specific" for T-cell receptors of the host should similarly increase with time.

The coselection model also leads to a new epidemiological prediction. The prediction is related to but distinct from an already documented MHC linkage of the rate of progression to AIDS, that is, the fact that with a given HIV infection, particular MHC-II alleles correlate with rapid progression to disease (41). If the selection of HIV variants recognized by many helper-T-cell idiotypes is the rate-limiting step in the pathogenic process, then we might expect to see progression of disease that is more rapid in cases when the "donor" and "recipient" of the virus share some HLA antigens than when they are completely disparate in the HLA genes. The fact that babies who inherit the virus from their mothers progress very rapidly to AIDS might perhaps be explained in terms of this concept of HLA-relatedness.

A long latency period can precede the HIV-triggered collapse of the immune system. The above coselection idea in the context of the MHC-image-anti-MHC-image model might again provide an explanation. There are many variants of the virus, and many different MHC haplotypes in humans. The initial perturbation of the immune system triggered by the virus is not necessarily "aligned" with the individual's MHC-image-anti-MHC-image major axis, and one can envision that during the latency period the coselection process could cause a gradual, systematic shift in the response toward the axis. This would mean that there is a positive selection of HIV variants that resemble the center pole, since the various virus particles would be under the same selective pressure as the suppressor T cells to recognize as many different helper T cells as possible. Positive selection could thus lead to the convergence of both HIV and the suppressor T cells to the same region of shape space. Anti-HIV immunity could then become, with time, cross-reactive immunity against the center pole as well, and disrupt this presumptively central element of immune-system regulation (2,3).

ACKNOWLEDGMENTS

This work was funded by the National Health Research and Development Program of Health and Welfare Canada and the Natural Sciences and Engineering Research Council of Canada.

REFERENCES

1. Martinez AC, Marcos MAR, de la Hera A, Marquez C, Alonso JM, Toribio ML, Coutinho A. Immunological consequences of HIV infection: advantage of being low responder casts doubts on vaccine development. Lancet 1988; i:454–457.

2. Hoffmann GW. On I-J, a network center pole and AIDS. In: Sercarz E, Celada F, Mitchison NA, Tada T, eds. The Semiotics of Cellular Communication in the Immune System. New York: Springer-Verlag, 1988:257–271.

3. Hoffmann GW, Kion TA, Grant MD. An idiotypic network model of AIDS immunopathogenesis. Proc Natl Acad Sci USA 1991; 88:3060–3064.

4. Shearer GM. Allogeneic leukocytes as a possible factor in induction of AIDS in homosexual men. N Engl J Med 1983; 308:223–224.

5. Lo SC, Shih JW, Newton PB III, Wong DM, et al. Virus-like infectious agent (VLIA) is a novel pathogenic mycoplasma: *Mycoplasma incognitus*. Am J Trop Med Hyg 1989; 41:586–600.

6. Lo S-C, Dawson MS, Wong DM, Newton PB III, et al. Identification of *Mycoplasma incognitus* in patients with AIDS: an immunohistochemical, in situ hybridization and ultrastructural study. Am J Trop Med Hyg 1989; 41:601–616.

7. Lo S-C, Tsai S, Benish JR, et al. Enhancement of HIV-1 cytocidal effects in CD4+ lymphocytes by the AIDS-associated mycoplasma. Science 1991; 251:1074–1076.

8. Montagnier L, Bernman D, Guetard D, Blanchard A, et al. Inhibition de l'infectiosité de souches prototypes du VIH par des anticorps dirigés contre une sequence peptidique de mycoplasme. CR Acad Sci (Paris) 1990; 311:425–430.

9. Chowdhury IH, Munakata T, Koyanagi Y, Kobayashi S, Arai S, Yamamoto N. Mycoplasma can enhance HIV replication *in vitro*: a possible cofactor responsible for the progression of AIDS. Biochem Biophys Res Commun 1990; 170:1365–1370.

10. Root-Bernstein R, Hobbs S. Homologies between mycoplasma adhesion peptide, CD4 and class II MHC proteins. Res Immunol 1991; 142:519–523.

11. Nelson DS. Studies on cytophilic antibodies: A mouse serum "antibody" having an affinity for macrophages and fast α-globulin mobility. Austr J Exp Biol Med Sci 1970; 48:329–341.

12. Benacerraf B. Genetic control of the specificity of T lymphocytes and their regulatory products. Prog Immunol 1980; 4:420.

13. Tada T. Help, suppression and specific factors. In: Paul WE, ed. Fundamental Immunology. New York: Raven Press, 1984:481–517.

14. Gunther N, Hoffmann GW. Qualitative dynamics of a network model of regulation of the immune system: A rationale for the IgM to IgG switch. J Theoret Biol 1982; 94:815–855.

15. Hoffmann GW, Grant MD. When HIV meets the immune system: network theory, alloimmunity, autoimmunity and AIDS. In: Castillo-Chavez C, ed. Mathematical and Statistical Approaches to AIDS Epidemiology. Lecture Notes in Biomathematics, Vol. 83. New York: Springer-Verlag, 1989:386–405.

17. Meuer SC, Hogdon JC, Hussey RE, Protentis JP, Schlossman SF, Rheinherz EL. Antigen-like effects of monoclonal antibodies directed at receptors on human T cell clones. J Exp Med 1983; 158:988.

18. Murphy DB, Herzenberg LA, Okumura K, Herzenberg LA, McDevitt HO. A new I subregion (I-J) marked by a locus (Ia-4) controlling surface determinants on suppressor T lymphocytes. J Exp Med 1976; 144:699–712.

19. Tada T, Taniguchi M, David CS. Properties of the antigen-specific T cell factor in the regulation of antibody response of the mouse. IV. Special subregion assignment of the gene(s) that codes for the suppressive T cell factor in the H-2 histocompatibility complex. J Exp Med 1976; 144:713–725.

20. Steinmetz M, Minard K, Horvath S, McNicholas J, Srelinger J, Wake C, Long E, Mach B, Hood L. A molecular map of the immune response region from the major histocompatibility complex of the mouse. Nature 1982; 300:35–42.

21. Sumida T, Sado T, Kojima M, Ono K, Kamisaku H, Taniguchi M. I-J as an idiotype of the recognition component of antigen-specific suppressor T-cell factor. Nature 1985; 316:738–741.

22. Uracz W, Asano Y, Abe R, Tada T. I-J epitopes are adaptively acquired by T cells differentiated in the chimaeric condition. Nature 1985; 316:714–745.

23. Flood PM, Benoist C, Mathis D, Murphy DB. Altered I-J phenotype in E_α transgenic mice. Proc Natl Acad Sci USA 1986; 83:8308–8312.

24. Waltenbaugh C. Regulation of immune responses by I-J gene products. I. Production and characterization of anti-I-J monoclonal antibodies. J Exp Med 1981; 154:1570.

25. Segel LA, Perelson AS. Computations in shape space: a new approach to immune network theory. In: Perelson AS, ed. Theoretical Immunology, Part 2. Redwood City, CA: Addison-Wesley, 1988:321–343.

26. Hoffmann GW, Cooper-Willis A, Chow M. A new symmetry: A anti-B is anti-(B anti-A), and reverse enhancement. J Immunol 1986; 137:61–68.

27. Lehner T, Brines R, Jones T, Avery J. Detection of cross-reacting murine I-J like determinants on a human subset of T8 + binding, presenting and contrasuppressor cells. Clin Exp Immunol 1984; 58:410–419.

28. Habeshaw J, Dalgleish A. The relevance of HIV env/CD4 interactions to the pathogenesis of Acquired Immune Deficiency Syndrome. J AIDS 1989; 2:457–468.

29. Kopelman RG, Zolla-Pazner S. Association of human immunodeficiency virus infection and autoimmune phenomena. Am J Med 1988; 84:82.

30. Ziegler JL, Stites DP. Hypothesis: AIDS is an autoimmune disease directed at the immune system and triggered by a lymphotropic retrovirus. Clin Immunol and Immunopathol 1986; 41:305–313.

31. Shearer GM. AIDS: An autoimmune pathologic model for the destruction of a subset of helper T lymphocytes. Mount Sinai J Med 1986; 53:609–615.

32. Andrieu JM, Even P, Venet A. AIDS and related syndromes as a viral-induced autoimmune disease of the immune system: an anti-MHC II disorder. Therapeutic implications. AIDS Res 1986; 2:163–174.

33. Hoffmann GW. A theory of regulation and self-nonself discrimination in an immune network. Eur J Immunol 1975; 5:638–647.

34. Hoffmann GW. Incorporation of a nonspecific T cell dependent helper factor into a network theory of the regulation of the immune response. In: Bell GI, Perelson AS, Pimbley GH, eds. Theoretical Immunology. New York: Marcel Dekker, 1978:571–602.

35. Hoffmann GW, Kion TA, Forsyth RB, Soga KG, Coooper-Willis A. The N-dimensional network. In: Perelson AS, ed. Theoretical Immunology, Part 2. Redwood City, CA: Addison-Wesley, 1988:291–319.

36. Grant MD, Weaver MS, Tsoukas C, Hoffmann GW. Distribution of antibodies against denatured collagen in AIDS risk groups and homosexual AIDS patients suggests a link between autoimmunity and the immunopathogenesis of AIDS. J Immunol 1990; 144:1241–1250.

37. Kion TA, Hoffmann GW. Anti-HIV and anti-anti-MHC antibodies in alloimmune and autoimmune mice. Science 1991; 235:1138–1140.

38. Friedman-Kien AE, Saltzman BR, Cao Y, Nestor MS, Mirabile M, Li JJ, Peterman TA. Kaposi's sarcoma in HIV-negative homosexual men. Lancet 1990; i:168.

39. Gatenby PA. Reduced CD4+ T-cells and candidiasis in absence of HIV infection. Lancet 1989; i:1027–1028.

40. Hansen ER, Lisby S, Baadsgaard O, Ho VO, de Villiers EM, Vejlsgaard GL. Abnormal function of CD4+ helper/inducer T lymphocytes in a patient with widespread human papillomavirus type 3-related infection. Arch Dermatol 1990; 126:1604–1608.

41. Pankhurst C, Peakman M. Reduced CD4+ T-cells and severe oral candidiasis in absence of HIV infection. Lancet 1989; i:672.

42. Jowitt SN, Love EM, Liu Yin JA, Pumphrey RSH. CD4 lymphocytopenia without HIV infection in patient with cryptococcal infection. Lancet 1991; 337:500–501.

43. Cozon G, Greenland T, Revillard JP. Profound CD4+ lymphocytopenia in the absence of HIV infection in a patient with visceral leishmaniasis. N Engl J Med 1990; 322:132.

44. Seligmann M, Aractingl S, Oksenhandler E, Rabian C, Ferchal F, Gonnot G. CD4+ lymphocytopenia without HIV in a patient with cryptococcal disease. Lancet 1991; 337:57–58.

45. Gautler V, Chanez P, Vendrell JP, et al. Unexplained CD4-positive T-cell deficiency in non-HIV patients presenting as a *Pneumocystis carinii* pneumonia. Clin Exp Allergy 1991; 21:63–66.

46. Daus H, Schwarze G, Radtke H. Reduced CD4+ count, infections, and immune thrombocytopenia without HIV infection. Lancet 1989; ii:559–580.

47. Castro A, Padreira J, Soriano V, et al. Kaposi's sarcoma and disseminated tuberculosis in an HIV-negative individual. Lancet 1992; 339:868.

48. Gupta S, Ribak CE, Gollapudl S, Kim CH, Salahuddin SZ. Detection of a human intracisternal retroviral particle associated with CD4+ T-cell deficiency. Proc Natl Acad Sci USA. In press.

49. Daar ES, Moudgil T, Ho DD. Persistently low T-helper (CD4 +) lympho-cyte counts in HIV-negative asymptomatic men. Western Society of Clinical Investigation meeting, February 1990.
50. Laurence J, Siegal FP, Schattner E, Gelman IH, Morse S. Acquired immune deficiency without evidence of infection with human immunodeficiency virus types 1 and 2. Lancet 1992. In press.
51. Kestler H, Kodama T, Ringler D, Mathas M, Pedersen N, Lackner A, Regier D, Sehgal P, Daniel M, King N, Desrosiers R. Induction of AIDS in rhesus monkeys by molecularly cloned simian immunodeficiency virus. Science 1990; 248:1109–1112.
52. Steel CM, Beatson D, Cuthbert RJG, Morrison H, Ludlan CA, Peutherer JF, Simmonds P, Jones M. HLA haplotype A1B8DR3 as a risk factor for HIV related disease. Lancet 1988; i:1185.

18

The Panergic Imnesia Hypothesis
Part I: Update of Current Findings

Michael S. Ascher and Haynes W. Sheppard

Viral and Rickettsial Disease Laboratory
California Department of Health Services
Berkeley, California

The failure of the conventional cytopathic model to account for the paradoxical features of HIV disease has spurred the development of alternative hypotheses for AIDS pathogenesis. Ideally, three key features of the HIV disease process should be accounted for in any successful model: 1) clinical signs of immune activation, 2) functional anergy of T cells, and 3) the gradual but complete loss of the CD4 lymphocyte population. The hypothesis discussed herein unifies these three phenomena under the effects of immune activation mediated by viral gp120 at the CD4 receptor and subsequent disruption of T-cell clonal dynamics. The model has gained credibility with the discovery of the viral nature of superantigens and further understanding of the mechanisms of programmed cell death, as discussed in Chapter 19. Strategies aimed at neutralizing excess immune activation deserve further study in the management of HIV disease.

INTRODUCTION: THE HYPOTHESIS

In 1988 we proposed that the key element in HIV-induced immunodeficiency is the fact that the virus is perceived by the T lymphocyte as a false or mimic physiological signal at the CD4 receptor (1). In the course of antigen-mediated activation, the HIV signal nonspecifically enhances T-cell responses leading to the clinical manifestations of HIV disease such as cachexia, lymphadenopathy, and nonspecific autoimmune phenomena, which we have called "panergy" to stand for both global activation and anergy. In addition, we proposed that the HIV signal causes CD4 cell loss by shifting T-cell clonal dynamics toward excess programmed cell death (PCD) and results in the recovery of fewer memory cells, a phenomenon we have labeled "imnesia" (2). In this model, HIV components circumvent critical regulatory controls of immune activation and lead to the broad spectrum of findings that make up the natural history of HIV disease independent of cytopathic effects (3). In this chapter, we discuss this hypothesis in light of new findings in immunology and HIV disease, and compare and contrast this model with subsequent hypotheses of others.

DOES HIV REALLY KILL T CELLS?

Although many experiments in which virus is added to T cells in vitro show "killing" of the cells, one intriguing set of experiments calls into question the relevance of such killing to HIV pathogenesis in vivo. Langhoff et al. (4) cloned T cells in the presence of HIV with identical cells and virus preparations that cause cell death in a standard bulk culture. Under cloning conditions, the cells grew normally (or a little better) and formed stable infected T-cell clones that produced virus. The interpretation is that virus does not kill T cells under physiological conditions but that the artificial in vitro milieu allows one to pack cells and virus together and get killing. It is also well known that other viruses whose disease manifestation does not include T-cell loss (5) show pathogenicity for T cells in vitro under crowded conditions (6).

ROLE OF CD4

When our hypothesis was first proposed, it relied on two observations in concluding that HIV was signaling at CD4: 1) that CD4 was a receptor for the virus and 2) that HIV infection was associated with many clinical and laboratory signs of generalized immune activation. This was a stronger interpretation of the functional role of CD4 than was current at the time, since CD4 was thought to be merely a cellular-adhesion receptor with no established signal-transduction capacity (7). Since then, the critical role of CD4-mediated signals in T-cell activation and in the induction of antigen-specific tolerance has been demonstrated (8).

HIV EFFECTS IN VITRO

If HIV is perceived as a signal by CD4 cells, it should be easy to demonstrate such effects in vitro, and, indeed, the ability of HIV to transduce signals through CD4 has been demonstrated (9). In a key paper (10), HIV signaling was used to establish a functional role for CD4. A number of other studies (11–13) have failed to demonstrate signal transduction. The problem is the same one that occurred in the early history of CD4: depending on the sequence and timing of signaling to T cells at the T-cell receptors and accessory molecules, one can get a spectrum of effects ranging from profound blocking to profound enhancement (see Chapter 19). In addition, the form and state of the gp120 preparation are critical to the result obtained (14,15). Despite these conflicting data, the overall consensus in the immunology community is that CD4-mediated signals participate positively in physiological T-cell activation, but in the HIV research community the current consensus is that the result of the interaction of gp120 with CD4 is neutral or negative. This is probably partly because of the bias that HIV disease is generally seen as "immune suppression." This is in spite of almost identical sets of data in the two different settings. The "aberrant metabolism" that is seen ex vivo in HIV infection has been interpreted as activation and is reversed by AZT (16). This is discussed further in the section on therapy below.

T-CELL MEMORY

Central to the second part of our hypothesis and critical to the development of T-cell loss in the model is the concept that the T-cell immune system depends on the recovery of daughter cells filed as memory from a previous immune response to retain the capacity to respond again and on a continuing basis. The nature and kinetics of T-cell memory are areas of great uncertainty and controversy. Experiments showing lifelong survival of resting "memory" T cells are contradicted by experiments showing rapid decay of responses in the absence of antigen (17). In the model, it is our contention that essentially all T-cell replacement in adults occurs through the progeny of clonal proliferation. If replacement by thymic maturation occurs at all, it is at a low level, is random with respect to antigen specificity, and cannot compensate for significant loss of T cells.

OCCAM'S RAZOR: WHY NOT A AND B AND C?

A key feature of our original idea for pathogenesis based on signaling and immune activation was that it integrated the three central and apparently disparate phenomena of HIV disease: clinical signs of immune activation, T-cell dysfunction, and T-cell loss (18). Others have clearly identified the same three central phenomena in HIV disease but attribute them, respectively, to three separate and unrelated mechanisms: a "graft-versus-host"-like disease, blocking of cellular activation, and infection during antigen presentation (19). Lewis Thomas wrote, "For every disease there is a single key mechanism that dominates all others. If one can find it, and think one's way around it, one can control the disorder" (20). We feel that the central concept of virus-mediated activation serves such a role in HIV disease.

RELATIONSHIP TO "AUTOIMMUNITY"

We object to the use of the term "autoimmunity" for the effects of HIV-mediated T-cell activation through molecular mimicry (21). Autoimmunity implies an inciting stimulus with self-specificity and/or a reaction to a particular tissue component in the response. In our view, although HIV obviously mimics self–class II MHC, the physiological ligands of CD4, there is neither a self-component inciting the response nor a specific self-component identified as the target of the response. It is a generalized activation of T cells with many specificities, but one whose effector functions are completely nonspecific, resulting in mediator disease with little evidence of tissue-specific reactions (22,23). More complex models of idiotype/anti-idiotype mimicry (24) are made less tenable by the failure to demonstrate such specificities in the sera of HIV-infected individuals (25).

COFACTORS

Our model considers HIV a mimic of costimulatory molecules acting at CD4 and requires the participation of antigen-specific activation in the overall pathogenetic process. In general, we feel that exposure to ubiquitous environmental antigens provides sufficient "first signal" to drive the system. This is also supported by data that suggest that the progression of HIV disease is independent of any specific cofactor experience. However, we allow that an environmental antigen with higher activation potential could contribute to weakening of the immune system. An interesting test of this idea is a case report on the clinical behavior of staphylococcal enterotoxin (SEB) disease in HIV-infected patients (26). Curiously, it was the behavior of the SEB disease that was modified and prolonged, not the course of HIV infection. This is consistent with a costimulatory role for HIV adding to the overall level of signaling and lowering the threshold for the SEB effects.

IMPLICATIONS FOR THERAPY

Any comprehensive theory of HIV pathogenesis should be evaluated on the basis of the new therapeutic approaches suggested by the model. Models of autoimmunity contribute little to treatment considerations, because the parent family of conditions—the autoimmune diseases—are notoriously difficult to treat specifically and have mainly responded to nonspecific measures at suppressing the immune system. A major suggestion deriving from our model is that targeted immunosuppression aimed at moderating the CD4-mediated signaling should be studied in more detail. The problem, however, is that immunosuppressive drugs have the potential to block normal immune functions as well as aberrant responses. We suggest that a derivative of cyclosporine, for example, which is selected on the basis of in vitro experiments assessing its ability to block HIV signaling at CD4, is worthy of a clinical evaluation. The cyclosporine trials that have been conducted to date show interesting results. An early trial in asymptomatic subjects showed dramatic elevations in CD4 numbers and no adverse effects (27). AIDS cases deteriorated at approximately the expected rate. Another trial used only AIDS cases and found general deterioration in the treatment group, with no untreated controls (28). A later unpublished trial in asymptomatic subjects showed a transient rise in CD4 counts, but the trial did not persist long enough to assess overall effects on natural history (Aboulker, personal communication). A great deal of concern exists in the immunological community as to the advisability of further work in this area, but there is considerable anecdotal evidence of the safety and apparently paradoxical results obtained with the approach in transplant patients, for example (29).

HOW AZT "WORKS"

A side issue that arises in this discussion is whether many of the positive effects of "antiviral" chemotherapy for HIV with azidothymidine (AZT) are really "antiactivation" effects. This idea must be considered seriously in light of a series of interesting findings with AZT treatment. First, many of the so-called "autoimmune" manifestations of HIV disease are responsive to AZT without clear changes in viral burden (30). Second, markers for immune activation decrease dramatically in response to AZT therapy (16,31,32). Third, an animal model of viral-induced leukemia has been described in which the virus and viral burden are not sensitive to AZT but the "disease" is prevented (33). Next, synergy has been demonstrated between AZT and cyclosporine in the treatment of murine AIDS (34). Our overall view of this situation suggests that "antiactivation" drugs deserve further evaluation and should not be selected for their "antiviral" activity, as was actually the case with cyclosporine (see above).

IS THE INFECTED CELL ANTIGEN-SPECIFIC FOR HIV?

One additional speculation made in our first paper (1) was the possibility that the infected lymphocyte reservoir was antigen-specific for HIV. The basis of the idea was that the frequency of cellular infection or burden is about the same as the number of cells one would expect to be specific for a given antigen. Although there is no obvious way to test this idea, the implications are very important in that, first, one could attack and eliminate infected cells by a combination of anti-idiotype (to the T-cell receptor) and a toxin, and second, increasing the population of antigen-sensitive cells by vaccination might increase the susceptibility of individuals to infection. One recent experiment on looking for $V\beta$ specificity of infection demonstrated a predilection for $V\beta$ 12 (35). Contrary to the prediction that these cells would preferentially be lost in infected individuals, they have actually been shown to be normal or somewhat elevated. This is consistent with a fixed reservoir of infected cells with some specificity. One continuing problem with the interpretation of viral-burden studies is that authors express the burden as a percentage of cells. Since the population of CD4 cells is dramatically decreasing in HIV disease, an increase in percentage of infected cells gives a relatively stable burden. In response to this problem, recent workers are beginning to express their data as infected cells per volume of blood as a more accurate reflection of viral burden (36,37).

REFERENCES

1. Ascher MS, Sheppard HW. AIDS as immune system activation: a model for pathogenesis. Clin Exp Immunol 1988; 73:165-167.
2. Ascher MS, Sheppard HW. AIDS as immune system activation. II. The panergic imnesia hypothesis. J AIDS 1990; 3:177-191.
3. Sheppard HW, Ascher MS. The natural history and pathogenesis of HIV infection. Annu Rev Microbiol 1992; 46:533-564.
4. Langhoff E, McElrath J, Bos HJ, Pruett J, Granelli-Piperno A, Cohn ZA, Steinman RM. Most CD4 + T cells from human immunodeficiency virus-1 infected patients can undergo prolonged clonal expansion. J Clin Invest 1989; 84:1637-1643.
5. Buchwald D, Cheney PR, Peterson DL, et al. A chronic illness characterized by fatigue, neurologic and immunologic disorders, and active human herpesvirus type 6 infection. Ann Intern Med 1992; 116:103-113.
6. Becker WB, Engelbrecht S, Becker MLB, Piek C, Robson BA, Wood L, Jacobs P. Isolation of a new human herpesvirus producing a lytic infection of helper (CD4) T-lymphocytes in peripheral blood lymphocyte cultures— another cause of acquired immunodeficiency? SAMJ 1989; 74:610-614.
7. Fleischer B, Schrezenmeier H. Do CD4 or CD8 molecules provide a regulatory signal in T-cell activation? Immunol Today 1988; 9:132-134.
8. Janeway CA. The co-receptor function of CD4. Sem Immunol 1991; 3:153-160.
9. Kornfeld H, Cruikshank WW, Pyle SW, Berman JS, Center DM. Lymphocyte activation by HIV-1 envelope glycoprotein. Nature 1988; 335:445-448.
10. Neudorf SML, Jones MM, McCarthy BM, Harmony JAK, Choi EM. The CD4 molecule transmits biochemical information important in the regulation of T lymphocyte activity. Cell Immunol 1990; 125:301-314.
11. Hofmann B, Nishanian P, Baldwin RL, Insixiengmay P, Nel A, Fahey JL. HIV inhibits the early steps of lymphocyte activation, including initiation of inositol phospholipid metabolism. J Immunol 1990; 145:3699-3705.
12. Horak ID, Popovic M, Horak EM, Lucas PJ, Gress RE, June CH, Bolen JB. No T-cell tyrosine protein kinase signalling or calcium mobilization after CD4 association with HIV-1 or HIV-1 gp120. Nature 1990; 348:557-560.
13. Kaufmann R, Laroche D, Buchner K, et al. The HIV-1 surface protein gp120 has no effect on transmembrane signal transduction in T cells. J AIDS 1992; 5:760-770.
14. Clouse KA, Cosentino LM, Weih KA, et al. The HIV-1 gp120 envelope protein has the intrinsic capacity to stimulate monokine secretion. J Immunol 1991; 147:2892-2901.
15. Cruikshank WW, Center DM, Pyle SW, Kornfeld H. Biologic activities of HIV-1 envelope glycoprotein: the effects of crosslinking. Biomed Pharmacother 1990; 44:5-11.

16. Nye KE, Knox KA, Pinching AJ. Lymphocytes from HIV-infected individuals show aberrant inositol polyphosphate metabolism which reverses after zidovudine therapy. AIDS 1991; 5:413–417.

17. Gray D, Matzinger P. T cell memory is short-lived in the absence of antigen. J Exp Med 1991; 174:969–974.

18. Ascher MS, Sheppard HW. A unified hypothesis for three cardinal features of HIV immunology. J AIDS 1990; 4:97–98.

19. Manca F, Habeshaw JA, Dalgleish AG. HIV envelope glycoprotein, antigen specific T-cell responses, and soluble CD4. Lancet 1990; 335:811–815.

20. Thomas L. The Medusa and the Snail: More Notes of a Biology Watcher. New York: Viking Press, 1979.

21. Dalgleish AG, Wilson S, Gompels M, Ludlam C, Gazzard B, Coates AM, Habeshaw J. T-cell receptor variable gene products and early HIV-1 infection. Lancet 1992; 339:824–828.

22. Solinger A, Adams L, Friedman-Kien A, Hess E. Acquired immune deficiency syndrome (AIDS) and autoimmunity—mutually exclusive entities? J Clin Immunol 1988; 8:32–42.

23. Alguilar JL, Berman A, Espinoza LR, Blitz B, Lockey R. Autoimmune phenomena in human immunodeficiency virus infection. Am J Med 1988; 85:283–284.

24. Hoffmann GW, Kion TA, Grant MD. An idiotypic network model of AIDS immunopathogenesis. Proc Natl Acad Sci USA 1991; 88:3060–3064.

25. Davis SJ, Schockmel GA, Somoza C, et al. Antibody and HIV-1 gp120 recognition of CD4 undermines the concept of mimicry between antibodies and receptors. Nature 1992; 358:76–79.

26. Cone LA, Woodard DR, Byrd RG, Schulz K, Kopp SM, Schlievert PM. A recalcitrant, erythematous, desquamating disorder associated with toxin-producing staphylococci in patients with AIDS. J Infect Dis 1992; 165:638–643.

27. Andrieu J-M, Even P, Venet A, et al. Effects of cyclosporin on T-cell subsets in human immunodeficiency virus disease. Clin Immunol Immunopathol 1988; 46:181–198.

28. Phillips A, Wainberg M, Coates R, et al. Cyclosporine-induced deterioration in patients with AIDS. Can Med Assoc J 1989; 140:1456–1460.

29. Jacobson SK, Calne RY, Wreghitt TG. Outcome of HIV infection in transplant patient on cyclosporin. Lancet 1991; 337:794.

30. Tongol JM, Gounder MP, Butala A, Rabinowitz M. HIV-related autoimmune hemolytic anemia: good response to zidovudine. J AIDS 1991; 4:1163–1164.

31. Hutterer J, Armbruster C, Wallner G, Fuchs D, Vetter N, Wachter H. Early changes of neopterin concentrations during treatment of human immunodeficiency virus infection with zidovudine. J Infect Dis 1992; 165:783–784.

32. Galli M, Ridolfo AL, Balotta C, Riva A, et al. Soluble interleukin-2 receptor decrease in the sera of HIV-infected patients treated with zidovudine. AIDS 1991; 5:1231–1235.

33. Morrey JD, Okleberry KM, Sidwell RW. Early-initiated zidovudine therapy prevents disease but not low levels of persistent retrovirus in mice. J AIDS 1991; 4:506–512.
34. Cerny A, Merino R, Fossati L, et al. Effect of cyclosporin A and zidovudine on immune abnormalities observed in the murine acquired immunodeficiency syndrome. J Infect Dis 1991; 166:285–290.
35. Laurence J, Hodtsev AS, Posnett DN. Superantigen implicated in dependence of HIV-1 replication in T cells on TCR V-beta expression. Nature 1992; 358:255–259.
36. Yerly S, Chamot E, Hirschel B, Perrin LH. Quantitation of human immunodeficiency virus, provirus and circulating virus: relationship with immunologic parameters. J Infect Dis 1992; 166:269–272.
37. Ascher MS, Sheppard HW, Arnon JM, Lang W. Viral burden in HIV disease. J AIDS 1991; 4:824–830.

19

The Panergic Imnesia Hypothesis

Part II: T-Cell Receptor Biology, AIDS, and Beyond

Haynes W. Sheppard and Michael S. Ascher

Viral and Rickettsial Disease Laboratory
California Department of Health Services
Berkeley, California

We present a general concept of T-cell activation and clonal dynamics that extends our model of AIDS pathogenesis (1) and unifies a number of apparently disparate immunological phenomena, including thymic selection, clonal anergy, and the response to alloantigens and superantigens. In this model, T-cell activation involves multiple cooperative signals at the $\alpha\beta$ T-cell receptor (TcR) ("signal 1") and at one or more costimulatory receptors, including CD4 ("signal 2"). The ultimate fate of a clone is determined by the combined effect of all signals it receives and the population dynamics, which determine how many progeny survive programmed cell death. Signal combinations that exceed a critical intensity threshold lead to clonal expansion in mature lymphocytes but clonal deletion of self-reactive thymocytes, which are developmentally trapped and cannot escape these signals. Clonal anergy occurs when subthreshold signals initiate an ineffective biochemical cascade that must be "reset" before new coordinate signals can cause a response. Alloantigens and particularly superantigens have acute but selective effects on the immune system because they deliver signal 1 by direct interaction with particular TcR β-chains. In contrast, human immunodeficiency virus (HIV) has widespread effects because it can deliver a costimulatory signal 2 to any CD4+ T cell. However, the effects of HIV are gradual because peripheral T cells are difficult to tolerize, and because the effects of HIV require the concomitant delivery of signal 1.

INTRODUCTION

The AIDS epidemic has occurred during a period of rapid development in the understanding of immune-system structure and function (particularly of T cells). The TcR has been cloned and characterized (2), the presentation of peptide antigens by MHC has been elucidated (3), costimulatory or coreceptor functions (particularly of CD4 and CD8) have been identified (4), superantigens have provided a model for tolerance (5), and experiments in transgenic mice have elucidated the mechanisms of thymic selection and T-cell activation (6,7). This progress has led to the paradox that positive and negative thymic selection and peripheral T-cell activation are all mediated through the same receptors (8).

Similarly, there has been rapid progress in the identification and characterization of HIV, but the initial model of pathogenesis, through direct cytopathology, conflicts with the observed natural history of HIV infection (see Chapter 18). This has led one scientist to conclude that HIV is not the cause of AIDS (9) despite unassailable epidemiological evidence that it is (10). We have proposed that these conflicts can be resolved by placing HIV-mediated activation of the immune system rather than cell-killing at the heart of HIV pathogenesis.

In considering these two apparently unrelated paradoxes, we noticed that some manifestations of HIV infection resemble events that occur during the development of self-tolerance. These include functional anergy (11), lymphocyte activation (12), selective loss of T cells (13), and programmed cell death (PCD) through apoptosis (14). This led us to propose that AIDS and tolerance occur through a common mechanism and that the interaction of the virus with CD4 provides important insights into both phenomena (15). The conceptual framework that integrates AIDS and tolerance also provides explanations for clonal anergy and the profound effects of immune responses to alloantigens or superantigens.

THE COMPLEXITY OF T-CELL SIGNALS

Over 20 years ago, the simplistic concept of activation through a single-antigen receptor was replaced by a two-signal model, requiring both antigen (signal 1) and signals from other cells (signal 2). Interaction with antigen alone was thought to be inhibitory (16). This model has proven to be essentially correct. T cells receive two primary signals, one through the $\alpha\beta$ TcR, which sees a foreign peptide presented by an MHC molecule (signal 1), and a second through the coreceptor activity of CD4 or CD8 (signal 2) (17-19). In addition, several other receptors for costimulatory signals have been identified (20,21). As predicted by Bretscher and Cohn, signal 1 alone induces paralysis, or "clonal anergy," which has been proposed as one mechanism for the induction and maintenance of self-tolerance (21-23). However, other types of partial or aberrant signals also induce anergy, and in some cases the paralysis can be reversed by providing additional signals (24,25). Paradoxically, the coordinate delivery of both signals activates peripheral lymphocytes but causes clonal deletion of thymocytes, the primary mechanism for self-tolerance. In our view, the synthesis of these paradoxical findings requires a new concept of how lymphocytes perceive receptor-mediated signals.

COOPERATION AND CONFLICT BETWEEN SIGNALS

The key concept that integrates these phenomena is that the fate of a T-cell population is determined by the overall intensity and/or duration of *all* the signals it receives. We propose that the initiation of clonal expansion and the expression of effector functions is all-or-none, but that multiple, biochemically additive or synergistic signals must cooperate to exceed a critical intensity threshold (25,26). Normally, the coordinate delivery of signal 1 and signal 2 exceeds the threshold, while each signal alone is insufficient to activate T cells.

The model also predicts that signals at different receptors can be additive, synergistic, or antagonistic, depending on the nature of the ligand, the timing and coordination of other signals, the degree of receptor cross-linking, and the activation state of the T-cell population. For example, costimulation through CD4 is dependent on its physical proximity to CD3, which is itself a function of prior activation (27,28). Such considerations can explain the apparent discrepancy between positive and negative effects of gp120 in vitro as described in Chapter 18.

This view is supported by a recent body of literature suggesting that many lymphocyte receptors share a common immunoglobulin-like multichain structure and initiate similar biochemical cascades involving activation of protein kinases, phosphorylation of a series of substrates, changes in calcium flux (29), and ultimately the activation or inhibition of nuclear transcription factors (30). These similarities provide the basis for interaction at the biochemical level (31). For example, exposure of immature thymocytes to glucocorticoid or to TcR ligation results in PCD, but simultaneous exposure to both results in cell survival (32). This paradoxical phenomenon appears to occur through the antagonistic interaction of two transcription factors (30).

CLONAL ANERGY

In this context, clonal anergy can be viewed as the consequence of "below-threshold" signals, which do not induce activation but nevertheless engage a sufficient number of receptors and induce biochemical events that temporarily prevent the coordinate delivery of new above-threshold signals. A period of rest may be required to reset biochemical pathways and receptor expression before responsiveness is recovered.

What is the purpose of anergy? Based on the immunopathological consequences of intense T-cell activation, we have proposed that the purpose of this complexity is to limit the destructive potential of T-cell responses to the tissue sites where antigens are being processed and presented in the "correct" form (8). As Lewis Thomas has asserted, immune effector mechanisms "are so powerful, and involve so many different defense mechanisms, that we are in more danger from them than from the invaders" (33). Reversible anergy in T cells that receive "inappropriate" signals may be a safeguard against such unrestricted antigen activation rather than a mechanism normally used for the induction or maintenance of self-tolerance.

CLONAL DYNAMICS

Unlike most other tissues, lymphoid cells undergo rapid proliferation and functional differentiation in response to receptor-mediated signals. It is axiomatic that most of the progeny of such activated cells must be eliminated to prevent net growth of the immune system. After antigen is eliminated, a small number of cells must return to a resting state but retain the capacity to repeat the response cycle (i.e., serve as memory cells). As discussed in Chapter 18, we contend that this is the primary mechanism for the maintenance of immunological memory and that appreciable de novo replacement of T-cell clones does not occur in the adult. Thus, it is the ability of cells to avoid elimination that is the critical feature of immune-system homeostasis. We have suggested that escape from signals is central in this process and that high-intensity or chronic signals will result in deletion (34). The regular cycles of stimulation and rest that are required to maintain antigen-specific T-cell lines in vitro may be a parallel of this phenomenon (35).

PROGRAMMED CELL DEATH

Recent work has shown that a common fate of cells in the immune system is PCD involving apoptosis, an active process characterized by nuclear condensation and DNA degradation (36–41). The in vitro induction of apoptosis, by receptor-mediated signals, has led to the concept of a unique death pathway (38), and the induction of this pathway by gp120 signals at CD4 has been proposed as a mechanism for CD4 + cell loss (42,43). This model could explain the cell loss but not the many signs of immune activation characteristic of HIV infection. Furthermore, the increased levels of PCD, in HIV-infected patients (14), are present in both CD4 + and CD8 + subpopulations (44), suggesting a general rather than CD4-specific process.

We feel that PCD, in all subpopulations, is a normal consequence of immune-system activation, driven by cytokines from HIV-amplified CD4 + helper-cell responses (panergy) (45). However, selective CD4 loss is caused by a shift in CD4 + population dynamics (i.e., the number that survive) mediated by HIV signals at CD4 (imnesia). This later process does not affect the CD8 + population. The progression of HIV disease is probably slow because the adult immune system is inherently resistant to the elimination of all progeny. It may require many cycles of clonal expansion, recovering fewer memory cells at each cycle, to cause clonal deletion.

TOLERANCE

In this context, a simple explanation for negative thymic selection is that self-reactive thymocytes are developmentally trapped in the presence of signal 1 and signal 2, cannot rest, and are driven to clonal deletion. Non-self-reactive thymocytes receive signal 2 but signal 1 is below-threshold, reducing activation to a level that permits maturation and migration to the periphery (i.e., positive selection) (46). One problem with this interpretation is that a peripheral immune response to antigen, which also provides both signals, might be expected to cause clonal deletion. One explanation is that some mature lymphocytes, unlike self-reactive thymocytes, can usually escape signals through elimination of the antigen or migration away from the local site of infection. In addition, activation signals may have a less intense effect on mature T cells so that escape from above-threshold signals is more easily achieved (25,47,48). In this model the net elimination of T cells, either self-reactive cells in the thymus or CD4 + T cells in HIV infection, is explained by a shift in the overall population dynamics after activation rather than the death of individual cells.

This parallel between HIV pathogenesis and tolerance implies that chronic antigenic stimulation in the presence of HIV infection could result in antigen-directed adult tolerance. Anecdotal support for this possibility can be found in an intriguing case report of a liver transplant, coincident with HIV infection, that was "accepted" despite the withdrawal of immunosuppressive therapy (49).

ALLOREACTIVITY

This view of superantigens may also explain the paradoxically intense response to alloantigens (50–52). Studies of thymic selection demonstrate that positive selection requires physical interaction of the TcR with MHC, independent of antigen peptide (46). Thus, MHC is, in a sense, a $V\beta$ binding protein with superantigen potential, and thymic selection should result in a repertoire of TcRs that recognize self-MHC at below-threshold intensity. Such a repertoire could contain many clones that recognize foreign MHC as an above-threshold signal 1, resulting in a superantigen-like response. This view predicts that self-MHC has a profound effect on selection of the non-self repertoire and may explain some of the variable patterns of $V\beta$ expression in different genetic backgrounds (53).

One caveat in this interpretation is the phenomenon of MHC restriction, in which foreign MHC is unable to present antigen to T cells that have been primed in the context of self-MHC. If the combination of antigenic peptide with MHC generally increases the intensity of signal 1, then foreign MHC would be expected to present antigen even better than self-MHC. An explanation may be found in the recent observation that protein antigens contain a limited number of peptides that can be processed and combined with MHC and that this subset of peptides that are "presentable" rather than "cryptic" is different in different genetic backgrounds (54). Therefore, MHC restriction may be as much a function of the ability to process the appropriate peptides as the interaction between MHC and TcRs.

SUPERANTIGENS

The term *superantigen* refers to a class of microbial components with much greater activity than conventional antigens, but with limited T-cell range compared to mitogens. A superantigen interacts directly with specific TcR β-chain variable regions (Vβ) and causes clonal deletion of thymocytes or polyclonal activation of mature lymphocytes that bear those Vβ molecules (55,56). In our model, a superantigen is simply an aberrant and broadly reactive form of signal 1 that is equivalent in biochemical intensity to the combination of self-MHC and antigenic peptide. The requirement for CD4/CD8 or other costimulatory signals is variable and may be a function of whether the superantigen can deliver an above-threshold signal by itself (57,58).

HIV AS SUPERANTIGEN?

When one of the best characterized "endogenous" superantigens (Mls-1) was identified as a retroviral gene product (59), it was suggested that HIV might also encode a Vβ-binding superantigen (5,60-62). Of particular relevance to this issue is the demonstration that MAIDS, a lymphoproliferative/immunodeficiency disease of mice (63,64), is caused by a virus with typical superantigen properties (65). Thus, the precedent for an "immunodeficiency" disease due strictly to excess activation signals is well established. However, a superantigen would be expected to cause acute illness (66) and deletion of a specific or limited number of Vβ families (67). In the one report of "selective" Vβ depletion in HIV disease (60), as many as 19 of 22 of the Vβs studied were deleted and the average Vβ level in infected individuals had a 0.63 correlation with levels in control subjects (our analysis of the published data). In our view, the natural history of HIV disease is more consistent with the effects of a costimulatory signal 2 which would be a less efficient toleragen and would require concomitant signal 1 (i.e., antigen), but would have more generalized effects than a superantigen because all helper T cells bear CD4. This would account for both the breadth of HIV-induced immunodeficiency and the length of the incubation period between HIV infection and AIDS.

REFERENCES

1. Ascher MS, Sheppard HW. AIDS as immune system activation. II. The panergic imnesia hypothesis. J AIDS 1990; 3:177–191.
2. Hedrick SM, Cohen D, Nielsen E, Davis M. Isolation of cDNA clones encoding T cell specific membrane-associated proteins. Nature 1984; 308:149.

3. Solbach W, Moll H, Rollinghoff M. Lymphocytes play the music but the macrophage calls the tune. Immunol Today 1991; 12:4–6.

4. Veillette A. Introduction: the functions of CD4 and D8. Sem Immunol 1991; 3:131–132.

5. Acha-Orbea, Palmer E. Mls—a retrovirus exploits the immune system. Immunol Today 1991; 12:356–361.

6. Kaye J, Hsu ML, Sauron ME, Jameson SC, Gascoigne NRJ, Hedrick SM. Selective development of CD4+ T cells in transgenic mice expressing a class II MHC-restricted antigen receptor. Nature 1989; 341:746–749.

7. Zhou P, Anderson GD, Savarirayan S, Inoko H, David CS. Thymic deletion of V-beta11+, V-beta5+ T cells in H-2E negative, HLA-DQbeta+ single transgenic mice. J Immunol 1991; 146:854–859.

8. Blackman M, Kappler J, Marrack P. The role of the T cell receptor in positive and negative selection of developing T cells. Science 1990; 248:1335–1341.

9. Duesberg PH. Human immunodeficiency virus and acquired immunodeficiency syndrome: correlation but not causation? Proc Natl Acad Sci 1989; 86:755–762.

10. Pinching AJ, Jeffries DJ, Harris JRW, Swirsky D, Weber JN. HIV and AIDS. Nature 1990; 347:324.

11. Lane HC, Depper JM, Greene WC, Whalen G, Waldmann TA, Fauci AS. Qualitative analysis of immune function in patients with the acquired immunodeficiency syndrome. N Engl J Med 1985; 313:79–84.

12. Fuchs D, Hausen A, Hoefler E, Schonitzer D, Werner ER, Dierich MP, Hengster P, Reibnegger G, Schultz T, Wachter H. Activated T cells in addition to LAV/HTLV-III infection: a necessary precondition for development of AIDS. Cancer Det Prev 1987; 1(suppl):583–587.

13. Nicholson JKA, McDougal JS, Jaffe HW, Spira TJ, Kennedy MS, Jones BM, Darrow WW, Morgan M, Hubbard M. Exposure to human T-lymphotropic virus type III/lymphadenopathy-associated virus and immunologic abnormalities in asymptomatic homosexual men. Ann Intern Med 1985; 103: 37–42.

14. Montagnier L, Guetard D, Rame V, Olivier R, Adams M. Virological and immunological factors of AIDS pathogenesis. Quatr Col Cent Gardes 1989; 11–17.

15. Sheppard HW, Ascher MS. The relationship between AIDS and immunologic tolerance. J AIDS 1992; 5:143–147.

16. Bretscher PA, Cohn M. Science 1970; 169:1042–1049.

17. Anderson P, Blue ML, Morimoto C, Schlossman F. Cross-linking of T3 (CD3) with T4 (CD4) enhances the proliferation of resting T lymphocytes. J Immunol 1987; 139:678.

18. Emmrich F, Strittmatter U, Eichmann K. Synergism in the activation of human CD8 T cells by cross-linking the T-cell receptor complex with CD8 differentiation antigen. Proc Natl Acad Sci USA 1986; 83:8298.

19. Turka LA, Linsley PS, Paine R, Schieven GL, Thompson CB, Ledbetter JA. Signal transduction via CD4, CD8, and CD28 in mature and immature thymocytes. J Immunol 1991; 146:1428–1436.
20. Mueller DL, Jenkins MK, Schwartz RH. Clonal expansion versus functional clonal inactivation: a costimulatory signalling pathway determines the outcome of T cell receptor occupancy. Annu Rev Immunol 1989; 7:445–480.
21. Schwartz RH. A cell culture model for T lymphocyte clonal anergy. Science 1990; 248:1349–1356.
22. Alters SE, Shizuru JA, Ackerman J, Grossman D, Seydel KB, Fathman CG. Anti-CD4 mediates clonal anergy during transplantation tolerance induction. J Exp Med 1991; 173:491–494.
23. Jenkins MK, Pardoll DM, Mizuguchi J, Chused TM, Schwartz RH. Molecular events in the induction of a nonresponsive state in interleukin-2 producing helper T-lymphocyte clones. Proc Natl Acad Sci USA 1987; 84:5409.
24. Jenkins MK, Ashwell JD, Schwartz RH. Allogenic non-T spleen cells restore the responsiveness of normal T cell clones stimulated with antigen and chemically modified antigen-presenting cells. J Immunol 1988; 140:3324–3330.
25. St.-Pierre Y, Watts TH. Characterization of the signaling function of MHC class II molecules during antigen presentation by B cells. J Immunol 1991; 147:2875–2882.
26. Janeway CA. The co-receptor function of CD4. Sem Immunol 1991; 3:153–160.
27. Ledbetter JA, June CH, Rabinovitch S, Grossman A, Tsu T, Imboden JB. Signal transduction through CD4 receptors: stimulatory vs. inhibitory activity is regulated by CD4 proximity to the CD3/T cell receptor. Eur J Immol 1988; 18:525–532.
28. Rivas A, Takada S, Koide J, Sonderstrup-MacDevitt G, Engleman E. CD4 molecules are associated with the antigen receptor complex on activated but not resting T cells. J Immunol 1988; 140:2912–2918.
29. Achsah DK, Paul WE. Multichain recognition receptors: similarities in structure and signaling pathways. Immunol Today 1992; 13:63–68.
30. Zacharchuk CM, Ashwell JD. Fruitful outcomes of intracellular cross-talk. Curr Biol 1992; 2:246–248.
31. Alexander DR, Cantrell DA. Kinases and phosphatases in T-cell activation. Immunol Today 1989; 10:200–205.
32. Zacharchuk CM, Mercep M, Chakraborti P, Simons SS, Ashwell JD. Programmed cell death: cell activation–and steroid-induced pathways are mutually antagonistic. J Immunol 1990; 145:4037–4045.
33. Thomas L. Lives of a Cell. New York: Viking Press, 1974.
34. Ascher MS, Sheppard HW. AIDS as immune system activation: a model for pathogenesis. Clin Exp Immunol 1988; 73:165–167.
35. Weyand CM, Goronzy J, Fathman CG. Human T cell clones used to define functional epitopes on HLA class II molecules. Proc Natl Acad Sci USA 1986; 83:762–768.

36. Alles A, Alley K, Barrett JC, Buttyan R, Columbano A, Cope FO, Copelan EA, Duke RC, Farel PB, Gershenson LE, Goldgaber D, Green DR, Honn KV, Hully J, Isaacs JT, Kerr JFR, Krammer PH, Lockshin RA, Martin DP, McConkey DJ, Michaelson J, Schulte-Herman, Server AC, Szende B, Tomei LD, Tritton TR, Umansky SR, Valerie K, Warner HR. Apoptosis: a general comment. FASEB J 1991; 5:2127-2128.

37. Kerr JFR, Wyllie AH, Currie AR. Apoptosis: a basic biological phenomenon with wide-ranging implications in tissue kinetics. Br J Cancer 1972; 26:239-257.

38. Russell JH, White CL, Loh DY, Meleedy-Rey P. Receptor-stimulated death pathway is opened by antigen in mature T cells. Immunology 1991; 88:2151-2155.

39. Smith CA, Williams GT, Kingston R, Jenkinson EJ, Owen JJT. Antibodies to CD3/T-cell receptor complex induce death by apoptosis in immature T cells in thymic cultures. Nature 1989; 337:181-184.

40. Wyllie AH, Kerr JFR, Currie AR. Cell death: the significance of apoptosis. Int Rev Cytol 1980; 68:251-306.

41. Zacharchuk CM, Mercep M, Chakraborti PK, Simons SS, Ashwell JD. Programmed T lymphocyte death. J Immunol 1990; 145:4037-4045.

42. Groux H, Torpier G, Monte D, Mouton Y, Capron A, Ameisen JC. Activation-induced death by apoptosis in CD+ T cells from human immunodeficiency virus-infected asymptomatic individuals. J Exp Med 1992; 175:331-340.

43. Ameisen JC, Capron A. Cell dysfunction and depletion in AIDS: the programmed cell death hypothesis. Immunol Today 1991; 12:102-105.

44. Meyaard L, Otto SA, Jonker RR, Mijnster MJ, Keet RPM, Miedema F. Programmed death of T cells in HIV-1 infection. Science 1992; 257:217-219.

45. Sheppard HW, Ascher MS. AIDS and programmed cell death. Immunol Today 1991; 12:243.

46. van Boehmer H, Kisielow P. Self-nonself discrimination by T cells. Science 1990; 248:1369-1373.

47. Pircher H, Rohrer UH, Moskophidis D, Zinkernagel RM, Hengartner H. Lower receptor avidity required for thymic clonal deletion than for effector T-cell function. Nature 1991; 351:482-485.

48. Speiser DE, Chvatchko Y, Zinkernagel RM, MacDonald HR. Distinct fates of self-specific T cells developing in irradiation bone marrow chimeras: clonal deletion, clonal anergy, or in vitro responsiveness to self-Mls-1a controlled by hemopoietic cells in the thymus. J Exp Med 1990; 172:1305-1314.

49. Vanhems P, Bresson-Hadni S, Vuitton DA, Miguet JP, Gillet M, Lab M, Brechot C. Long-term survival without immunosuppression in HIV-positive liver-graft recipient. Lancet 1990; 337:126.

50. Benoist C, Mathis D. Demystification of the alloresponse. Curr Biol 1991; 1:143-144.

51. Demotz S, Sette A, Sakaguchi K, Buchner R, Appella E, Grey HM. Self-peptide requirement for class II major histocompatibility complex allorecognition. Proc Natl Acad Sci USA 1991; 88:8730–8734.

52. Rotzschke O, Falk K, Faath S, Rammensee HG. On the nature of peptides involved in T cell alloreactivity. J Exp Med 1991; 174:1059–1071.

53. Sprent J, Gao EK, Webb SR. T cell reactivity to MHC molecules: immunity versus tolerance. Science 1990; 248:1357–1363.

54. Gammon G, Klotz J, Ando D, Sercarz EE. The T cell repertoire to a multideterminant antigen. Clonal heterogeneity of the T cell response, variation between syngeneic individuals, and in vitro selection of T cell specificities. J Immunol 1990; 144:1571–1577.

55. Kappler JW, Staerz U, White J, Marrack PC. Self-tolerance eliminates T cells specific for Mls-modified products of the major histocompatibility complex. Nature 1988; 332:35–40.

56. McDonald HR, Schneider R, Lees RK, Howe RC, Acha-Orbea H, Festenstein H, Zinkernagel RM. T-cell receptor V-beta use predicts reactivity and tolerance to Mls-1a encoded antigens. Nature 1988; 332:40–45.

57. Quaratino S, Murison G, Knyba RE, Verhoef A, Londei M. Human CD4 – CD8 – alpha-beta + T cells express a functional T cell receptor and can be activated by superantigens. J Immunol 1991; 147:3319–3323.

58. Sekaly RP, Croteau G, Bowman M, Scholl P, Burakoff S, Geha RS. The CD4 molecule is not always required for the T cell response to bacterial enterotoxins. J Exp Med 1991; 173:367–371.

59. Marrack P, Kushnir E, Kappler J. A maternally inherited superantigen encoded by a mammary tumour virus. Nature 1991; 349:524–526.

60. Imberti L, Sottini A, Bettinardi A, Puoti M, Primi D. Selective depletion in HIV infection of T cells that bear specific T cell receptor V-beta sequences. Science 1991; 254:860–862.

61. Janeway C. Mls: makes a little sense. Nature 1991; 349:459–461.

62. Yagi J, Rath S, Janeway CA. Control of T cell responses to staphylococcal enterotoxins by stimulator cell MHC class II polymorphism. J Immunol 1991; 147:1398–1405.

63. Aziz DC, Hanna Z, Jolicoeur P. Severe immunodeficiency disease induced by a defective murine leukaemia virus. Nature 1989; 338:505–508.

64. Huang M, Simard C, Jolicoeur P. Immunodeficiency and clonal growth of target cells induced by helper-free defective retrovirus. Science 1989; 246:1614–1617.

65. Hugin AW, Vacchio MS, Morse HC. A virus-encoded "superantigen" in a retrovirus-induced immunodeficiency syndrome of mice. Science 1991; 252:424–427.

66. Marrack P, Kappler J. The staphylococcal enterotoxins and their relatives. Science 1990; 248:705–711.

67. Marrack P. Superantigens and immune system design. Clin Immunol Spectr 1991; 3:8–10.

INDEX

ABOUT THE EDITORS

LUC MONTAGNIER, codiscoverer of HIV, is Head of the AIDS and Retrovirus Department at the Pasteur Institute and a Director of Research at the Centre National de la Recherche Scientifique, Paris, France. The author of numerous important papers in the field of AIDS research, he is a member of the French Academy of Medicine, the Academy of Sciences of Madrid, and the European Molecular Biology Organization, and a corresponding member of the French Academy of Sciences and the Royal Academy of Medicine of Belgium. An Officer of the French Legion of Honor, Dr. Montagnier is the recipient of many awards, including the Albert Lasker Clinical Medical Research Award, the Louis Jeantet Prize, and the Japan Prize. He received the B.S. degree (1955) from the University of Paris and the University of Poitiers, and the M.D. degree (1960) from the University of Paris.

MARIE-LISE GOUGEON is Head of the Immunology Laboratory in the AIDS and Retrovirus Department at the Pasteur Institute and Associate Professor of Immunology at the University of Paris VII, France. A member of the French Society of Immunology, she is the author or coauthor of numerous journal articles in the field of immunodeficiency and AIDS research. Dr. Gougeon received the B.S. (1972) and M.S. (1974) degrees in biochemistry from the University of Paris XI, and the Ph.D. degree (1978) in immunology from the University of Paris VII.